BIOTECHNOLOGY
An Introduction

BIOTECHNOLOGY
An Introduction

S. Ignacimuthu, s.j.

Alpha Science International Ltd.
Oxford, U.K.

Biotechnology
378 Pages/51 Tables/47 Figures

Rev. Fr. Dr. S. Ignacimuthu, s.j.
Entomology Research Institute
Loyola College (Autonomous)
Chennai, India

Alpha Science International Ltd.
7200 The Quorum, Oxford Business Park North
Garsington Road, Oxford OX4 2JZ, U.K.

www.alphasci.com

ISBN 978-1-89265-451-4

Published by N.K. Mehra for Narosa Publishing House Pvt. Ltd.,
22 Delhi Medical Association Road, Daryaganj, New Delhi 110 002

Printed in India

To
The Society of Jesus
for making me
what I am

Preface

Biotechnology refers to any technological application that uses biological systems, living organisms, or derivatives thereof, to make or modify products or processes for specific use. Biotechnology is a very useful technology that is being exploited by many different sectors. The applications of biotechnology offer enormous potential for agricultural, pharmaceutical, environmental, healthcare and developmental purposes.

With the sequencing of the human genome, the researchers are moving to the next level, which involves understanding the genetic basis of diseases. Benefits for human development are already experienced. Breakthrough applications in medicine have huge potential for accelerating human development.

Apart from the usual topics related to biotechnology, aspects related to Polymerase Chain Reaction, Microarray, Gene targeting, Gene silencing, Animal cloning, Human Cloning, Stem cells, Genetically modified food, Fermentation technology, Enzyme technology, Bioinformatics, Drug Discovery, Nano-medicine, Biosensors and Bioremediation have been elaborated

I am confident that the students and teachers will benefit much from this book.

Rev. Fr. Dr. S. Ignacimuthu, s.j.

Acknowledgements

I am grateful to all those who have helped me to prepare this book. My failure to list their names individually does not detract from my indebtedness to them. I must thank Sisters Anne Xavier, Sarguna, and Regi, and Miss Parvathy, Holy Cross College (Autonomous), Tiruchirapalli for correcting the manuscript and giving the finishing touches. I would also like to specially thank Messrs Albert Rabara, D. Amalraj, and S. Arockiasamy, St. Joseph's College (Autonomous), Tiruchirapalli and Mr C. Muthu, Entomology Research Institute, Loyola College, Chennai, for their constant and generous help in typing the manuscript. I am grateful to Rex Johnson for embellishing the book with beautiful illustrations.

I thank my dear students for inspiring me to write this book and also for their constructive suggestions to improve it. I also thank Dr C.R. Babu, Department of Botany, University of Delhi, for his guidance and help.

My sincere thanks are due to the following publishers for granting me permission to use some of their diagrams, explanations, and tables:

Academic Press, New York
Blackwell Scientific Publications, Oxford
Cambridge University Press, Cambridge
Holt, Reinhart and Winston Inc., New York
John Wiley and Sons, New York
Jones and Bartlett Publishers, Massachusetts
Prentice-Hall, International, New Jersey
Springer Verlag, Berlin
W.H. Freeman and Company, New York
Wiley Eastern Limited, New Delhi

Let me thank and compliment the publishers for having published the book in a neat and excellent manner. Finally, I must acknowledge with deep appreciation the indispensable help and encouragement received from my dear friends.

Contents

Introduction

The most significant achievement of biologists is the rediscovery of biotechnology. As a subject, biotechnology is not a new area of scientific endeavour. Microorganisms have been used to produce food such as beer, vinegar, yoghurt, and cheese for over eight millennia. Certainly the ancient Sumerians were familiar with beer; alehouses were an established part of Roman civilization. Romans tried to introduce grapevines for wine-making. References to wine and vinegar are scattered throughout the Bible.

Biotechnology is an area of multidisciplinary science, involving a variety of distinct subjects, where living organisms or their useful parts are put into effective use to cater to the welfare of humanity. It can conveniently be grouped under two major headings, namely, 'conventional biotechnology' and 'modern biotechnology'.

In the early days, biotechnologists used living organisms for the manufacture of a variety of useful materials. Whatever by-products were obtained during normal cell growth, were used by people. For example, during the normal growth of yeast cells in grape juice, sucrose is converted to ethanol and this fermented juice containing alcohol is used as wine. Similarly, *Penicillium notatum* and *P. chrysogenum* produce the antibiotic penicillin as a by-product of their secondary metabolism and this compound is used to fight microbial diseases. Microbial production of glycerol by yeast, acetone, and butanol fermentation using *Clostridium acetobutylicum,* citric acid production by *Aspergillus niger,* and streptomycin production using *Streptomyces griseus* are some of the fields developed under conventional biotechnology. Mutation, recombination and strain selection were employed to increase the yield of the product.

Modern biotechnology enables an organism to produce a totally new product, which the organism does not or cannot produce in its normal course of life. Since we are able to engineer a new genetic potential in an organism, this technology is also called genetic engineering. Basic techniques which stimulate the progress of modern biotechnology are: (1) recombinant DNA manipulation—genetic engineering, (2) plant and animal tissue culture, (3) protoplast fusion, (4) monoclonal antibodies, (5) protein engineering, (6) immobilized enzymes and cell catalysis, (7) biosensors, (8) computer-aided bioprocess, (9) new reactor design, (10) DNA transfer into living cells, (11) polymerase chain reaction, and (12) chromosome engineering. Without these techniques, the growth of biotechnology would have been impossible. All these techniques are used in most industries either to engineer a new capability or to reduce the cost of production or to introduce a safer industrial practice.

This book aims at providing some basic and relevant information on important applications of biotechnology, namely (1) fermentation industry, (2) healthcare, (3) food processing industry, (4) agriculture, (5) chemical industry, (6) waste treatment, and (7) energy and environment. The major advancement in fermentation industry deals with reactor design and computer aided process control. This technology has its application in food, agriculture, alcoholic beverages, pharmaceuticals, and chemicals. New reactor designs such as air lift fermentors, fluid bed reactors and other systems designed to grow animal and plant cells in large quantities have revolutionised bio-technological applications.

In relation to healthcare, biotechnology has helped in the production of (a) small molecules such as antibiotics, hybrid antibiotics, amino acids, vitamins etc. (b) macromolecules such as interferons, insulin, hormones, vaccines, etc. (c) drug detecting agents, monoclonal antibodies, and magnetic microspheres, (d) purification agents such as immobilized monoclonal antibodies, (e) new catalysts, e.g. immobilized enzymes and cells, (f) diagnostic reagents like enzymes and monoclonals, (g) biomaterials like artificial skin, and (h) biomedical equipment like artificial kidney machines.

In the field of agriculture, biotechnology has contributed to crop improvement by developing salt and drought resistant crops, developing crop varieties which can fix atmospheric nitrogen, improving crop varieties for higher photosynthetic efficiency, improving the quantity and quality of storage proteins, and production of high yielding hybrid seeds. Further, it has contributed to crop protection by development of disease resistant varieties of transgenic plants which offer protection against virus, bacteria, fungi and insects, development of herbicide resistant plants and development of recombinant DNA based diagnostic reagents for early identification and treatment of viral, bacterial and fungal diseases. Tissue culture techniques have helped in the propagation of forest plants such as bamboo, teak, *Eucalyptus*, sandalwood, etc. and economically important plants such as cardamom, banana and brassica. Biotechnology has also helped in the production of single cell proteins and biofertilizers.

In the field of animal husbandry, biotechnology has helped to increase milk production in cattle, to achieve faster growth in farm animals and to produce disease resistant animals through transgenesis.

In the field of energy, biotechnology has helped in the conversion of cellulosic and agricultural waste to produce fuels such as ethanol and butanol by cloning active enzyme systems for their efficient degradation and subsequent fermentation. Biotechnology has helped in the production of biogas from agricultural and animal wastes by engineering methanogenic bacteria. It has also helped in the production of oil producing bacteria.

Biotechnology has also played an important role in waste treatment by developing high capacity bacteria to degrade cellulose and lignin, to degrade metals and cyanide, to clean up oil, to destroy TNT, to degrade chlorinated organic wastes, etc.

Thus, biotechnology has contributed to the welfare of humanity in many and varied ways. Biotechnology has become an important and integral part of any life-science today. This book has been written in as concise and simple a manner as possible with a view to help the students and teachers in many universities and colleges. It is hoped that undergraduate and postgraduate students would find it useful as a textbook as well as for research purposes.

Suggestions for further improvement of the book are welcome.

Rev. Fr. Dr. S. Ignacimuthu, S.J.

1
Biotechnology—An Overview

Introduction

Biotechnology has been defined in various ways. In simple terms, biotechnology refers to the use of living organisms or their products for the welfare of humanity. One rather vague definition says that biotechnology is the application of biological organisms, systems or processes to manufacturing and service industries. In other words it simply means biology applied for use.

According to the definition adopted by the European Federation of Biotechnology, created in 1978, 'biotechnology makes it possible, through an integrated application of knowledge and techniques of biochemistry, microbiology, genetics and chemical engineering, to draw benefit, at the technological level, from the properties and capacities of microorganisms and cell cultures. Biotechnology offers the possibility of producing, from widely available renewable resources, substances and compounds essential to life and the greater well-being of human beings.' In short, biotechnology comprises technical processes that enable us not only to manipulate the DNA, but also to use in other ways living organisms for specific purposes. Biotechnology is defined as the application of current scientific methods and techniques to improve the biological systems, be they plants, animals, microorganisms, for the betterment of human beings.

The term biotechnology was brought into popular use in the mid-1970s as a result of the increased potential for the application of the emerging techniques of molecular biology. The word itself seems to have been first employed by the Leeds City Council in the United Kingdom in the early 1920s, when they set up an Institute of Biotechnology. In fact, biotechnological processes are nearly 5000 years old. It began with the discovery of fermentation and the consequent production of alcoholic beverages. Present interest in biotechnology has been stimulated by the potential that can result from the marriage of biological processes and techniques—some old, some new—with production engineering, electronics and bioprocessing.

1.1 History

Probably the oldest biotechnological processes are found in microbial fermentations, as borne out by a Babylonian tablet dated around 6000 B.C., unearthed in 1981, depicting the preparation of beer. The Sumerians were able to brew as many as 20 different varieties of beer in the third millennium B.C. The perfecting of fermentation processes, their increased efficiency, and the discovery of a large number of microbial bioconversions, along with the isolation of substances of bacterial and fungal origin to replace synthetic products has led to the discovery of more effective drugs and medicines. Recent biotechnological processes rely on genetic recombination techniques as well as the use of immobilized enzymes, cells or cell organelles.

At this stage, a brief history of various events that led to the present-day knowledge of biotechnology will be useful. The foundation of modern biotechnological applications can be traced to 1866 when Czech monk Gregor Mendel published the results of his experiments on garden pea. He suggested the involvement of some factors in the transfer of traits from one generation to another. Later this factor was determined as the gene. After the rediscovery of Mendelism in 1900, biologists were concerned mainly with the inheritance of structural or other visible variations. Later, A.E. Garrod (1902) recognized a class of defects in human beings such as diabetes, phenylketonuria, tyrosinosis cretinism, albinism etc., which were caused by a fault in the metabolism within the body.

O.T. Avery, C.M. MacLeod and M. McCarty (1940) were the pioneers in studying the chemical nature of the substance that was responsible for bacterial transformation. G.W. Beadle and E.C. Tatum (1941) carried out genetic experiments with the breadmould *Neurospora crassa* with a biochemical slant, and established that genes worked through biochemical pathways. They also postulated that each gene was responsible for the synthesis of one particular enzyme.

The whole structure of a protein, insulin, was established by Sanger (1953). Crick and Watson (1953) showed that deoxyribonucleic acid (DNA) had a double-stranded structure. Nirenberg (1963) deciphered the genetic code that was applicable from bacteria to man. Merrifield (1963) manufactured and marketed the first automatic polypeptide synthesizing machines. Edman and Begg (1967) developed methods for protein degradation. Arber, Smith and Nathans (1972) discovered the restriction enzymes which cut out DNA at specific points. Gilbert, Maxam and Sanger (1976) developed rapid methods for chemical analysis of DNA. Itakura and his co-workers (1977) synthesized the genes of human somatostatin and insulin. N. Goodon and M.D. Chilton (1977) proved that the transfer of genes was possible using the bacterium *Agrobacterium tumefaciens* as a carrier H.G. Khorana (1979) succeeded in synthesizing, for the first time, an entirely artificial gene capable of functioning within a living cell. Itakura (1980) also constructed the first gene assembler. Hood (1981), who invented the protein micro-analyser, built another automated machine for the same purpose.

Kary Mullis (1983) invented Polymerase Chain Reaction (PCR) which revolutionized biotechnological applications. Alec Jeffrey (1984) developed genetic fingerprinting technique which can be used to identify individuals by analysing the varying sequences (polymorphisms) in the DNA. The human genome project was initiated in 1986. In 1995 M. Sehena developed complementary DNA microarray system to monitor gene expression; also the

Institute for Genomic Research reported the first complete DNA sequence of the genome of a free-living organism. In 1997 Dolly the sheep was cloned using somatic cell by Ian Wilmut and his colleagues. Also the complete sequence of the genome of the yeast *Saccharomyces cerevisiae* was reported. In 1999 human chromosome 22 was sequenced. In 2000, the genome sequence of *Adabidopsis thaliana* was completed. In 2001, complete map of the genome of rice was reported. Also annotations and analysis of human genome was published. In 2002, cloned pigs were reported. In 2003 human stem cells were used to treat diseases. Mouse genome was also sequenced.

In the field of tissue culture, isolation of protoplast was carried out by Klercker (1892). Haberlandt (1902) demonstrated the totipotency of cells. White (1934) showed the possibility of growing excised tomato root tips *in vitro* for an indefinite period. Gauthert (1937) succeeded in cultivating undifferentiated carrot tissues. Van Overbeek and his group (1941) isolated embryos of *Datura* which could grow and develop on a chemical medium supplemented with coconut milk. The possibility of regenerating plants *in vitro* from the shoot apex of certain angiosperms was first demonstrated by Ball (1946). Skoog and Tsui (1948) showed that shoot initiation, also termed as caulogenesis, in tobacco stem segments and callus could be chemically regulated by manipulating the nutrient medium. La Rue (1949) managed to grow immature maize endosperm in culture.

Morel and Wetmore (1951) were the first to achieve success with monocot cultures. Tulecke (1953) obtained the first haploid callus from the pollen grains of *Ginkgo biloba*. Munir, Hildebrandt and Riker, (1954) reported the growth of isolated cell cultures in a liquid medium. Skoog's group (1955) identified 6-furfurylaminopurine, a degraded product of herring sperm DNA, as a chemical capable of stimulating cell divisions. Skoog and Miller (1957) showed that shoot and root initiation in tobacco callus cultures could be regulated by maintaining a subtle ratio between auxin and cytokinin in the medium, paving the way for the chemical regulation of organogenesis. Carew and Schwarting (1958) were the first to get callus cultures from rye, a monocot. Steward (1958) discovered the differentiation of somatic bipolar embryos in carrot using cell suspension techniques. Reinert (1959) reported the use of a nutrient medium solidified with agar for embryogenesis.

Cocking (1960) isolated plant protoplasts enzymatically. Morel (1960) developed the techniques of shoot apex culture of orchids for clonal propagation. Guha and Maheshwari (1964) obtained direct embryos from cultured anthers of *Datura* which led to the development of haploid plants. Nishi and his colleagues (1968) were the first to induce differentiation in monocot callus culture of rice.

Binding and his colleagues (1970) isolated streptomycin resistant callus of *Petunia hybrida*. Carlson and his group (1972) were the first to fuse the protoplast of *Nicotiana glauca and Nicotiana langsdoiffti,* two sexually compatible species of tobacco, and regenerated a parasexual hybrid.

1.2 Biotechnological Processes

The development of biotechnology relies to a large extent on the existence of effective research in microbiology, biochemistry, enzymology and microbial genetics as well as on the existence of culture collections, perfectly recorded and regularly studied. The use of animal cells also plays an important role, such as in the culture of viruses for producing vaccines, in the production of interferons and in the synthesis of monoclonal antibodies by hybridomas. Plants also have contributed in the production of plant clones and synthesis of various alkaloids and other secondary metabolites. Microbiology, genetics, molecular biology and biochemistry are the roots of biotechnology.

Activity in biotechnology may be conveniently broken down into eight areas of endeavour, namely, (i) Recombinant DNA and genetic engineering, (ii) cell cultures (iii) waste treatment and utilization, (iv) enzymes and biocatalysts, (v) fuels, (vi) nitrogen fixation (vii) fermentation and pharmaceuticals and (viii) healthcare (Table 1.1).

Table 1.1

Areas in biotechnology and the principal products

	Technology	Products
(i)	Recombinant DNA and Genetic Engineering	Enzymes, Vaccines, Interferons, hormones, antibodies, blood factors.
(ii)	Cell cultures	Biomass production, single cell proteins, fine chemicals, interferons, vaccines, blood products, monoclonal antibodies.
(iii)	Waste treatment and utilization	Byproduct utilization, e.g. cheese whey, waste cellulose, recovery of catalyst, water recycling.
(iv)	Enzymes and biocatalysts	Food processing, fine chemicals, diagnostic kits, chemotherapy, biosensors, isoglucose, glucose syrups, ethanol.
(v)	Fuels	Alcohol, hydrogen, methane, gasohol
(vi)	Nitrogen Fixation	Reduction of nitrogenous fertilizers
(vii)	Fermentation and Pharmaceuticals	Alcohols, fine chemicals, antibiotics, vitamins, enzymes, amino acids, nucleotides, steroids, alkaloids, diagnostic reagents, citric acid, biopolymers, biopesticides, ethanol, acetone, butanol, biogas.
(viii)	Healthcare	Antibiotics, hormones, DNA probes, gene therapy.

The ability to isolate a gene coding for a desired product and transfer it to another organism has opened the way either to the more effective production of useful proteins, or to the introduction of novel characteristics in the host organism. Thus the large-scale production of hormones, vaccines, blood clotting factors or enzymes by some friendly bacterium has become possible.

1.2.1 Recombinant DNA and Genetic Engineering

The ability to isolate a gene coding for a desired product and transfer it to another organism has opened the way either to the more effective production of useful proteins, or to the introduction of novel characteristics in the host organism. Thus the large-scale production of hormones, vaccines, blood clotting factors or enzymes by some friendly bacterium has become possible.

There is also an additional possibility with this form of technology, i.e. the production of truly novel proteins. By selectively modifying the gene coding for an enzyme before it is introduced into the host organisms, its structure, and hence the properties of the enzyme may be advantageously modified.

Modification of the genome of economically important plants is also very promising. The levels of storage proteins in seeds could be increased to give high protein seeds. It is also possible that crops could be engineered for a greater resistance to herbicides or infection.

1.2.2 Cell Cultures

The problem of culturing mammalian cells on a large scale will become a major preoccupation of cell biologists and biochemical engineers in the near future. Monoclonal antibodies, due to the complexity of the transcription and translation of their genetic material, and interferons, due to the cost and effectiveness, are likely to become more important in future both for therapeutical, preparative and analytical applications.

Plants are an important source of many valuable raw materials and high-value drugs. The ability to culture plant cells on a large scale, either for the production of biomass *per se* or in order to extract the desired product from cell cultures, is becoming a highly desirable technology. Immobilization technology has come in handy to synthesize complex compounds and to produce greater amounts of secondary metabolites.

1.2.3 Waste Treatment and Utilization

Sewage disposal is a problem long faced by human beings. There are many forms of wastes which cannot only be more easily disposed of, but can perhaps be turned into a useful commodity. For example, cheese production starts with the curdling of milk to form the solid curds and liquid whey. An average size cheese making plant produces thousands of litres of whey a day, and letting it go waste in the sewers is not only problematic but also costly. Whey is composed of a few proteins, minerals and about 4% lactose. If these could be broken down to useful compounds with the help of engineered enzymes, then it would help in waste disposal.

Cellulose is another abundant waste material, particularly in the form of straw from cereal crops. Traditionally, it is either ploughed back into the fields or burnt. In theory, this waste cellulose could be biologically degraded and used as a feedstock for the production of microbial proteins. It has been estimated that sufficient protein could be produced in this way from agricultural wastes alone to feed the entire world's population. Also other waste materials like herbicides, pesticides, chemicals etc. used in agriculture could be degraded into useful by-products.

1.2.4 Enzymes and Biocatalysts

Enzymes are nature's supreme catalysts, exhibiting great specificity and enormous catalytic power. They have been in use for many centuries, particularly in food processing (for example cheese making, removal of hair from hide etc.) and represent one of the oldest forms of biotechnology. More recently, great interest has been shown in extending the use of enzymes (whether purified, as dead or partially viable cells) in food processing, chemical production, analytical and diagnostic systems, and in the treatment of diseases. The elucidation of the structure and functions of certain enzymes as well as their use, in an immobilized form, in a variety of industrial production processes has opened great avenues for human endeavour and curiosity.

1.2.5 Fuels

The world is running short of combustible fuels, particularly, mineral oils. Biotechnology might offer new fuels and alternative carbon feedstocks. Soon we may use methane, biodiesel and hydrogen as important fuels. Biophotolytic production of hydrogen from water has already been achieved, and is based on the combination of the photosystems of plants with bacteria-derived hydrogenase enzymes and light. This seems to be the ideal combustible fuel since it produces no pollution and regenerates its source material.

1.2.6 Nitrogen Fixation

The introduction into crops the ability to fix nitrogen from the atmosphere would not only save on the cost of applying nitrogenous fertilizers, but would eliminate the potential problems of water pollution from nitrates washed off from agricultural land. The achievement of such associations between nitrogen-fixing bacteria and cereals would have important agricultural applications. Attempts are being made to increase the efficiency of nitrogen fixation and assimilation by acting on the genetic mechanisms regulating the process. Research is going on to develop new nitrogen fixing systems by means of somatic hybrids between the desired cultivars and nitrogen-fixing plants; or by introducing the *nif* genes into symbiotic or free living microorganisms; also to transfer the nitrogen-fixing ability to plants by using viruses or self-transmissible plasmids as vectors of the *nil genes*; or by recombining these genes with mitochondrial or chloroplast DNA.

1.2.7 Fermentation and Pharmaceuticals

Fermentation along with biocatalysts shares the distinction of being the oldest form of biotechnology. Traditionally, fermentation has meant the production of potable alcohol from carbohydrates. However, fermentation, that is, the application of microbial metabolism to transform simple raw materials into valuable products can produce an amazing array of useful substances; for example, chemicals such as citric acid, antibiotics, biopolymers, single cell proteins, vitamins, alkaloids, steroids, vaccines and other diagnostic reagents can be produced using the fermentation technology.

It is one thing for the laboratory scientist to clone a novel gene, discover a new antibiotic or invent an enzyme catalysed process, but it is quite another to transfer this knowledge to the scale of operation required to make a useful product in significant amount. Process engineers play a vital role in this transfer by employing various techniques such as harvesting, pretreatment, filtration of the raw material, reactor design, reuse of biocatalyst or organisms, product extraction and analysis. And this makes biotechnology worth billions of dollars by contributing to the gross domestic product of the economy in many developed countries. In terms of national economic growth as a result of the introduction of biotechnology, the greatest potential lies in the food and chemical industries.

1.2.8 Healthcare

Biotechnological inputs have been helpful in i) preventing diseases through various therapeutic products like antibiotics, antibodies, vaccines, hormones, regulatory products, etc., ii) prenatal diagnosis of genetic diseases and genetic counselling, iii) immunodiagnostic tools and probes aiding disease identification, iv) correction of diseases, v) personalized medicine, vi) gene therapy, vii) cloning, etc.

1.3 Products

Biotechnology has promoted the production of monoclonal antibodies, DNA probes, antibodies, antibiotics, recombinant vaccines, human insulin, interferons, human growth hormones, which are helpful in the treatment of various diseases and metabolic disorders. On the industrial front, production of ethanol, lactic acid, citric acid, glycerine, acetone, penicillin, streptomycin, erythromycin, cycloheximide, immunotoxins, amylase, protease, lipase, single cell proteins has been taken up in a large-scale. On the agricultural front, production of many transgenic plants and clonal multiplication has been done. On the environmental front production of biosensors and bioplastics has been going on.

In the year 2000, the global revenues of biotechnology industry were estimated to be more than US$ 70 billion, with biopharmaceuticals forming the largest chunk accounting for 60% of the market followed by diagnostics (14%) and industrial enzymes (4%). Therapeutic proteins accounted for 10% of the global pharmaceutical market. In India, the revenue of biotech industries for

2004-2005 is as follows: Biopharma-35700 million; Bioservices- 4250 million; Bioagri-3300 million; bioindustrial-3200 million and bioinformatics-800 million.

The development of biotechnology will be a long-term affair, dependent on the needs of market forces, the acceptability of the products and developments in competing technologies. The key to the successful development of biotechnology lies either in producing a product which can be made by no other means, or by producing an existing product more cheaply and abundantly. The latter approach involves catching up on existing technology, which itself may be advancing, and thus involves considerable risk. Some possible medium-term products such as vaccines for common cold, safer tobacco substitutes, cheap wines, reliable self-diagnosis kits, site specific drugs etc. which are possible only through biotechnology may eventually fulfil many dreams.

The spectacular development of biotechnology is full of promises. In addition to the contribution at the family, village and industrial levels biotechnology offers some solutions to humanity as a whole by tackling the problems of food and protein deficiencies. It may also contribute to the therapeutic revolution that will rely on the progress of cellular biochemistry, molecular biology and immunology, and will call more upon biological substances to fight against diverse pathological problems. Biotechnology also contributes to the preservation of genetic diversity as well as to technological innovations.

1.4 Biotechnology and IPR

Intellectual Property Rights (IPR) are essential part of todays business. IPR's are the means to protect any intangible asset. Examples of IPR are patent, copyright, trademark, geographical indication and trade secret. A patent is an exclusive monopoly granted by the government to an inventor over his invention for limited period of time. Some examples are given below:

Bayer CropScience GmbH (Frankfurt, Germany) has patented nucleic acid molecules which encode enzymes involved in starch synthasis in plants. These enzymes are wheat isoamylases. The invention furthermore relates to vectors and host cells which contain the above-described nucleic acid molecules, in particular to transformed plant cells and plants which can be regenerated from these and which have an increased or reduced activity of the isoamylases according to the invention. (US 6,951,969)

Columbia University (New York, NY) has patented antibodies directed to OLD-35 protein, the product of the OLD-35 gene, which displays enhanced expression during cellular senescence and terminal cell differentiation. (US 6,951,923)

Ruan, et al. has patented a "cocktail" combination of two monoclonal antibodies respectively acting on different sites of the platelet GPIIb-IIIa complex. This "cocktail" combination can completely block receptor function of the GPIIb-IIIa complex, inhibit platelet aggregation and thereby efficiently inhibit thrombosis. (US 6,951,645)

University of California (Oakland, CA) and Chiron Corporation (Emeryville, CA) has patented gene delivery vectors, such as, for example, recombinant adeno-associated viral vectors, and methods of using such vectors for use in treating or preventing diseases of the eye. (US 6,943,153)

Deltagen, Inc. (San Carlos, CA) has patented nucleotide constructs and methods for making DNA constructs useful for introducing sequences into and disrupting the function of a gene in a cell, particularly an embryonic stem cell. (US 6,942,995)

Study Outline

Biotechnological Processes

Biotechnology is the application of biological organisms, systems or processes to manufacturing and service industries. The major areas of interest in this field are genetic engineering, Recombinant DNA, culture techniques, waste treatment, utilization of enzymes and biocatalysts, fuel, nitrogen fixation, fermentation and pharmaceuticals and healthcare. The extraction and transfer of a gene with the desired characters, has been a fascinating field of achievement and this has resulted in the production of useful proteins and novel characters. Large scale production of hormones, vaccines and bacteria are noteworthy achievements. Microbial fermentation is considered to be one of the oldest biotechnological processes and has captured the attention of modern biotechnologists who had given this a highly industrial status due to the various products that are formed as a result of it.

Cell Culture

The ability to culture plant cells on a large scale and protoplast isolation and fusion have given a boost to agriculture. Newer varieties which are early fruiting and which supply better fruits, owe their credit to biotechnology. Immobolization technology has come in handy to synthesize complex compounds and to produce greater amount of secondary metabolites. Technological selection and modification of genome and its introduction into crops have helped to synthesize novel proteins and increased the nitrogen fixing ability of plants.

Waste Treatment and Utilization

Sewage disposal is a problem long faced by mankind. Today there are many forms of waste which are turned into useful products with the help of biotechnology. Whey, which results from cheese industry is considered to be a waste product. It is composed of proteins, minerals and about 4% lactose. With the help of engineered enzymes these could be broken down to useful compounds. Similarly cellulose is biodegraded and is used as a feedstock for the production of microbial proteins. Enzymes are nature's supreme catalysts and exhibit great specificity. Recently great interest has been aroused in using these in food processing, chemical production, analytical and diagnostic systems and in the treatment of diseases. Biotechnology has offered new fuels and alternative carbon feedstocks.

Nitrogen Fixation

Introduction of nitrogen fixing ability into nonleguminous crops through transfer of *nif* genes is another field and if it achieves total success, it will be a great boon to agriculture. Research is going on to develop new nitrogen fixing systems by means of somatic hybrids between the desired cultivars and nitrogen fixing plants; or by introducing the nif genes into symbiotic or tree living microorganisms.

Fermentation, Pharmaceuticals and Healthcare

Application of microbial metabolism to transform simple raw materials into valuable products can produce an amazing range of useful substances; e.g., chemicals such as citric acid, antibiotics, biopolymers, single cell proteins, vitamins, alkaloids, steroids and other diagnostic reagents. The development of biotechnology, therefore, relies to a large extent, on the existence of effective research in microbiology, biochemistry, enzymology, microbial genetics, cell cultures and molecular biology. Biotechnological inputs have been helpful in preventing diseases and in identifying and treating many diseases.

Biotechnology and IPR

Intellectual Property Rights (IPR) are essential part of today's business. They are a means to protect any intangible asset. Examples are patent, copyright, trademark, geographical indication and trade secret.

Questions

(1) Define biotechnology?
(2) What is recombinant DNA technology?
(3) What are the roles played by enzymes and biocatalysts in biotechnological process?
(4) What role does biotechnology play in waste treatment and utilization?
(5) What are the various fermentation products?
(6) What is IPR?

2
Genetic Engineering and Gene Cloning

Introduction

Genetic engineering involves a manipulation of the genetic material towards a desired end in a directed and pre-determined way. This is alternately called recombinant DNA technology or gene cloning. Strictly to 'engineer' means to design, construct and manipulate according to a set plan. Genetic engineering aims at isolating DNA fragments and recombining them. The basic technique is quite simple. Two DNA molecules are isolated and cut into fragments by one or more specialized enzymes and then the fragments are joined together in a desired combination and restored to a cell for replication and reproduction. The term recombinant DNA is also used specifically to refer to composite DNA molecules, that result from the physical combination of DNA segments derived from different sources.

Genetic engineering started developing in the mid-1970s when it became possible to cut DNA and to transfer particular pieces of DNA containing specific bits of information, from one type of organism into a second type of organism. As a result, the characteristics of the second organism (recipient) could be changed in a specific and pre-determined way. When the recipient organism is a microbe, such as a single celled bacterium, the specific fragment of transferred DNA is also multiplied many times as the recipient microbe multiplies. Millions of identical cells, i.e. a clone of cells, eventually arise. Consequently, it is possible to obtain millions of copies of a specific region of DNA inside a bacterial cell by allowing the cell (and the piece of DNA) to multiply millions of times.

Current interest in genetic engineering is due to its varied applications such as: 1. isolation of a particular gene, part of a gene, or region of a genome, 2. production of a particular RNA and protein molecules in quantities formerly thought to be unobtainable, 3. improvement in the production of biochemicals (such as enzymes and drugs) and commercially important organic chemicals, 4. production of varieties of plants having particular desirable characteristics (e.g., requiring less fertilizer or resistant to disease etc.), 5. correction of genetic defects in higher organisms, and 6. creation of organisms with economically important features (e.g., plants capable of maturing faster or having greater yield). All these are made possible by some basic methodologies which form the essential ingredients of genetic engineering. They are:

(i) a method for physically joining two DNA segments together,

(ii) a self-replicating segment of DNA (a cloning vehicle or vector) that is able to propagate in the host organism, and which can be linked to the DNA segment to be cloned,

(iii) a procedure for introducing the composite DNA molecules into a biologically functional recipient cell, and

(iv) a means of selecting those organisms that have acquired the desired composite molecule.

In short, gene cloning or genetic engineering is essentially the insertion of a specific piece of 'foreign' DNA into a cell, in such a way that the inserted DNA is replicated and handed on to daughter cells during cell division. The main factors involved in gene cloning are the following:

(1) Isolation of the gene (or other piece of DNA) to be cloned.

(2) Insertion of the gene into another piece of DNA called a vector, which will allow it to be taken up by bacteria and replicated within them as the cells grow and divide.

(3) Transfer of the recombinant vectors into bacterial cells, either by transformation or by infection using viruses.

(4) Selection of those cells which contain the desired recombinant vectors.

(5) Growth of the bacteria, that can be continued indefinitely, to give as much cloned DNA as needed.

(6) Expression of the gene to obtain the desired product.

2.1 Outline Of A Genetic Engineering Procedure

Genetic engineering requires two types of knowledge, namely, a grasp of the concepts of molecular biology and a familiarity with laboratory manipulations. The major steps in genetic engineering are briefly outlined in Figure 2.1.

(a) The first step is to break open living cells. A number of methods are available to accomplish this. One popular way is to shear the cells in a blender and then treat them with a detergent.

(b) The next step is to remove genetic information from cells. This is an easy and straight-forward process; the information is stored in a chemical form as part of DNA. Since DNA molecules are much longer than most other large molecules found in cells, it has been possible to develop techniques of purifying DNA. The DNA can be isolated and purified using different techniques

(c) The third step is to cut away specific genes of interest from the rest of the DNA. DNA is divided into segments which correspond to the letters in the genetic code. When a number of segments or genetic letters are organized in a specific combination, they create a gene. The molecular scissors used to cut DNA into gene-sized pieces are called restriction endonucleases and they recognize and cut at specific DNA sequences.

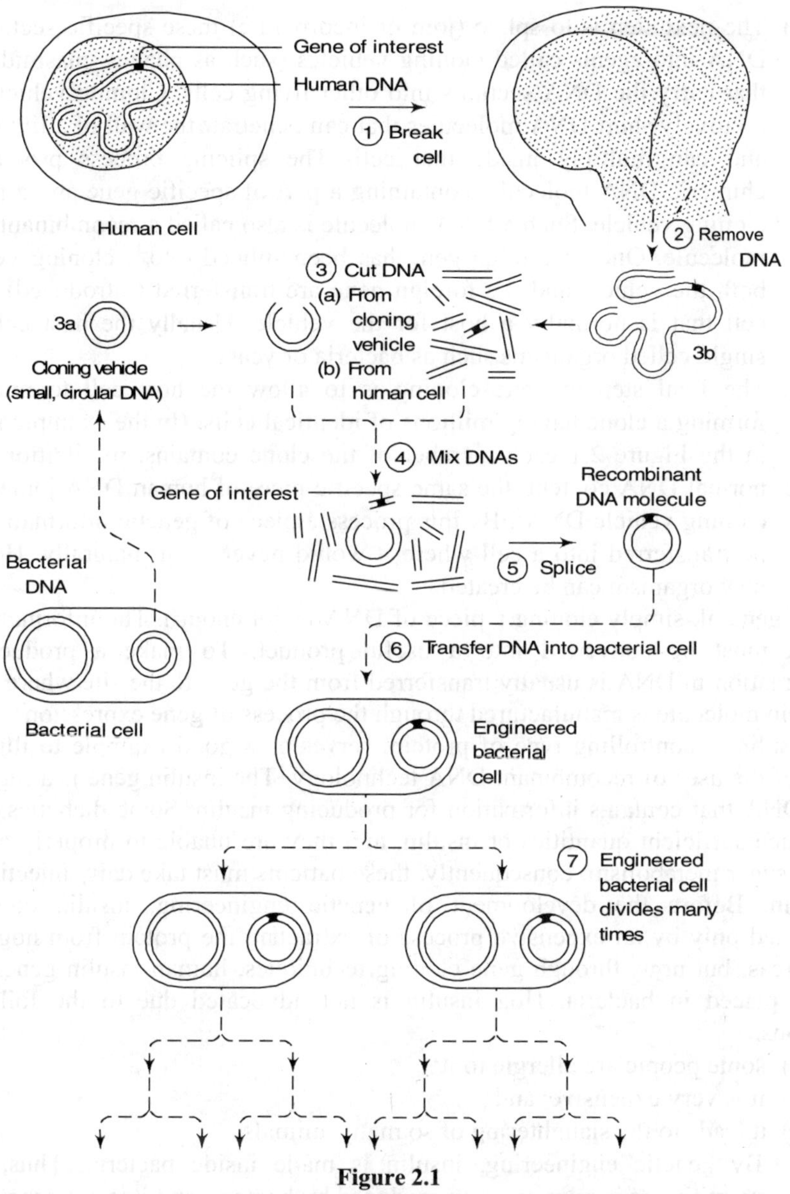

Figure 2.1

Major steps involved in gene cloning. 1. Human cells are broken (for clarity only one cell is shown) 2. DNA containing the gene of interest is removed from human cells. 3. The DNA from a cloning vehicle and human DNA are cut in specific places. The cloning vehicleDNA is obtained from bacterial cells. 4. The two types of DNA are mixed. 5. The DNA fragments are spliced together, yielding a recombinant DNA molecule. 6. The recombinant DNA molecule is transferred into a bacterial cell, which has its own DNA. 7. The engineered cell created by step 6 is allowed to reproduce millions of times to form a clone. of identical cells.

(***Source:*** *Drilica, K. Understanding DNA and Gene Cloning.* © 1984 *New York, John Wiley and Sons Inc. Reprinted by permission.*)

(d) The next step is to splice (join or incorporate) these specific sections of DNA into agents called cloning vehicles (such as phages, plasmids etc.) that carry the DNA sections into other living cells. Cloning vehicles are relatively short DNA molecules that can penetrate the wall of a living cell and can multiply inside that cell. The splicing process produces a chimeric DNA molecule, containing a part of specific gene and a part of cloning vehicle. Such a DNA molecule is also called a recombinant DNA molecule. Once a foreign gene has been spliced into a cloning vehicle, both the vehicle and the foreign gene are transferred (introduced) into a cell that is normally a host for the vehicle. Usually the host cells are single-celled organisms such as bacteria or yeast.

(e) The final step in gene cloning is to allow the host cell to multiply, forming a clone having millions of identical cells. (In the example shown in the Figure 2.1 each member of the clone contains, in addition to its normal DNA content, the same specific piece of human DNA joined to a cloning vehicle DNA). By this process a piece of genetic information can be transferred into a cell where it would never occur naturally. Hence a new organism can be created.

In general, simply cloning a piece of DNA is not enough. The information in DNA must be converted into a useful product. To make a product, the information in DNA is usually transferred from the gene to the site where a new protein molecule is manufactured through the process of gene expression.

Insulin, a controlling type of protein, serves as a good example to illustrate one of the uses of recombinant DNA technology. The insulin gene is a region in the DNA that contains information for producing insulin. Some diabetics fail to produce sufficient quantities of insulin, and they are unable to properly control their sugar metabolism; consequently, these patients must take daily injections of insulin. Before the development of genetic engineering, insulin could be obtained only by an expensive process of extracting the protein from hog (pig) pancreas, but now, through gene cloning techniques, human insulin genes have been placed in bacteria. Hog insulin is not advocated due to the following reasons:

(i) some people are allergic to it;
(ii) it is very expensive; and
(iii) it leads to the slaughtering of so many animals.

By genetic engineering, insulin is made inside bacteria. Thus, large quantities of insulin are now produced by bacteria and it is easier to obtain insulin from bacteria than from pancreas tissue. Moreover, the engineered bacteria produce human insulin, an important feature for diabetics who have become allergic to hog insulin.

To summarize, genetic engineering is a strategy for transferring small bits of genetic information (DNA) from one organism to another. Certain pieces of DNA will permanently alter the chemistry of the recipient organism in useful, predictable and permanent ways.

2.2 Restriction Endonucleases

2.2.1 Nature

Enzymes that cut the phosphodiester bonds of polynucleotide chains are called nuclease. Those nucleases that preferably break internal bonds are known as endonuclease. During the 1970s, it was found that bacteria contained nucleases that would recognize short nucleotide sequences with duplex DNA and cut the phosphodiester backbone at highly specific sites on both strands of duplex. These enzymes are called restriction endonucleases or simply restriction enzymes.

The discovery of a variety of restriction endonucleases is one of the reasons for the rapid development of recombinant DNA. technology. Enzyme that cuts the phosphodiester bonds of polynucleotide chains is called nuclease. The nuclease that preferably breaks internal bonds is known as endonuclease. The enzyme makes two incisions, one through each of the phosphate backbones of the double helix without damaging the bases. Different endonucleases found in different organisms recognize different nuclecotide sequences and therefore cut DNA at different cleavage sites as depicted in Figure 2.2. Table 2.1 gives the list of some restriction endonucleases and the site at. which they cleave DNA.

In nature, these restriction enzymes are used by the bacteria to destroy various viral DNAs that might enter the cell, thereby restricting the potential growth of the virus. Thus restriction enzymes serve as a defense mechanism. The bacteria protect their own DNA from nucleolytic attack by ethylating the bases at susceptible sites, a chemical modification that blocks the action of the enzyme. Restriction enzymes are molecular scissors that are used to recognize and cut DNA at specific sequences. The sites recognized by them are called recognition sequences or recognition sites. By locating the positions of the cleavage sites of a number of restriction enzymes in a DNA segment, restriction maps can be prepared.

Sometimes restriction enzymes cleave both DNA strands at precisely opposite points on the two strands, yielding blunt ended fragments. In some cases the two DNA strands are not cut directly opposite each other. Instead, the cuts are staggered forming cohesive ends(sticky ends). Figure 2.3 depicts the two types of cleavages. Most restriction enzymes recognize only one short base sequence in a DNA molecule and make two single-strand breaks, one in each strand, generating 3′-OH and 5′-P groups at each position. The sequences recognized by restriction enzymes are often palindromes—i.e. inverted repetitious sequences which are symmetrical.

In a palindrome with rotational symmetry, the base sequence in the first half of one strand of a DNA double helix is the mirror image of the second half of its complementary strand. Restriction enzymes can cleave the DNA in three ways, generating blunt ends, cohesive/ sticky ends with 3' tails and cohesive/ sticky ends with 5' tails. The way of breaking the DNA solely depends on the restriction enzyme. Each enzyme is named by a three letter (or four letter) abbreviation (letters are italicized) that identifies its origin. Roman numerals (I, II, III) are added to distinguish several enzymes with same origin (e.g., *Eco*RI).

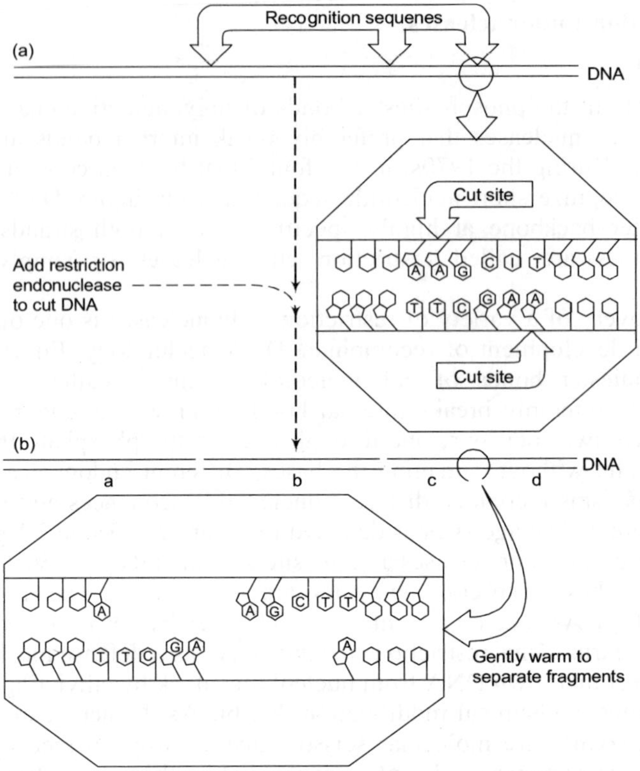

Figure 2.2

Cleavage of DNA by a Restriction Endonuclease. (a) A DNA molecule depicted as two parallel lines, may contain many- short nucleotide sequences recognized by restriction endonucleases. (b) When a restriction endonuclease is added to the DNA, it binds to the DNA and cuts it. Some of these enzymes produce staggered cuts. The DNA molecule in the example is converted into four shorter molecules, a, b, c, d each with staggered ends that can form base pairs with each other.

(***Source:*** *Drilica, K. Understanding DNA and Gene Cloning.* © 1984 *New York, John Wiley and Sons Inc. Reprinted by permission.*)

2.2.2 Properties

Many restriction enzymes have been isolated so far. All of these enzymes have been found in prokaryotes; no similar enzymes have been identified in the few eukaryotic organisms that have been examined.

The restriction enzymes fall into three types designated as Type I, Type II and Type III. In Type I and III, both the methylase and restriction activities are carried out by a single large enzyme complex. In Type II, the restriction enzyme is independent of its methylase and cleavage occurs at very specific sites that are within or close to the recognition sequence. Some enzymes recognize a specific nucleotide pair sequence and then cleave the DNA at a non-specific site away from that recognition site. Some enzymes cleave the DNA at the specific

Table 2.1

Some restriction endonucleases, their source, recognition sequences and sites of cleavage (indicated by arrow).

Enzyme	Source	Recognition sequence and clearage site
Eco RI	*Escherichia coli* Ry13	↓ G AATTC GTTAA G ↑
Hind II	*Haemophilus influenzae*	↓ GTPy PuAC CAPu PyTG ↑
Hind III	*Haemophilus influenzae* Rd	↓ A AGCTT TTC GA A ↑
Hpa I	*Haemophilus parainfluenzae*	↓ GTT AAC CAA TTG ↑
Hpa II	*Haemophilus parainfluenzae*	↓ CC GG GG CC ↑
Bam HI	*Bacillus amyloliquefaciens*	↓ G GATCC CCTAG G ↑
Bgl III	*Bacillus globigi*	↓ A GATCT TCTAG A ↑
Hae II	*Haemophilus aegyptius*	↓ PuGG GC Py PyCG CGPu ↑
Hae III	*Haemophilus aegyptius*	↓ GG CC CC GG ↑

Contd...

Table 2.1 Contd…

Enzyme	Source	Recognition sequence and clearage site
Hha I	*Haemophilus haemolyticus*	↓ G CGC CGC G ↑
Pst I	*Providencia stuartii*	↓ C TGCAG GACG TC ↑
Sma I	*Serratia marcescens*	↓ CCC GGG GGG CCC ↑
Taq I	*Thermus aquaticus*	↓ T CGA AGC T ↑
Bal I	*Brevibacterium albidum*	↓ TGG CCA ACC GGT ↑
Sal I	*Streptomyces albus* G	↓ G TCGAC CAGCT G ↑
Xor II	*Xanthomonas oryzae*	↓ C GAT CG GCTAG C ↑
Alu I	*Arthrobacter luteus*	↓ A GCT TCG A ↑
Msp I	*Moraxella* sp.	↓ CC GG GG CC ↑ Contd…

Enzyme	Source	Recognition sequence and clearage site
		↓
Mbo I	*Moraxella bovis*	G ATC CTA G ↑
Sau 3 Al	*Staphylococcus aureus* 3A	↓ GA TC CT AG ↑

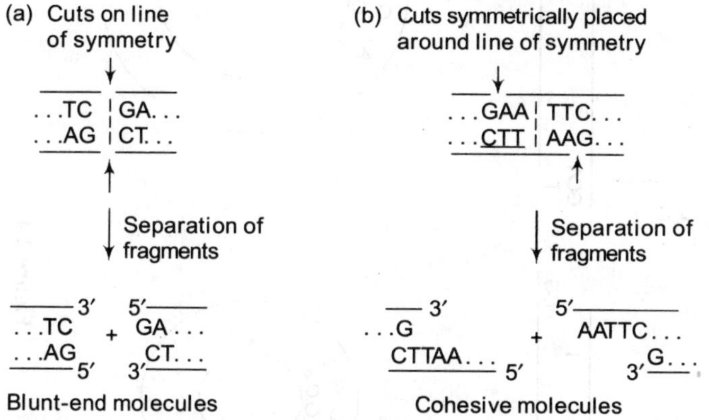

Figure 2.3

Two types of cuts made by restriction enzymes. The arrows indicate the cleavage sites. The dashed line is the centre of symmetry of the sequence.
(***Source:*** *Hartl, D.L.; Freifelder, D.; Snyder, I.A. Basic Genetics. © 1988 Boston: Jones and Bartlett Publishers. Reprinted by permission.*)

recognition site. All the enzymes are sequence specific, and thus the number of cuts they make in a particular DNA molecule or population of molecules is dependent upon the number of times the particular sequence is present in the DNA.

The sequences recognized by restriction enzymes are 4 to 8 nucleotides long and characterized by a particular type of internal symmetry. Besides cleavage, modification in the form of methylation is also brought about by some enzymes. They are called modification enzymes (methylases). This methylation distinguishes genes in different states of functioning. There are also enzymes which perform the function of restriction and modification. Based on these attributes restriction enzymes have been grouped into different types: type II restriction enzymes systems (e.g. *Eco*RI), which have different enzymes for modification and restriction; type I (*Eco*K) and type III (*Eco*PI) enzyme systems, in which the

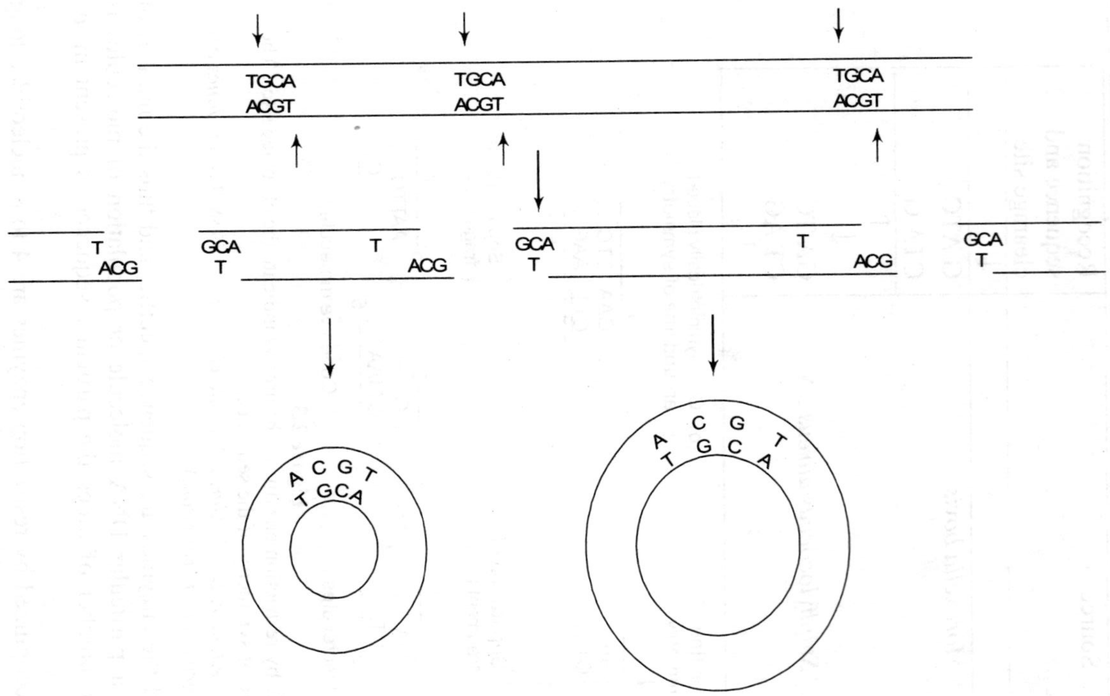

Figure 2.4

Circularization of DNA fragments produced by a restriction enzyme.
Arrows indicate cleavage sites.
(***Source:*** *Hartl, D.L.; Freifelder, D.; Snyder, L.A. Basic Genetics. © 1988 Boston: Jones and Bartlett Publishers. Reprinted by permission.*)

same enzyme possesses both activities although the restriction and modification sites differ in position.

Of the above two classes of restriction enzymes, type II are most important for cloning purposes. Enzymes with 4 bp target sites are used when frequent cuts are desired to get small DNA fragments and those with 8 bp are used when rare cuts are desired to get long DNA segments. Otherwise majority of the enzymes have 6 bp target sites. Some of them can cleave both methylated as well as unmethylated targets, but majority of them cleave only unmethylated targets.

One of the most important events in the study of restriction enzymes was the observation by electron microscope that fragments produced by many restriction enzymes spontaneously circularize. Figure 2.4 depicts this phenomenon. The circles could be relinearized by heating, but if after circularization they were also treated with *E. coli* DNA ligase, which joins 3′-OH and 5′-P groups, circularization became permanent. The Eco Rl enzyme, discovered in the laboratories of Dussoix and Boyer, was also able to cleave a circular DNA molecule to form a linear duplex with complementary ends. Figure 2.5 illustrates this.

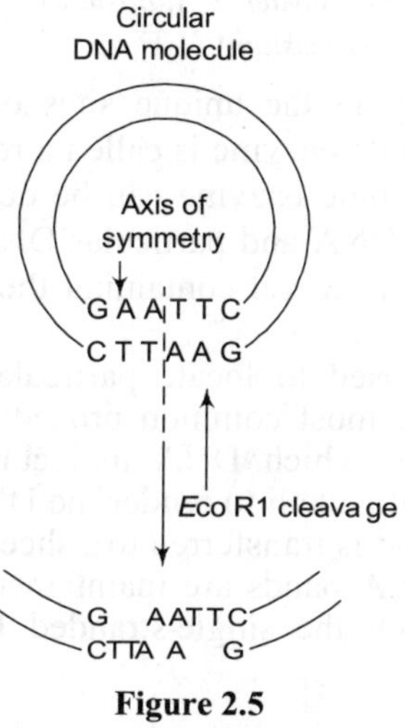

Figure 2.5

A circular DNA molecule with a single recognition site for Eco Rl restriction enzyme is cleaved to a linear duplex with complementary ends. Note the symmetry in recognition site and cleavage pattern.

Most restriction enzymes recognize one base sequence without regard to the source of the DNA. Thus, fragments obtained from a DNA molecule from one organism have the same cohesive ends as the fragments produced by the same enzyme acting on DNA molecules from another organism. This property is one of the foundations of the recombinant DNA technology. Since most restriction enzymes recognize a unique sequence, the number of cuts made in the DNA from an organism, by a particular enzyme is limited. Of special interest are the smaller DNA molecules, such as viral or plasmid DNA, which may have only 1–10 sites of cutting (or even none) for particular enzymes. Plasmids having a single site for a particular enzyme are especially valuable.

Because of the sequence specificity, a particular restriction enzyme generates a unique set of fragments for a particular DNA molecule. Another enzyme will generate a different set of fragments from the same DNA molecule. Figure 2.6 shows the sites of cutting of *E. coli* phage lambda DNA by the enzymes Eco R1

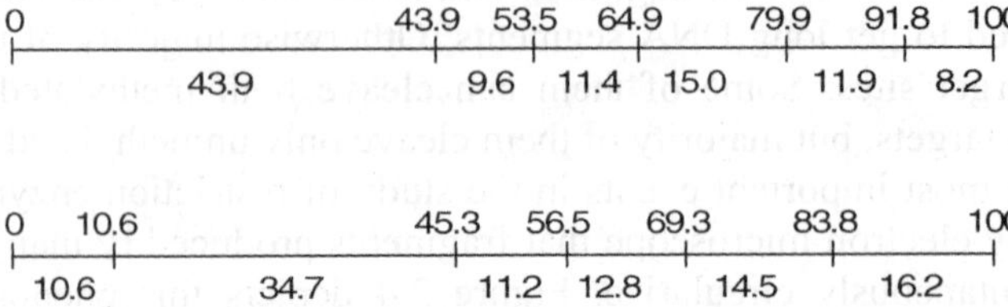

Figure 2.6
Restriction maps of a DNA for the restriction enzymes Eco Rl and Bam Hl. The vertical bars indicate the sites of cutting. The numbers above the line indicate the percentage of the total length of DNA measured from the end of the molecule arbitrarily designated as the left end. The numbers below the line are the length of each fragment, again expressed as percentage of the total length.
(***Source:*** *Hartl, D.L.; Freifelder, D.; Snyder, L.A. Basic Genetics. © 1988 Boston: Jones and Bartlett Publishers. Reprinted by permission.*)

and Bam HI. A map showing the unique sites of cutting of the DNA of a particular organism by a single enzyme is called a restriction map. The family of fragments generated by a single enzyme can be detected easily by gel electrophoresis of enzyme-treated DNA and particular DNA fragments can be isolated by cutting out the portion of the gel containing the fragment and removing the DNA from the gel.

Several techniques are used to locate particular genes on fragments of a restriction map. One of the most common procedures is Southern blotting. In Southern blotting, a gel in which DNA molecules have been separated by electrophoresis is treated with alkali to render the DNA single stranded (denature the DNA) and then the strand is transferred to a sheet of nitrocellulose so that the relative positions of the DNA bands are maintained. Figure 2.7 illustrates this. The nitrocellulose, to which the single-stranded DNA tightly binds, is then

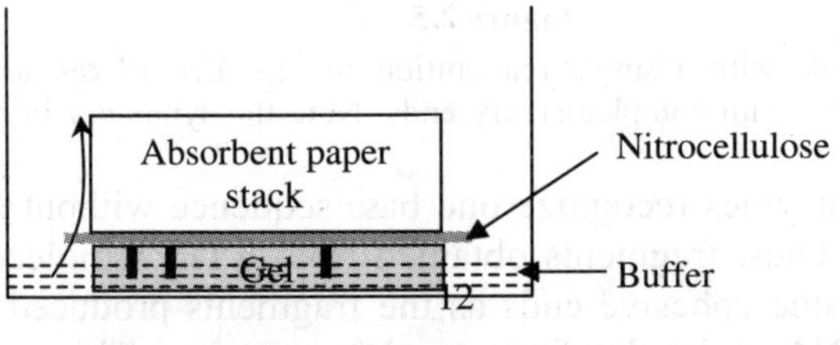

Figure 2.7 Southern Blotting

exposed to radioactive RNA or DNA probe which leads to renaturation. Radio labeled probe becomes stably bound (resistant to removal by washing) to the DNA only at positions at which base sequences complementary to the radio labeled probes are present. The radioactivity is located by placing the paper in contact with X-ray film; after development of the film, blackened regions indicate positions of radioactivity. If a radioactive mRNA species transcribed from a particular gene is used (e.g., mRNA isolated from a specialized cell that predominantly makes one type of RNA), it will hybridize only with the restriction fragment containing that gene.

2.3 Cloning Vehicles or Vectors

Cloning vehicles are small plasmid, phage, or animal virus DNA molecules used to transfer a DNA fragment from a test tube into a living cell. Cloning vehicles are also called vectors. Vectors have the ability to replicate by themselves. There can be cloning vectors and expression vectors. Cloning vectors are used for multiplying DNA inserts in a suitable host Transcription or translation of cloned gene does not occur. Cloning vectors are used in creating genomic library or gene bank, in the preparation of probe etc. Expression vector is used to express the cloned gene, i.e. transcription and translation of the cloned gene occurs, due to which a protein is produced. Expression vectors are used in producing transgenic plants or animals.
Southern blotting. Due to capillary action of absorbent paper stack, buffer travels through gel into absorbent paper stack. The DNA fragments will also be carried from the gel along with the buffer, which can't cross the membrane and adhere to it.

To be useful, a vector must have the following properties:

(1) It should have the ability of self-replication so that many copies of the DNA insert can be formed as the vector replicates.
(2) It should get introduced into the host cell very easily.
(3) It should contain unique target sites for restriction enzymes so that foreign DNA can be inserted without disrupting its function
(4) It should have promoter, operator etc., if the expression of foreign DNA is to be verified.

One of the most important uses of recombinant DNA technology is the cloning of (i) random DNA or cDNA segments, often used as probes or (ii) specific genes, which may be either isolated from the genome or synthesized either organochemically or in the form of cDNA from mRNA. This cloning of DNA is possible only with the help of another DNA molecule, which is capable of replicating in the host. This other DNA molecule is often used in the form of a vector, which could be a plasmid, a bacteriophage, a derived cosmid, a phagemid (phage + plasmid) or even a virus. Sometimes vectors are modified by inserting a DNA segment to locate unique site(s) for one or more restriction enzymes to facilitate its use in gene cloning. This inserted DNA is sometimes called 'poly linker'.

Certain types of small DNA molecules are infectious. Once inside a living cell, they can utilize the machinery of the cell for reproduction. According to the biochemist's definition of life, these DNA molecules are not alive; they cannot reproduce by themselves. Among other things they need RNA polymerase from their host (the infected bacterium) to transcribe their DNA into messenger RNAs. They also need host ribosomes to translate the messages into proteins. But even with these deficiencies, infectious DNAs can have profound effects on living cells. Some types take over a cell and kill it, while other types can be beneficial to a cell.

These infectious DNA molecules fall--++++++++++++++++ into two general types, the viruses and the plasmids. Viruses surround their DNA molecules with a protective shell of protein; thus, they can sometimes survive for many years outside their host cell. Plasmids, on the other hand, are naked, circular DNA molecules, generally found inside cells only. It is possible to cut DNA molecules from plasmids and bacteriophages (viruses that attack bacteria) at a specific place, insert a piece of DNA from another source, and still retain all the information necessary for infection by the plasmid or phage. Thus these infectious DNA molecules are useful as tools to transfer DNA from one type of cell to another.

2.3.1 Plasmids

Plasmids are small, circular, double-stranded, autonomously replicating, covalently bonded DNA molecules (Fig 2.8) that occur naturally in bacteria. Like all natural DNA molecules, plasmids contain a special region in their DNA called an origin of replication. The origin serves as a start signal for DNA polymerase and ensures that the plasmid DNA molecule will be replicated by the host cell.

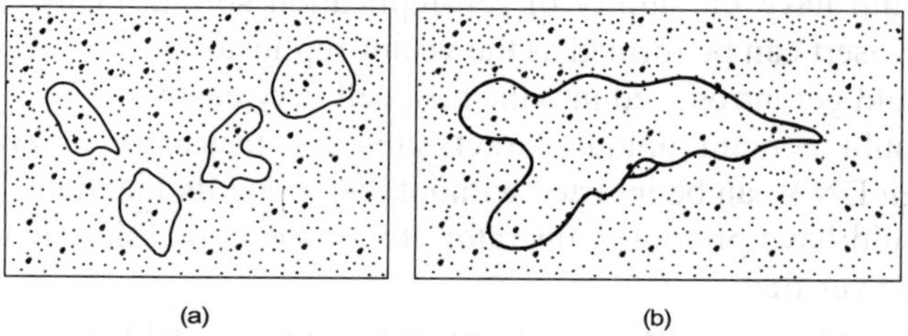

Figure 2.8

Magnified plasmids as observed under electron microscope (diagramatic) (a) Four DNA molecules of the type called Col El. These small, circular DNAs are only 0.001 times the length of *E. coli* DNA. (b) Enlargement of plasmid similar to col El showing a small portion with separation of strand.

(***Source:*** *Drilica, K. Understanding DNA and Gene Cloning. © 1984 New York, john Wiley and Sons Inc. Reprinted by permission.*)

Many kinds of plasmids have been discovered. Plasmids differ in length and in the genes contained in their DNA. Some of the smaller plasmids which are popular in gene cloning, have about 5000 nucleotide pairs, enough DNA to code for about five average-sized proteins. In comparison, *E. coli* contains slightly more than four million nucleotide pairs in its DNA, and we have about four billion nucleotide pairs in our DNA. There are plasmids which are larger and are difficult to handle (e.g. transmissible plasmids). They are generally not used in gene cloning. Some plasmids have the ability to integrate into the host's chromosome, and these are called episomes. The F factor that is involved with conjugation of *E. coli* is an example of an episome.

An important aspect of plasmid DNA molecules is that they often contain genes that make their host bacterial cell resistant to antibiotics. These plasmids carry antibiotic resistant genes that play an important role in the identification and selection of recombinant DNA molecules. In general the plasmid vehicles have different buoyant density than that of the host DNA and thus they can be easily purified. A plasmid that has been used extensively for molecular cloning is pBR 322 (Fig 2.9). This plasmid is of the non-conjugal type; it will not promote conjugation, and each *E. coli* cell transformed with it will have six to eight copies per host chromosome. pBR 322 is a plasmid that has been engineered in the laboratory from natural plasmids so that it has features which are useful for molecular cloning experiments. Its replication in the *E. coli* cell is dependent upon the presence of *rep.* the origin of replication sequence. pBR 322 is 4363 base pairs long, weighing 2.7×10^6 daltons.

Another series of plasmids that are used as cloning vectors belong to pUC series. They are available in pairs with reversed orders of restriction sites relative to *lac*Z promoter. pUC8 and pUC9 make one pair. These plasmid vectors are often used for cloning DNA segments of small size (upto 10 kilobases).

pSC 101 derived from plasmid *R-6-5* is the first cloning vehicle to be described. It has a single Eco R1 substrate site. It specifies tetracycline resistance and can replicate autonomously. Insertion of foreign DNA into this plasmid does not alter its other functions, specially those of resistance and replication. This has been successfully used for the cloning of antibiotic resistant genes, ribosomal DNA from the toad *Xenopus* and histone genes from the sea-urchin. The only disadvantage with pSC 101 is that the wild type cannot be distinguished from the recombinant derivatives.

This is a tumour inducing plasmid carried by the bacterium *Agrobacterium tumefaciens.* The bacterium transfers the plasmid into plant cells where it induces the formation of crown galls. Modified forms of the Ti plasmid are now being used for genetic engineering of plants. More details are given in chapter 4. pUC 18 is a popular and widely used plasmid first prepared in the University of California. It has 2686 bp, ampicillin resistant gene and Lac Z gene. It has multiple cloning sites.

Several plasmids were found to carry genetic factors for fertility, resistance to antibiotics, ability to ferment sugars and even hydrocarbons like petroleum, and for the production of bacteriocins and haemolysins. All these kinds of plasmids have duly been altered to yield smaller plasmids suitable as small vehicles. They are classified on the basis of their compatibility characteristics. Plasmids are considered incompatible when they fail to establish themselves due to competition for essential replication sites on the cell membrane.

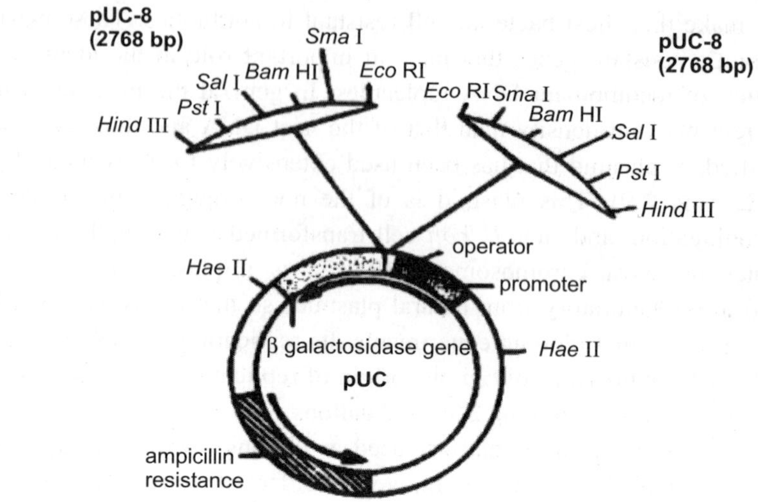

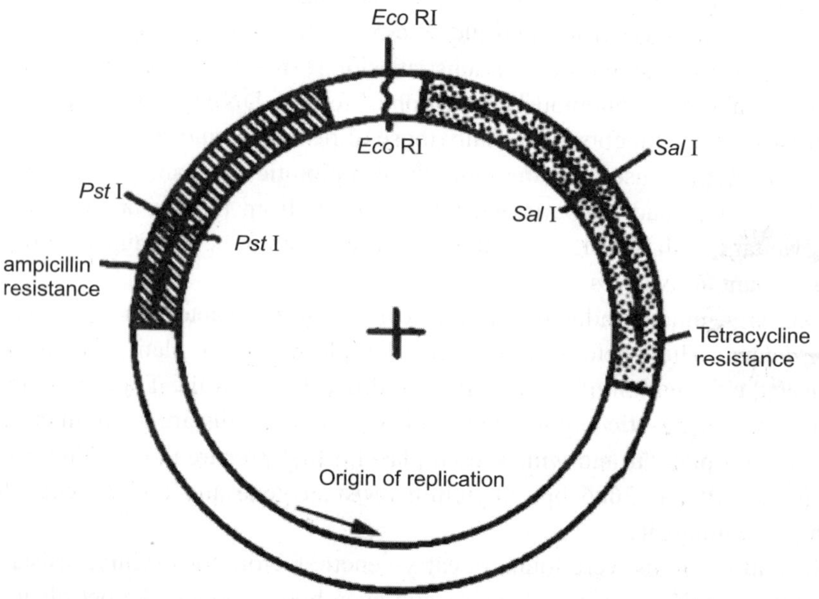

Figure 2.9

Physical map of the pBR 322 and pUC cloning vehicles.

Some plasmids belonging to group P exhibit promiscuity and are able to infect a wide range of gram-negative bacteria. Therefore they are used to introduce new genes. F plasmids are naturally occurring sex-factor plasmids which induce conjugation. These are not used in cloning experiments.

2.3.2.1 Lambda Phages (Temperate bacteriophage)

One of the phages used for cloning is called lambda. Lambda is slightly more sophisticated than other phages. When lambda DNA is injected into a bacterial cell, it has two choices. It can multiply and destroy the bacterium, or it can take up residence in the cell. This is referred to as a lysogenic cycle. When the latter choice is made the lambda DNA inserts into the bacterial chromosome; it becomes part of the bacterial chromosome (Fig. 2.11). The phage genes that normally would produce the proteins to kill the cell are turned offby a repressor protein made from phage gene. Thus every time the bacterial DNA replicates, lambda replicates. In this dormant state lambda DNA does a little more than produce repressor protein to keep its genes shut down. At the same time, the repressor protects the bacterial cell from infection by other lambda phages; when

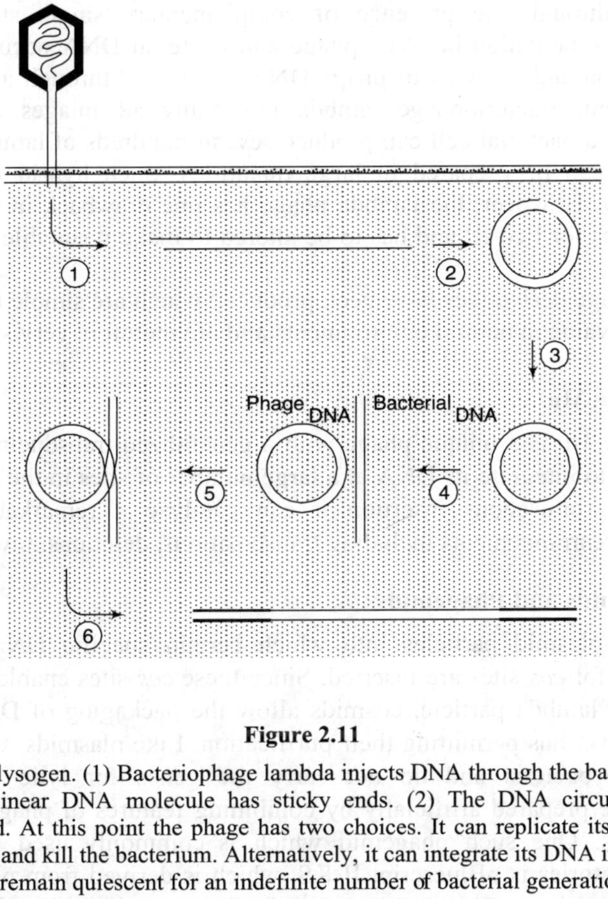

Figure 2.11

Formation of a lysogen. (1) Bacteriophage lambda injects DNA through the bacterial cell wall. The resulting linear DNA molecule has sticky ends. (2) The DNA circularizes and (3) becomes ligated. At this point the phage has two choices. It can replicate its DNA, produce progeny phage, and kill the bacterium. Alternatively, it can integrate its DNA into the bacterial DNA (4-6) and remain quiescent for an indefinite number of bacterial generations. Both phage and bacterial proteins play important roles in the integration process.

(***Source:*** *Drilica, K. Understanding DNA and Gene Cloning. © 1984 New York, John Wiley and Sons Inc. Reprinted by permission.*)

the newcomers inject their DNA, it is soon bound by a repressor produced from the resident lambda DNA. Thus the incoming DNA is unable to initiate a lytic infection that would kill the cell. Consequently, one can easily find lysogens (bacterial cells that are being protected by a resident phage).

When a lysogen is made with a phage carrying a cloned gene, a situation arises in which a gene is spliced onto a plasmid; the bacterial cell will carry the cloned fragment forever. By constructing the proper regulatory regions on the cloned gene through splicing, it is possible to control when the gene is turned on. Thus, either plasmids or phages can be used to insert genes into bacteria. Cloned genes can be retrieved from lysogens by destroying the phage repressor; the phage DNA then removes itself from the bacterial chromosome and directs the cell to make phage particles.

For lysogenization, the infected genome must be converted into a circle which is achieved through the presence of complementary single stranded ends. Reciprocal recombination between phage and bacterial DNA occurs at specific loci. Integration and excision of phage DNA is effected through a phage coded enzyme system. Bacteriophage lambda has many advantages as a cloning vehicle. Since a bacterial cell can produce several hundreds of lambda particles, hybrid DNA can be prepared in large quantities. Such hybrid DNA can be purified easily. However, the lambda phage has one drawback in that it carries five target sites for Eco Rl and has to be altered to make it suitable for a cloning vehicle.

Several phage derivatives have been produced which are simple to use, have a poor survival value in natural environments and are therefore very safe.

2.3.2.2 Phage Mu

Bacteriophage *Mu* is a unique phage with a generalized transducing ability and with capacity to integrate its DNA at a large number of sites in the host genome. Through its promiscuous insertion it can catalyze a remarkable range of chromosome rearrangements including transpositions, deletions, inversions etc.

2.3.2.3 Cosmids and Phagemids

Cosmids are plasmid particles into which certain specific DNA sequences, namely those for *cos* sites are inserted. Since these *cos* sites enable the DNA to get packed in lambda particle, cosmids allow the packaging of DNA in phage particle *in vitro*, thus permitting their purification. Like plasmids, these cosmids perpetuate in bacteria and do not carry the genes for lytic development. Phagemids are prepared artificially by combining features of phages (eg. M13) with plasmids. One such phagemid which is commonly used in molecular biology laboratories is pBluescript II KS, which is derived from pUC19, and is 2961 base pairs long. This is an expression vector, since the cloning site is flanked by T_3 and T_7 promoters to be read in opposite directions.

2.3.3 Transposable Genetic Elements

Gene cloning technologies allow us to insert small, discrete fragments of DNA into specific places in other DNA molecules. Nature also has this ability. Transposable genetic elements are structurally and genetically discrete segments of DNA capable of moving from one position in the genome to another. They are also called mobile genetic elements or jumping genes.

2.3.3.1 Insertion Elements

For many years, the corn plant provided the only genetic system in which such movable elements were observed. Later there was some preliminary evidence that several highly mutable genetic loci in *Drosophila* might be associated with movable control elements. But most geneticists paid little attention to such loci until it was discovered, in the late 1960s, that certain highly pleiotropic mutations (mutations affecting several functions) in *E. coli* resulted from the insertion of large segments of DNA called insertion sequences (IS).

An insertion element or insertion sequence is a short length of DNA duplex, ranging from 768 to 5700 base pairs, that has no origin of replication and must therefore be inherited in an integrated form. Quite a few insertion sequences have been identified in *E. coli* like IS I, IS 2, IS 3, IS 4, IS 5. Multiple copies of the IS 1 and IS 3 elements are scattered throughout the *E coli* chromosome. Not only are the individual IS elements capable of movement, but when present in closely spaced pairs they can move as a unit, carrying along the genes lying between them (Fig 2.12.A).

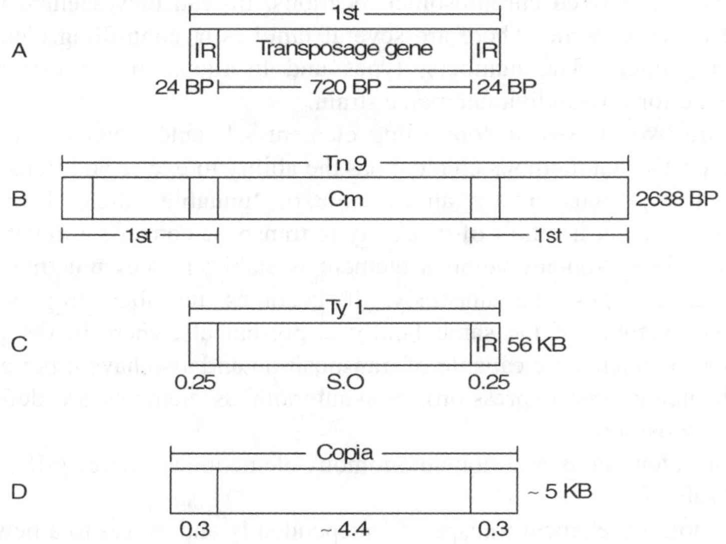

Figure 2.12

Different kinds of transposable elements. A. Insertion element; B. Transposon; C. Yeast T_Y element; D. *Drosophila* copia element.

2.3.3.2 Transposons

Transposon is another type of mobile genetic element encountered in many bacteria. Transposons, which are more complex than insertion sequences are short segments of DNA that lack the ability to self-replicate. They persist because they insert themselves into a pre-existing chromosome or plasmid and are replicated along with the host DNA. They are able to move from one site of insertion to another. Hence they can move from one plasmid to another or from one site to another within the same plasmid. A typical transposon carries one or more genes for antibiotic resistance and two inverted repeats at its termini (Fig. 2.12.B). More than 35 transposons have been characterized: e.g, Tn 3, Tn 4, Tn 5, Tn 9, Tn 10, Tn 903. There are three classes (Calss I, II and III) of transposons. Class III transposons are also known as miniature inverted repeat Transposable elements or MITES.

2.3.3.3 Maize Elements

Transposable elements or controlling elements are another type of mobile genetic elements encountered in maize plants. These elements alter the expression of standard genes and their activities are developmentally regulated. These elements transpose and promote genetic rearrangements at characteristic times and frequencies during plant development.

They have been studied in detail in bacteria but were first discovered in the maize plant, *Zea mays,* by Barbara McClintock. These genetic elements inhibited the expression of other maize genes with which they came into close contact; they did not have fixed chromosomal locations. Instead they seemed to move about the maize genome. There are several families of controlling elements in the maize genome. The numbers, types and locations of the elements are characteristic for each individual maize strain.

There are two classes of controlling elements: 1. autonomous and 2. Non-autonomous. The autonomous element has the ability to excise and transpose; its insertion at any locus creates an unstable or 'mutable' allele. Loss of the autonomous element itself, or of its ability to transpose converts a mutable allele to a stable allele. Non-autonomous element is stable; it does not transpose or suffer other changes spontaneously. It becomes unstable only when an autonomous member of the same family is present elsewhere in the genome. Autonomous elements are capable of transposition and also have other activities (e.g., influencing gene expression). Non-autonomous elements are deficient at least in transposition.

Pairs of autonomous and non-autonomous elements can be classified into 4 families (Table 2.2).

An autonomous element transposes independently and moves to a new site. A non-autonomous element requires the help of an autonomous element to move to a new site.

Table 2.2
Pairs of autonomous and non-autonomous elements

Autonomous	*Nonautonomous*
Ac (activator)	Ds (dissociation)
Mp (modulator)	Ds (dissociation)
Spm (supressor-mutator)	dspm (defective spm)
En (enhancer)	1 (inhibitor)
Dotted	Unnamed
Mu (mutator)	Not known
Cin	Not known
8s-1	Not known
Tz-86	Not known

2.3.3.4 Ty Elements in Yeast

A Ty element is another type of mobile genetic element. It is a family of dispersed repetitive DNA sequences that are found at different sites in different strains of yeast. Ty is the abbreviation for 'transposon yeast'. 5bp of target DNA are repeated on either side of the inserted Ty element (Fig.2.12.C). The frequency of Ty transposition is less than that of bacterial transposon. There are two major classes: Ty 1 and Ty 917. The development of yeast artificial chromosome (YMC) cloning vectors capable of carrying several hundred kilobase-pairs of DNA insert, has made it possible to study complex genomes, and the cloning of large genes of single fragments. Since YMCs can contain large inserts, contigs (sets of overlapping clones or sequences) of upto several megabases can be assembled facilitating the construction of maps over large chromosomal regions.

2.3.3.5 Copia Elements

P.x. copia elements are another type of mobile genetic elements. (Fig. 2.12.D). They are encountered in *Drosophila.* Other elements such as FB (fold back) and P elements are also seen in *Drosophila*.

2.4 Insertion of A Particular DNA Molecule into A Vector

We have already discussed restriction enzymes and cloning vehicles. Now let us see how these two can be employed to prepare recombinant DNA molecules. A collection of fragments obtained by digestion with a restriction enzyme can be made to anneal with a cleaved vector molecule, yielding a large number of hybrid vectors containing different fragments of foreign DNA (Fig. 2.13). However, if a particular DNA segment or gene is to be cloned, the vector possessing that segment must be isolated from the set of all vectors possessing foreign DNA.

For many genes, simple selection techniques are adequate for the recovery of a vector containing that gene. One method is that if the DNA of interest is known to be contained in a particular restriction fragment, that fragment can be isolated from a gel after electrophoresis and joined to an appropriate vector. However, eukaryotic cells contain about a million cleavage sites for a typical restriction enzyme; so direct isolation of a eukaryotic gene from a mixture of fragments separated by electrophoresis is not feasible.

One other technique for cloning a particular DNA molecule depends on an unusual polymerase, reverse transcriptase, which can use a single-stranded RNA molecule (such as mRNA) as a template and synthesize a double-stranded DNA copy, called complementary DNA or cDNA. If the template RNA molecule is a mRNA molecule (i.e., if the introns have been removed from the primary transcript), the corresponding full-length cDNA will contain an unintermpted coding sequence. This sequence will not be that of the original eukaryotic gene; however, if the purpose of forming the recombinant DNA molecule is to synthesize a eukaryotic gene product in a bacterial cell, and if such processed RNA can be isolated, then cDNA formed from processed mRNA is the material of choice to be inserted.

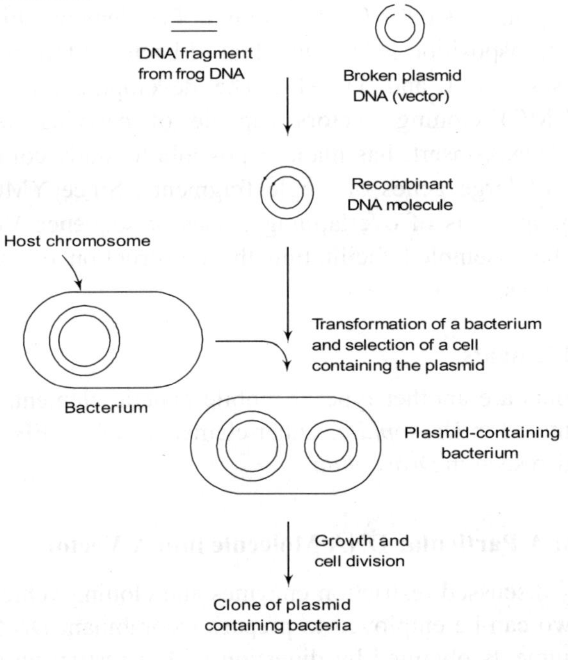

Figure 2.13

An example of cloning. A fragment of frog DNA is joined to a cleaved plasmid. The hybrid plasmid then transforms a bacterium, and thereafter frog DNA is present in all progeny bacteria.

(***Source:*** *Hartl. D.L.; Freifelder, D.; Snyder, L.A. Basic Genetics. © 1988 Boston: Jones and Bartlett Publishers. Reprinted by permission.*)

Foreign DNA can be cut into segments by a restriction enzyme that also makes one cut in the plasmid vehicle (e.g., pBR 322) converting the latter to a linear molecule. Figure 2.14 illustrates this for Eco Rl. By the very fact that Eco R1 cleaves at a specific site in this way, the single-stranded ends of the linear plasmid vehicle are complementary to the single-stranded ends of the Eco R1 generated segments of foreign DNA. In solution the two DNAs can come together to produce a larger circular DNA held together by hydrogen bonding of the complementary ends. In the presence of the enzyme polynucleotide ligase, the single-stranded gaps in the sugar-phosphate backbones are sealed and the structure is stabilized. The result is a recombinant DNA molecule. Since the ends of the DNA pieces produced by Eco R1 digestion are all identical, the foreign DNA can insert into the plasmid vehicle in two orientations, and this will occur in a random way. This orientation may have effects on transcription of the genes or gene fragments on the foreign DNA since the initiation of transcription is likely to depend on the location of promoter and other controlling sites on the vehicle.

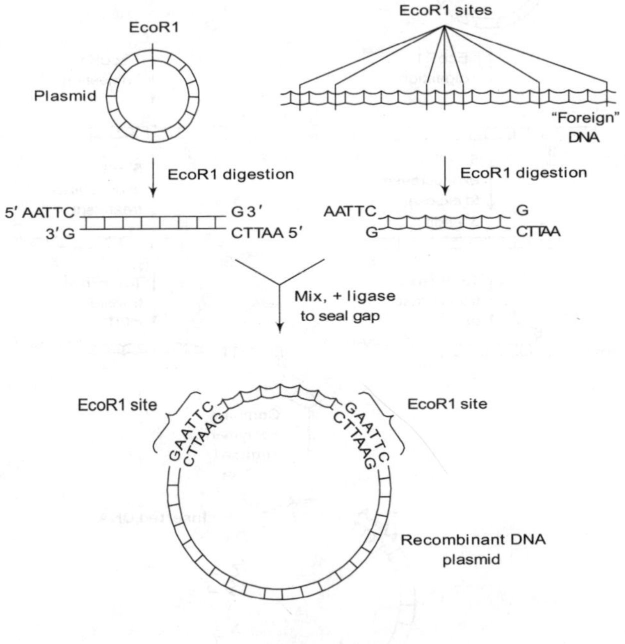

Figure 2.14

Construction of a recombinant DNA plasmid through the use of the restriction enzyme Eco R1. The Eco R1 cuts both the plasmid and the foreign DNA and by mixing, we get recombinant DNA plasmid.

(***Source:*** *Russel, P.J. Essential Genetics. © 1987 Oxford, Blackwell Scientific Publications. Reprinted by permission.*)

Practically, the number of single-stranded nucleotides on the DNA after digestion with a restriction enzyme that makes a staggered cut is small, and thus the probability of the complementary sequences finding one another in solution is relatively small. Further, some restriction enzymes do not make staggered cuts, and some methods for producing the DNA fragment to be cloned result in completely double-stranded (blunt ended) DNA. In these cases it is possible to synthesize a single-stranded polynucleotide chain on the DNA molecules using the enzyme terminal deoxynucleotidyl transferase. Thus, for example, in the presence of dATP, this enzyme will catalyze the production of a poly (dA) tail on each 3′ end of the DNA. To apply this to the insertion of a DNA fragment into the plasmid vehicle, poly (dA) tails (approximately 100 nucleotides long) can be polymerized on the linearized plasmid, and poly (d/T) tails of the same length can be polymerized on to the foreign DNA (Fig. 2.15). Then, by mixing the DNAs in solution and adding polynucleotide ligase, a recombinant DNA molecule can be produced.

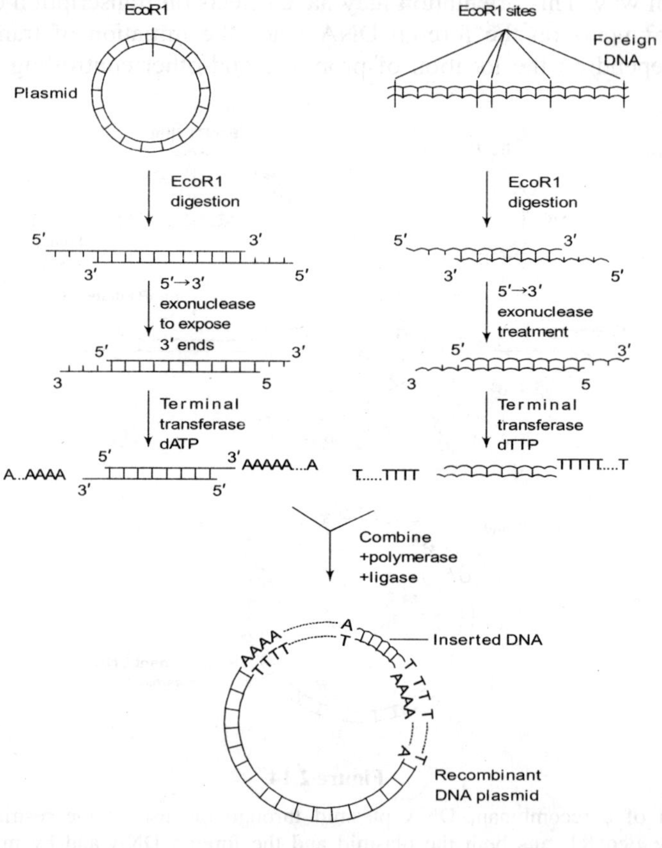

Figure 2.15

Construction of a recombinant DNA plasmid using the enzyme terminal transferase to synthesize complementary ends on the linearized plasmid and a restriction enzyme generated fragment of foreign DNA.

(***Source:*** *Russel, P.J. Essential Genetics.* © 1987 *Oxford, Blackwell Scientific Publications. Reprinted by permission.*)

The enzyme ligase forms a phosphodiester linkage between free 5′ phosphoryl and 3′ hydroxyl groups, thus joining two DNA molecules together, or circularizing a single, linear molecule. The main source of ligase is T4 phage, and this enzyme requires ATP to drive the ligation. An important feature of T4 DNA ligase is its ability to join blunt ends of DNA together, provided the concentrations of enzymes and DNA are high enough. A technique known as homopolymer tailing can be used to join blunt-ended molecules, and has the advantage that only intermolecular bonds, between vector and insert, can occur. Vector and insert are treated separately with terminal transferase and either dATP or TTP, so that poly dA tails are built up on the 3′ termini of one and poly T tails on the other. On mixing, the complementary tails will result in stable, hybrid molecules which can be used for transformation. The disadvantage of this method is that since it does not automatically create restriction sites on either side of the inserted DNA, the recovery of inserts may be difficult.

2.5 Transformation And Growth Of Cells

Before the recombinant DNA can be bulked up by cloning, it must be taken up by a suitable bacterial host cell, which is then said to be transformed; i.e. a host bacterial cell must accept the plasmid with the foreign gene, get it incorporated into its genome and start transcribing that gene. Usually a strain of *E. coli* lacking the restriction system which would normally degrade foreign DNA is used for this purpose. Untreated cells will not take up DNA to any significant extent, and so they must be pre-treated to make them 'competent.' This pre-treatment usually involves incubation of exponentially growing cells with $CaCl_2$ at low temperatures, after which the DNA is added; a mild heat shock then results in the uptake of the DNA.

The selection of transformed cells usually depends on their resistance to an antibiotic. So it is important to incubate the cells in a medium without antibiotic for about an hour, to allow the plasmid antibiotic resistant genes to be expressed. The cells can then be plated on a solid medium containing antibiotic for the selection of colonies containing recombinant DNA.

2.6 Detection of Recombinant Molecules

When a vector is cleaved by a restriction enzyme and renatured with a mixture of all restriction fragments from a particular organism, many types of molecules result e.g. a self-joined vector that has not acquired any fragments, a vector with one or more fragments, a molecule consisting only of many joined fragments. To facilitate the isolation of a vector containing a particular gene, some means is needed to ensure, first, that a vector established after $CaCl_2$ transformation does possess an inserted DNA fragment, and second, that it is the DNA segment of interest.

In using the $CaCl_2$ transformation procedure to establish a plasmid in a bacterium, the initial goal is to isolate bacteria that contain the plasmid from a mixture of plasmid-free and plasmid-containing colonies. A common procedure is to use a plasmid possessing an antibiotic-resistance marker and to grow the transformed bacteria on a medium containing the antibiotic; only cells in which a plasmid has become established will form a colony. A useful plasmid is pBR322. It has two different antibiotic-resistance markers—resistance to tetracycline *(tet-r)* and to ampicillin *(amp-r).* Thus plasmid-containing transformants are easily detected by the growth of a transformed culture on medium containing either one of these antibiotics. pBR 322 is also very useful because it contains only one copy of each of the seven different types of restriction-enzyme cleavage sites at which DNA can be inserted, so that the position of inserted DNA is always known.

In addition to a screening procedure for identifying plasmid-containing cells, a method is needed to identify plasmids in which DNA has been inserted. The presence of two antibiotic-resistance markers in pBR 322, allows the use of a procedure for detecting insertion called insertional inactivation. This is carried out as follows: In pBR 322 the *tet* gene contains sites for cutting by the restriction enzymes Bam HI and Sal I. Thus, insertion at either of these sites will yield a plasmid that is *amp- r tet-s,* because insertion interrupts and hence inactivates the *tet* gene. If the wild type (*Amp-s, Tet-s)* cells are transformed with a DNA sample in which the cleaved pBR 322 and restriction fragments have been joined, and the cells are plated on a medium containing ampicillin, all surviving colonies must be *amp-r* and hence must possess the plasmid. Some of these colonies will be *Tet-r* and some *Tet-s,* and these can be identified by replica-plating on to a medium containing tetracycline. Because unaltered pBR 322 carries the *tet-r* allele, an *Amp-r* colony will also be *Tet-r* unless the *tet-r* allele has been inactivated by the insertion of foreign DNA. Thus, an *Amp-r Tet-s* cell must contain pBR 322 DNA as well as donor DNA.

2.7 Selection and Screening of Particular Recombinants

From the large number of colonies produced by transformation, how is it possible to pick out those few which contain a particular fragment of DNA? One of the most useful methods is known as colony hybridization (Fig. 2.16). The colony hybridization assay allows detection of the presence of any gene for which radioactive mRNA is available. Colonies to be tested are replica-plated from a solid medium on to a nitrocellulose filter paper. A portion of each colony remains on the medium, which constitutes the reference plate. The paper is treated with NaOH, which simultaneously breaks open the cells and denatures the DNA. The paper is then saturated with ^{32}P-labelled mRNA, complementary to the gene being sought, and DNA-RNA renaturation occurs. After washing to remove unbound (^{32}P) mRNA, the positions of the bound radioactive phosphorous, usually detected by autoradiography, desired colonies are located. A similar assay is done with phage vectors; in this case, plaques are replica-plated.

If the protein product of a gene of interest is synthesized, immunological techniques allow the protein producing colony to be identified. In one test, the colonies are transferred, as in colony hybridization, and the transferred copies are exposed to a radioactive antibody directed against the particular protein. The colonies to which the radioactivity adheres are those containing the gene of interest. The radioactivity is detected by autoradiography.

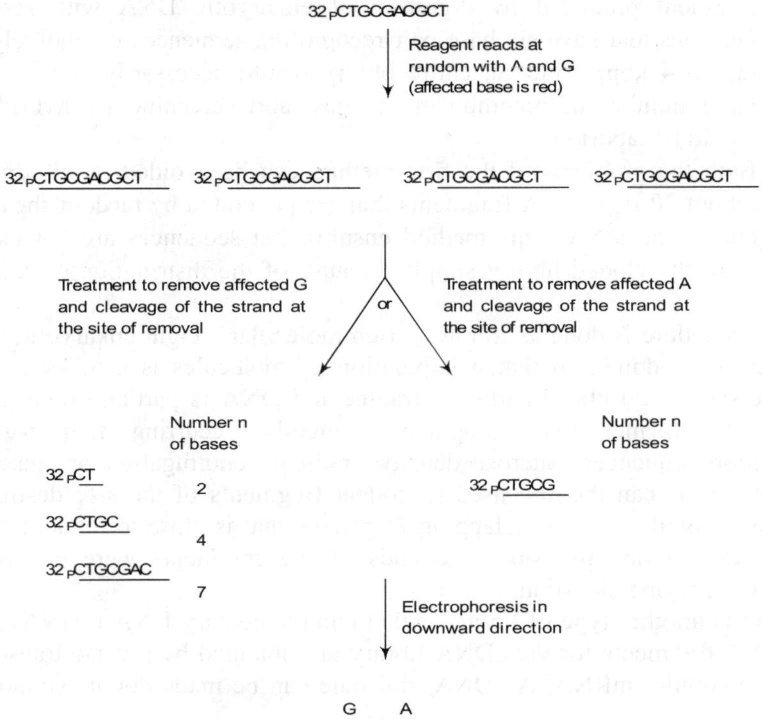

Figure 2.16

(***Source:*** *Hartl, D.L.; Freifelder, D., Snyder, L.A. Basic Genetics. © 1988 Boston: Jones and Bartlett Publishers. Reprinted by permission.*)

2.8 Genomic DNA and cDNA Libraries

A genomic DNA library is a collection of independently isolated vector-linked DNA fragments derived from a single organism. It contains at least one copy of every DNA sequence in the genome. An ideal library is one that represents all of the sequences with the smallest possible number of clones.

Genomic DNA libraries of eukaryotes may be prepared in two ways:

(1) Genomic DNA is digested to completion with a restriction enzyme and the fragments are inserted into a suitable vector, usually lambda. One drawback of this method is that if the sequence of interest contains recognition site for the restriction enzyme used, the sequence will be cut into two or more pieces. Another drawback is that the average size of the fragment produced by digestion of eukaryotic DNA with restriction enzymes that have six base pair recognition sequences is relatively small (about 4 kbp). Thus an entire library would necessarily contain a very large number of recombinant phages, and screening by hybridization would be laborious.

(2) Both the problems of the first method can be avoided by cloning large (about 20 kbp) DNA fragments that are generated by random shearing of eukaryotic DNA. This method ensures that sequences are not excluded from the cloned library simply because of the distribution of restriction sites.

The procedure is done as follows: High molecular weight eukaryotic DNA is fragmented randomly so that a population of molecules is produced with an average size of 20 kbp. Randomly fragmented DNA is partially digested with restriction enzymes that recognize frequently occurring four base pair recognition sequences. Sucrose density gradient centrifugation or agarose gel electrophoresis can then be used to collect fragments of the size desired. The result is a population of overlapping fragments that is close to random and that can be cloned directly, since the ends of the fragments were produced by restriction enzyme digestion.

There is another type of library called complementary DNA (cDNA) library. The DNA fragments for the cDNA library are obtained by reverse transcription from the cellular mRNA. A cDNA molecule can be made double stranded and cloned.

2.8.1 Chromosome Walking

When we wish to analyze several hundred kilobases of contiguous information from a eukaryotic genome, we cannot obtain that much DNA on a single phage or cosmid. However, one recombinant phage or cosmid can be used to isolate another recombinant that contains overlapping information from the genome. This technique is known as chromosome walking and it depends on isolating a small segment of DNA from one end of the first recombinant and using this piece of DNA as a probe to re-screen the phage or cosmid library in order to obtain a recombinant containing that piece of DNA and the next portion of the genome. The second recombinant is used to obtain a third, and so on, to yield a set of overlapping cloned segments.

2.9 Sequencing DNA

The sequence of DNA refers to the order of nucleotide bases along its sugar-phosphate backbone. Through the specificity of base pairing a double helix of DNA maintains a constant structure irrespective of its particular sequence. The difference between individual molecules of DNA lies in their particular sequences of base pairs, not in gross changes of structure. DNA exists in the form of very long chains (5,000 base pairs long in one bacteriophage; 2,40,0001000 bp long in human chromosome).

No technique can determine the sequence of bases in an entire chromosome in a single experiment; so it is necessary to cut the chromosomes into fragments of manageable size (a few hundred base pairs long) and purify each fragment type. This is done by cloning the fragment into a plasmid or viral DNA vector. After amplification, the cloned DNA segments are released for sequencing by cleavage with a restriction endonuclease.

Firstly, a series of single stranded DNA molecules are generated, each molecule one base longer than the last. DNA molecules of the same sequence, but differing in length by as little as one base at one end, can be separated by electrophoresis on acrylamide gels. This extraordinary sensitivity to size is made use of in the base sequencing procedure. Two types of approaches have been used to obtain these sets of bands. One is to use chemical reactions that cleave DNA at individual bases. The other is to use an enzymatic reaction in which DNA is synthesized *in vitro* in such a way that the reaction terminates specifically at the position corresponding to a given base. To determine the sequence of the molecule by either approach, it is subjected to the appropriate protocol in four separate reactions, each reaction specific for one of the four bases, by which a cut is made in the DNA next to a G, an A, any pyrimidine (i.e. T or C) and a C.

Maxam and Gilbert's chemical degradation method

This method was developed by Allan Maxam and Walter Gilbert of Harvard University. In this method chemical reagents are used to destroy specific nucleotide bases and thus break the DNA molecule at specific sites. The steps involved are:

(i) The strands of the DNA molecule are radioactively labelled by the addition of ^{32}P-dATP at one end (usually the 5'end).

(ii) Two strands of DNA are separated to yield the complementary single strands.

(iii) Each complementary single strand, which is end-labelled is treated with four different chemical reagents that break the strand at one end or at two specific nucleotides. The cleavage is allowed to occur at C, G+A, C+T, or T.

(iv) The digest from the four reaction mixtures are then separately subjected to gel electrophoresis simultaneously to separate the fragments by their size. The shortest fragments are those that move the fastest and farthest.

(v) Each complementary strand is sequenced independently and then the sequences are compared for confirmation.
(vi) The bands can be located by placing an autoradiographic (responding to radioactivity) film on the gel.

The procedure for sequencing a DNA fragment is given in Figure 2.17.

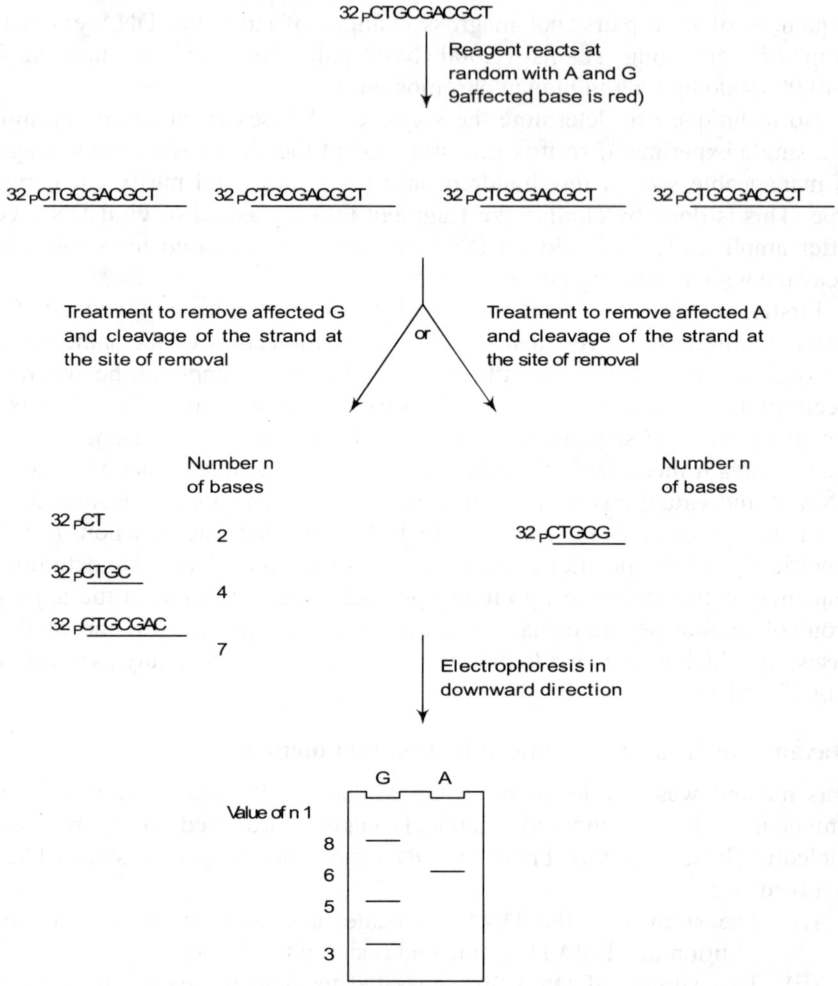

Figure 2.17

Determination of the positions of G and A in a DNA fragment containing ten bases. The value of n + 1 for all four bases would be determined by noting positions in all four bands in a gel containing the A, C, G, and C + T samples.
(***Source:*** *Hartl, D.L.; Freifelder, D.; Snyder, L.A. Basic Genetics. © 1988 Boston: Jones and Bartlett Publishers. Reprinted by permission.*)

The positions of A and G in the single strand are determined by the following rules:

(1) If a fragment containing *n* nucleotides is generated by a chemical treatment that causes cleavage at the site of a particular base, then that base is present in position n + 1 of the DNA strand, the position being counted from the 5′ ends.

(2) If a band containing *n* nucleotides is present in the A, G, C, or only in T + C parts, then a A, G, C, or T respectively, exists at position n + 1 in the original molecule.

Sanger Dideoxyribonucleotide synthetic method

This technique was developed by Fredrick Sanger and A.R. Coulson of the Medical Research Council, Cambridge. In this method an enzyme (polymerase) is used to insert the complementary deoxyribonucleoside triphosphate (dNTP) into the DNA chain and dideoxyribonucleoside triphosphate (ddNTP) is used to terminate the DNA chain elongation since it cannot form a phosphodiester bond with next incoming dNTP. There are four dNTPs (dATP, dGTP, dCTP and dTTP). Similarly there are four ddNTPs (ddATP, ddGTP, ddCTP and ddTTP). The basic steps are:

(vii) Cut the DNA with restriction enzyme to get different DNA fragments of about 500 base pairs.

(viii) Denature the DNA fragments (by heating and cooling or alkali treatement)

(ix) Divide them into 4 different groups in separate tubes

(x) Add to each tube a radioactively labelled oligonucleotide (acting as primer) that is complementary to the 3'end of the single stranded DNA, DNA polymerase enzyme, all the four dNTPs (dATP, dGTP, dCTP and dTTP), and a low amount of ddATP in one tube, ddGTP in the second tube, ddCTP in the third tube, ddTTP in the fourth tube (these bring about termination at specific bases (A, G, C, T)).

(xi) Incubate the reaction mixture at appropriate conditions. The labelled oligonucleotide binds to the 3' end of single-stranded DNA and serves as a primer for addition of dNTPs into a growing complementary chain. When ddNTP is incorporated in the place of normal dNTP, chain termination occurs. The result is the formation of incomplete, radioactively labelled different length DNA fragments

(xii) Load the four reaction mixtures into separate wells on high resolution poly acrylamide gel electrophoresis

(xiii) The gel is used for autoradiography to visualize the band in each lane and from their position the sequence of the DNA fragment can be noted.

2.10 Gene Identification and Mapping

Restriction fragment length polymorphism (RFLP), random amplified polymorphic DNA (RAPD), and DNA fingerprinting techniques are widely used in gene mapping and identification of different systems. RFLPs have especially increased the efficiency of mapping the quantitative trait loci. New technologies such as ribozymes and gene tagging are promising in gene cloning. Polymerase Chain Reaction (PCR) has become a widely applicable tool in biology, agriculture and medicine and may be replaced with a new method called Ligase chain reaction (LCR). The analysis of molecular markers can accomplish the characterization, gene mapping and identification, certification and patent protection of products.

2.10.1 Restriction Fragment Length Polymorphism (RFLP)

The use of cloned fragments of chromosomal DNA as genetic markers is usually termed RFLP. This technique is dependent on a natural variation in DNA base sequence and digestion of DNA with a restriction enzyme. Homologous restriction fragments of DNA which differ in size, or length, can be used as genetic markers to follow chromosome segments through genetic crosses. Using this technique, RFLP linkage maps can be prepared. These molecular maps and markers have provided a direct method for selecting desirable genes such as disease resistant, variety identification and so on. Extremely high saturation of RFLP markers around genes of interest can be achieved with near isogenic lines. The basic advantage of this technique is that a probe can be identified to be linked to a gene just by comparison of the RFLP patterns of the donor parent, the recurrent parent and one or more lines isogenic for that trait of interest.

The continuous variation for most of the traits in nature is a result of the concept that the quantitative traits can arise from segregation of multiple genes, modified by environmental effects. The linkage and accurate systematic mapping of quantitative trait loci was not possible because the inheritance of an entire genome could not be studied with genetic markers. The use of RFLPs has increased the efficiency of mapping quantitative trait loci, because of the greater number of markers that can be scored in a single population relative to other markers such as isozymes or morphological markers. It is also possible to examine the effects of environment upon the expression of individual gene loci involved in a complex trait, and determine functionally a genotype-environment interaction. In agriculture, quantitative trait loci analysis can help in locating useful quantitative traits harboured in wild species, including resistance to diseases and pests, tolerance to drought, heat, cold and other adverse conditions, and efficient use of resources and nutritional quality.

2.10.2 Random Amplified Polymorphic DNA (RAPD)

The technical complexity of RFLP analysis, coupled with the widespread use of shortlived radioisotopes in the detection method, questions the suitability of the routine use of RFLPs on a large-scale. Williams *et al.* (1990) described a new DNA polymorphism assay based on the polymerase chain reaction (PCR) amplified random segments with single primers of arbitrary nucleotide sequence.

They suggested that these polymorphisms may be called RAPD markers, after random amplified polymorphic DNA. The RAPD method is technically simple, quick to perform, requires small amounts of DNA, involves no radioactivity, and is well suited for use in large sample-throughput systems required for breeding, population genetics and bio-diversity.

Every organism is marked by some polymorphic changes at the DNA level. RAPD technique is a DNA polymorphism assay which involves the amplification of random segments using Primers with arbitrary nucleotide sequences (about 10 nucleotide sequences). RAPD allows the random amplification of DNA sequences throughout the genome. The banding patterns in the amplified fragments show polymorphism and help in genetic finger printing of individuals within a population or a species. This technique also helps to distinguish between organisms that exhibit similar biochemical properties. RAPD is a relatively simple technique which requires only a small amount of DNA.

Simple Sequence Repeats

Simple Sequence repeats (SSR) or microsatellites are 1-6 nucleotides length tandem repeats scattered throughout the genomes of most organisms. Inter simple sequence repeats (ISSR) are designed from dinucleotide or trinucleotide simple sequence repeats of 1-3 nucleotides that are anchored to either the 5' or 3' nucleotides. Primer matches found on opposite stands on the template DNA molecule, when within an amplifiable distance, give rise to discrete products. SSR and ISSR markers are generated by single primer PCRs similar to RAPD method. However, SSR and ISSR markers exhibit higher degrees of polymorphism compared to RAPD and are more reproducible.

2.10.3 DNA Fingerprint Analysis

In genomic DNA of various species, mini satellite and micro satellite DNA sequences have been found to detect several loci consisting of tandem repeats of a short nucleotide sequence (10-60 based pairs). Analysis of these sequences yields very high levels of polymorphism. This is due to tandem repeats, presumably resulting from unequal mitotic or meiotic exchanges or by DNA slippage during replication. At a given locus, numerous alleles differing in the number of repeats, may thus occur. Probes that hybridize to fragments from several variable loci simultaneously have been found, producing an autoradiograph with a complex fragment pattern called a DNA fingerprint. These fragments are inherited in a Mendelian fashion, and they therefore provide a technique suitable for genetic analysis. DNA fingerprints are highly individual-specific and are applicable in: genetic variation studies, forensic and ecological studies, breeding programmes, and population genetics and in the analysis and characterisation of genome and variety identification.

DNA fingerprinting is also used extensively in identifying victims of murder, accident, etc., in confirming criminals in cases of rape, murder etc., and to solve parental disputes.

2.10.4 Ligase Chain Reaction (LCR)

The ligase chain reaction is an offshoot of polymerase chain reaction (PCR). This may prove to be more effective than PCR. This is helpful to discriminate between two individuals who differ by a single base pair substitution.

2.10.5 Ribozymes

Ribozymes are RNA molecules that act as enzymes and exhibit intramolecular catalysis (e.g. self-cleavage or self-splicing). Ribozymes are of two types that can cleave RNA in a sequence-specific manner. In the first type, the self-splicing reaction occurs to remove an intron from the nuclear pre-ribosomal RNA. These ribozymes have a four base recognition sequence and they are useful for specific cleavages of RNA *in vitro*. The second type of ribozymes depends on the self-cleavage reactions that occur during the replication of certain virioids and satellite RNAs. Ribozymes can be targetted to different regions of a virus genome.

2.11 Analysis of Integration and Expression of Cloned Genes

The integration of cloned genes can be analyzed with Southern blot analysis, the position of the gene can be determined using *in situ* hybridization. The expression of a gene can be analyzed using Northern analysis.

2.11.1 Southern Blot Analysis

This method (proposed by E.M.Southern) utilizes the hybridization of complementary DNA fragments to identify integrated foreign DNA. Total DNA of the organism is isolated, digested with restriction enzymes and the resulting double stranded DNA (dsDNA) fragments are resolved on the basis of molecular weights by electrophoresis on agarose gel. The dsDNA are denatured to generate single stranded DNA fragments with the help of an alkali solution and then are transferred and fixed to a nitrocellulase filter and is incubated with the radioactively labelled cloned inserts (the probe). For example, the probe can be labelled with ^{32}P. The probes specifically bind to cDNA present on the filter and can be visualized on an autoradiograph of the filter. Non-radioactively probes are also used.

2.11.2 Northern Blot Analysis

This method is employed to identify RNA that has been resolved by gel electrophoresis. It involves the analysis for transcribed mRNA. mRNA can be transferred to nitrocellulose membrane and hybridized. Radioactively labeled DNA will hybridize only with transcribed RNA.

2.11.3 Western Blotting Analysis

This technique is used to detect proteins of a particular specificity. When a transferred gene expresses in transformed cells, the translated product in the form of protein can be identified by this technique. The extracted proteins are subjected to electrophoresis and then transferred to nitrocellulose membrane. This membrane is probed with a specific labelled antibody (which will not hybridize but bind) to bind with protein. Using autoradiography, the binding can be visualized. This technique is also called immunoblotting.

2.11.4 Dot Blot Analysis

In dot blot cloned or pure DNA to be tested is spotted on a nitrocellulose membrane adjacent to each other as dots. The DNA is immobilized and denatured to form single strands. This is hybridized with a probe and signals are identified using autoradiography.

2.11.5 *In Situ* Hybridization (ISH)

The position of a particular gene on the cytological map of the organism can be determined directly with *in situ* hybridization (ISH). A radioactive probe representing a gene (a labelled cDNA clone derived. from the mRNA) is hybridized with the denatured DNA of the polytene chromosomes *in situ.* By autoradiography, the position or positions of the corresponding genes can be identified. Fluorescence *in situ* hybridization (FISH) enables us to perform specific detection of unique sequences of varying length, chromosomal regions or entire chromosomes within metaphase or interphase cells, and rapid mapping and ordering of DNA fragments on single metaphase chromosome bands. A modification of this method is genomic *in situ* hybridization (GISH) which is used to identify alien chromatin in chromosome spreads.

2.12 Gene Amplification and screening

2.12.1 Polymerase Chain Reaction (PCR)

The polymerase chain reaction (PCR) is an *in vitro* method for replicating a defined DNA sequence so that its amount is increased exponentially. Even a single gene copy can be amplified to a million copies within a few hours by PCR.

PCR consists of repetitive cycles of DNA denaturation through melting at elevated temperature to convert double stranded DNA to single stranded DNA, annealing oligonucleotide primers to the target DNA and extension of the DNA by nucleotide addition from the primers by the action of DNA polymerase.

The target region for amplification is defined by unique oligonucleotide primers that flank a DNA segment. The oligonucleotide primers are designed to hybridize to regions of DNA that flank a desired target gene sequence, annealing to complementary strands of the target sequence. The primers are then extended across the target sequence by using a heat-stable DNA polymerase in the presence of free deoxynucleoside triphosphates (dNTPs), resulting in a doubled replication of the starting target material.

By repeating the three stage process many times, a nearly exponential increase in the amount of target DNA is obtained. The product of each PCR cycle is complementary to and capable of binding the primers, and so the amount of DNA is potentially doubled in each successive cycle.

PCR products can be tagged with fluorescent dyes that would help in mapping the gene of interest when we screen large number of individuals. This can be accomplished by synthesizing the primer for each locus by incorporating a fluorescent tag on the 5' end of the new primer. There are many PCR dyes: 6-FAM (blue), VIC (green), NED (yellow) PET (red) and LIZ (orange).

The progress of a PCR reaction is monitored in a real time PCR (RTPCR). Even very small amounts of PCR products can be quantified. RTPCR is based on the detection of fluorescence produced by a reporter molecule which increases as the reaction proceeds. The fluorescent reporter molecules include dyes that bind to the double stranded DNA or sequence specific probes.

Taq DNA polymerase

Taq DNA polymerase ia thermostable DNA-dependent DNA polymerase. It was originally purified from the extreme thermophile bacterium *Thermus aquaticus* from hotspring. Now it is available in a genetically engineered form. These enzymes have a 5'→3' polymerization – dependent exonuclease activity. For nucleotide incorporation, the enzyme works best at 75-80°C, depending on the target sequence. This enzyme can use either genomic DNA or single stranded cDNA as the original template and produce 10^6-fold amplification of specific sequences. It is very useful in mapping and sequencing mutations in uncloned genomic DNA or mRNA and for cloning desired genomic DNA or mRNA sequences

Several other thermostable Taq DNA polymerases have been isolated. Three of the most used polymerases are the following:

Polymerase	5'→3' Exonuclease	Source
Taq	No	*Thermus equaticus*
Pfu	Yes	*Pyrococcus furiosus*
Vent	Yes	*Thermococcus litoralis*

Applications:

PCR provides a relatively simple method for cloning genes. By amplifying gene sequences, PCR produces sufficient amounts of a target gene to increase the probability of successful cloning of the target gene. Besides simply making sufficient amounts of a gene for cloning, PCR can be used to make new gene sequences to add expression sequences and to insert or delete sequences into DNA for gene cloning. PCR can be used for gene cloning even when only limited or virtually no specific sequence information is known. PCR products can either be cloned prior to sequencing or can be sequenced directly. PCR can be used for site-directed mutagenesis.

2.12.2 DNA chips and Microarrays

During mid 1990s, DNA chips and Microarrys loaded with DNA samples became available to achieve very fast speeds in generating information about DNA sequences. These microarrays are prepared on solid surfaces (glass plates, slides) and represent high-density miniaturized arrays of molecular samples, thus facilitating the screening of genomic DNA or cDNA samples for the presence of 1 in 100,000 or even more DNA sequences in a single hybridization. The sequences on DNA chips may be oligonucleotides of known sequences or these may be cDNA sequences with known function. These microarrays are hybridized with an unknown labelled DNA sample, and the hybridization patterns are analyzed with computer devices. The major uses are; i.) DNA sequencing by hybridization leading to the detection of single nucleotide polymorphisms as has been done for human genome project, ii) diagnostics and genetic mapping, iii) gene expression studies and iv) proteomics.

2.13 SPECIAL TECHNIQUES

2.13.1 Gene Targeting

Gene targeting is achieved through the precise replacement of a gene by (partially) homologous foreign DNA via homologous recombination. Gene targeting can result from homologous recombination between an introduced DNA molecule and the homologous genomic locus. In this case, a reciprocal exchange of genetic sequences occurs between the two DNA molecules. Alternatively, it may result from a gene conversion event, which leads to the adaptation of the sequence of one strand to the sequence of another strand. Gene conversion involves local copying of genetic information from one strand to another and is not necessarily associated with cross-overs. A targeted and specific gene inactivation system will facilitate stable and heritable gene silencing with more reliablility than conventional systems such as anti-sense RNA and cosuppression.

The ability to inactivate target genes in an efficient manner, will also obviate the need for generating large populations of insertionally inactivated plants for each crop to evaluate gene function. Secondly, targeted modification of gene sequences will make *in vivo* protein engineering a reality, in essence enabling engineering of new genetic variation in a directed and predictable fashion.

Thirdly, gene targeting will enable facile replacement and exchange of genes and promoters in the genome. Novel gene could be placed adjacent to a promoter driving a desirable expression pattern in its normal chromosomal context resulting in predictable levels and patterns of gene expression. This will make conventional transgenic modifications obsolete because the current techniques result in random integration into the genome and wide variation in transgene expression levels due to position effects.

2.13.2 Antisense RNA Technique

The central dogma of molecular biology consists of the flow of genetic information from DNA through mRNA to protein assisted by transcription and translation. In the double stranded DNA, the strand that codes for the gene is called 'sense' strand. Antisense RNA is a single stranded nucleic acid, which is complementary to coding 'sense' strand. It is also complementary to mRNA. It has the opposite sense to mRNA. The flow of genetic information, from DNA to mRNA and to protein can be blocked by the introduction of antisense RNA sequence complementary to the sequence of the target mRNA. A RNA duplex is formed between mRNA and antisense RNA which blocks mRNA from its normal function. Antisense RNA for specific gene sequence can be generated by reversing the coding sequence of a gene under the control of promoter in normal orientation. Inhibition of particular genes can be achieved by directly introducing antisense RNA or antisense RNA oligonucleotides into cell.

2.13.3 Ribozyme constructs

Ribozymes are catalytic RNA molecules that carry out site-specific cleavage and ligation reactions on RNA substances. The incorporation of ribozyme catalytic centers into antisense RNA allows the ribozyme to be targeted to particular mRNA molecules, which are then cleaved and degraded.

2.13.4 Cosuppression

Cosuppression refers to the ability of a sense transgene to suppress the expression of a homologous endogenous gene. The integration of multiple copies of the transgene leads to the suppression of some or all of the transgenes and the cosuppression of homologous endogenous genes. Cosuppression involves silencing at either the transcriptional or post-transcriptional levels.

2.13.5 Transgene silencing

Transgene silencing is a complex phenomenon, occurring in all eukaryotes. It is caused by the introduction of foreign nucleic acid into the cell. Typically, the expression of the affected transgene is reduced or abolished with increased methylation at the transgenic locus. Position-dependent silencing, sequence-dependent silencing and homology-dependent silencing at the transcriptional or post-transcriptional levels are reported. Gene silencing may be a defense mechanism against 'invasive' nucleic acids.

2.13.6 RNA interference

RNA interference (RNAi) is useful tool for gene silencing. When both antisense and sense RNA are simultaneously introduced into an organism, an increased and specific inhibitory effect is seen.

2.13.7 Insertional Mutagenesis

If naturally occurring transposable elements can be mobilized at a sufficient frequency, they can be used to deliberately interrupt functional genes and generate insertional mutants. Foreign DNA introduced into a cell may occasionally integrate into existing gene and disrupt its expression.

2.13.8 Gene tagging

When insertional mutagenesis takes place the interrupted locus becomes 'tagged' with a unique sequence. This is helpful in identifying the interrupted gene. PCR-based analysis can be used to directly amplify the genomic DNA flanking a transgene tag.

Study Outline

Genetic Engineering

Manipulation of genetic material towards a desired end in a pre-determined way is otherwise known as recombinant DNA technology. Genetic engineering aims at isolating DNA fragments and recombining them outside a cell. It has varied applications such as isolation of a particular gene, part of a gene, region of a genome, production of particular RNA and protein molecules in quantities formerly thought to be unobtainable.

Genetic engineering is essentially the insertion of a specific piece of foreign DNA into a cell, in such a way that the inserted DNA is replicated and handled on to daughter cells during cell division. It is a strategy for transferring small bits of genetic information (DNA) from one organism to another.

Restriction Endonucleases

A group of enzymes known as restriction enzymes plays a big role in recombinant technology. These are enzymes that recognize specific nucleotide sequences in DNA and cut these at different sites, thus helping in cutting unique sets of fragments from a DNA molecule. To transfer these portions of DNA, cloning vehicles such as vectors are used. These are plasmids, phages—such as lambda and M 13.

Cloning Vehicles

Plasmids are small, circular, double stranded DNA molecules that occur in bacteria. They differ in length and the gene contained in the DNA. These are used in gene cloning. They possess genetic factors for fertility, antibiotic resistance, ability to ferment sugars, for production of bacteriocins, haemolysines etc. Bacteriophages are complicated than plasmids. Phage DNA contains genes coding for proteins that form a protective shell around the DNA; they lack the machinery necessary to make protein, hence they reproduce only inside living bacterial cells. These are highly efficient in producing progeny particles, which are potentially infectious. One of the phages used for cloning is called lambda. When it is injected into the bacteria it can either destroy the bacteria or it can reside in it (lytic or lysogenic). In the latter case it becomes part of the bacterial chromosome. The bacterial cell produces several hundreds of lambda particles. Thus it can act as a cloning vehicle.

Transposable Genetic Elements

They are otherwise known as jumping genes. These are capable of moving at any position of DNA segments; they lack the ability to self duplicate but can insert themselves into pre-existing chromosomes or plasmid and are replicated along with the host DNA. These can move from one site to another, from one plasmid to another and from one site to another within the same plasmid. Another type of mobile genetic elements found in maize is the transposable element or controlling element. This can alter the expression of standard genes and promote genetic rearrangements. Retroviruses are RNA viruses that multiply through conversion into duplex DNA. This has the capacity to insert DNA copies of an RNA viral genome into the chromosomes of the host cell. A major achievement of biotechnology is the possibility of inserting a particular fragment of DNA molecule from donor to a vector, through which desired characters are translocated.

Genomic DNA Libraries

It is a collection of independently isolated vector linked DNA fragments derived from a single organism. It contains at least one copy of every DNA sequence in the genome. There is another type called cDNA library. The DNA fragments for cDNA library are obtained by reverse transcription from the cellular RNA.

DNA Sequencing

Sequence of DNA refers to the order of nucleotide bases along its sugar-phosphate back bone. For studying DNA sequencing, it is subjected to the appropriate protocol in four separate reactions, each reaction specific for one of the four bases, by which a cut is made in the DNA next to a G and A, any pyrimidine (that is T or C) and a C. All the four parts are then electrophoresed and the bands are located by placing an autoradicigraphic film (a film that responds to radioactivity) on the gel. All four samples are electrophoresed simultaneously enabling all bands to be seen in a single gel. The sequence is read directly from the gel. The shortest fragments are those that move the fastest and farthest. Each fragment contains the original $5'-{}^{32}p$ group; the sequence can therefore be read from the bottom to the top of the gel.

Gene Identification and Mapping

The use of cloned fragments of chromosomal DNA as a genetic marker is usually termed RFLP. This technique is dependent on natural variation in DNA based sequence and digestion of DNA with restriction enzyme. RFLPs are used to systematically mapped and characterise genes conferring quantitative trace. RAPD is a new DNA polymorphism assay based on the polymerase chain reaction amplified random DNA segments with single primers of arbitrary nucleotide sequence. DNA fingerprints refer to probes that hybridize to fragments from several variable loci simultaneously producing an autoradiograph with a complex fragment pattern.

Analysis of Integration and Expression of Cloned Genes

Southern blot analysis, *in situ* hybridization and Northern blot analysis are used to locate different fragments of DNA, RNA in electrophoresis and autoradiography. Western blot analysis is used to locate proteins.

Gene Amplification

Polymerase chain reaction is an *in vitro* method for replicating DNA sequence so that its amount is increased exponentially. It consists of repetitive cycles of DNA denaturation, annealing and extention. A thermostable enzyme called DNA polymerase plays a vital role in this. PCR has many uses in gene cloning, gene sequencing, etc.

DNA chips and microarrays are helpful in the screening of genomic DNA or cDNA samples.

Special Techniques

Gene targeting is the precise replacement of a gene by homologous foreign DNA via homologous recombination. A targeted and specific gene inactivation system will facilitate stable and heritable gene silencing with more reliability than conventional systems such as antisense RNA and cosuppression.
Antisense RNA has the opposite sense to mRNA. The flow of genetic information can be blocked by the introduction of antisense RNA sequence complementary to the sequence of the target mRNA. Ribozymes are catalytic RNA molecules that carry out site-specific cleavage and ligation reactions on

RNA substances. Cosuppression refers to the ability of a sense transgene to suppress the expression of a homologous endogenous gene. Transgene silencing is caused by the introduction of foreign nucleic acid into the cell. RNA interference is useful for gene silencing.

Questions

(1) What are the basic methodologies in genetic engineering?
(2) How gene cloning technique helps in insulin production?
(3) What are the important features and properties of restriction endonucleases?
(4) State few examples of cloning vehicles and how are they used in gene cloning?
(5) What are plasmids? Differentiate them from cosmids?
(6) What is the importance of lambda phage?
(7) What are transposable genetic elements? Give examples?
(8) What do you understand by insertion sequence?
(9) What are retroviruses? Give their structural properties?
(10) What is cDNA? What is the function of reverse transcriptase?
(11) What is colony hybridization? What is its purpose?
(12) What are genomic libraries?
(13) Briefly explain DNA sequencing.
(14) Distinguish between RFLP and RAPD?
(15) What is DNA fingerprint analysis?
(16) Discuss ligase chain reaction and ribozymes?
(17) Distinguish between Southern blot, Northern blot and *in situ* hybridization analysis?
(18) What are the methods used for gene amplification and screening?
(19) How are the special techniques like gene targeting, antisense RNA, RNA interference and gene tagging useful?

3

Gene Transfer Mechanisms in Bacteria

Introduction

Gene recombination, a short generation time, the numerous conveniently recognized mutants, and the ease with which recombinant colonies could be scored among very large parental populations gave bacteria special advantages for recombinational studies over those of eukaryotes. A bacterium has only a single (major) DNA molecule, which almost never encounters another complete molecule. Instead, crossing over usually occurs between a chromosomal fragment and an intact chromosome. Furthermore, a clear donor-recipient relation exists; that is, a donor cell is the source of the DNA fragment, which is transferred to the recipient cell by one of several mechanisms whereby the exchange of genetic material occurs in the recipient.

There are three major gene transfer mechanisms by which bacterial donor genes are transferred into bacterial recipients:

1. Transformation: Transfer of genetic information into recipient cells in the form of exogenous (extracellular) DNA extracted from donor cells. It is the uptake of DNA from the environment. (In genetic engineering, this term is used for the transfer of extracted plasmid DNA into the host cells).
2. Conjugation: Gene transfer occurs by means of cell-to-cell contact promoted by a sex factor (conjugative plasmid) that can become incorporated into the bacterial donor chromosome. Usually only the plasmid itself is transferred from the donor to the recipient by this process. Sometimes the entire bacterial chromosome may be mobilized for transfer into the recipient, although not all of it is necessarily transferred. (When an independent sex factor incorporates one or more bacterial genes into its own chromosome, the subsequent transfer of such genes to recipient cells as part of the sex factor chromosome itself is called sexduction).
3. Transduction: Transfer of donor genes into recipient bacteria by bacterial viruses that act as intermediary carriers. (Viruses that can transfer almost any part of their cellular host chromosome engage in generalized transduction, and viruses that usually transfer only a specific part of their host chromosome engage in specialized transduction).

3.1 Transformation

This was the first mechanism of bacterial genetic exchange to be discovered. F. Griffith's classical experiment in 1928 showed that injection of mice with an avirulent (not capable of causing disease) strain of *Streptococcus pneumoniae* (pneumococcus) together with heat-killed cells of a virulent strain killed the mice, although injection of mice with either culture alone caused no disease. On autopsy, these mice were found to contain live virulent cells of S. *pneumoniae*. This experiment showed that there was a genetic exchange. Later it was presumed to be due to a transforming principle. In 1944, O.T. Avery, C.M. MacLeod and M.McCarty purified the pneumococcal transforming principle and identified it as being DNA. Recent studies have shown that during the process of extraction, the donor DNA is broken into smaller transforming molecules or fragments which are about 1/200 of the total donor DNA. These transforming molecules usually contain on the average about 20,000 nucleotide base pairs. Smaller DNA pieces can also be absorbed by the recipient cell, but a minimum length of about 450 base pairs seems to be essential for transformation to occur.

3.1.1 Stages in the Transformation Process

There are three general stages in the transformation process, with details in each stage differing between bacterial groups that have different cell wall structures. Cells that are in a state in which they can be transformed by DNA in their environment are said to be competent. Competence i.e. the ability of cells to take up DNA through changes in the cell wall is the first stage. This involves the formation or activation of special DNA receptor proteins that can be induced by polypeptide 'competence factors' in some species, or by special growth conditions in others. A set of about 12 proteins is synthesized that mediate the process of transformation.

The second stage is DNA binding and uptake. This involves direct interaction between the cell wall receptors and donor DNA. This sequence is at first reversible, but as more cell membrane proteins become involved, DNA attachment to the cell wall is considerably increased.

The last major stage which is the third stage begins with the intracellular transport of the transforming DNA to the recipient chromosome in some protected form, either complexed with a specific DNA—binding protein or in small vesicles derived from the recipient cell surface, or both. During the culmination of this last stage, (integration), a single strand of donor DNA is incorporated into the recipient chromosome by displacing a homologous section of one of the recipient DNA strands, which is then excised and degraded. The integrated donor strand then replicates forming a double helix while the remaining unpaired recipient strand is excised. Thus transformation seems to arise from some form of recombination mechanism which produce a gene exchange similar to that produced by sexual recombination.

3.1.2 Types of Transformation Mechanisms

In a significant number of bacteria, entry into the competent state is encoded by chromosomal genes and signaled by certain environmental conditions. Such bacteria are said to be capable of undergoing natural transformation. Many other bacteria do not become competent under ordinary conditions of culture but they can be made competent by a variety of highly artificial treatments such as exposure of cells to high concentrations of divalent cations. Such systems are termed artificial transformation.

In the laboratory, purified solutions of DNA are usually employed in studies on transformation. This raises the question of how DNA becomes available for transformation in nature. Curiously, the role of the donor cell has received very little attention. It has been assumed by many bacterial geneticists that the role of the donor cell is completely passive and the donation of DNA depends on the occasional and random lysis of certain cells in the population. However, recent experiments suggest that DNA might be actively extruded from certain complement cells by a genetically encoded pathway.

3.1.3 Establishing Gene Linkage

To establish gene linkage by transformation the following considerations are made. If two genes, A and B, are closely linked, there is a good likelihood that transformation at the A locus produced by a single DNA molecule would also produce transformation at the B locus. This process where both A and B genes are transformed is referred to as double transformation. Double transformation can arise either because a cell receives two separate DNA fragments, one with A and the other with B, or because a cell receives a single fragment carrying both A and B. If these two genes are distantly linked, then the probability of double transformation is remote. Thus closely linked genes will produce a much higher frequency of double transformants than those that are distantly linked or not linked, especially if low concentrations of transforming DNA are used.

Based on transformation experiments, we can readily define whether two markers are linked or not. Moreover, by determining that marker A is linked to B and that B is linked to C, a marker order of AB.C can be deduced. Using this we can deduce the order of genes along a chromosome and construct the transformation map of an entire chromosome.

3.2 Conjugation

As described earlier, conjugation is a process by which DNA can be transferred from a donor cell to a recipient cell by cell-to-cell contact. It was first discovered in *E. coli* by J. Lederberg and E.L. Tatum in 1951. When bacteria conjugate, a clear donor-recipient relation exists: DNA is transferred to a recipient cell from a donor cell which possesses a contiguous set of genes called the transfer genes that give the cell its donor properties; it occurred even if DNAse was present in the medium.

Transfer genes may be present either in a nonchromosomal circular DNA molecule called a plasmid or as a block of genes in the chromosome. In the latter case the plasmid is said to have been integrated into the chromosome.

Conjugation begins with physical contact between a donor cell and a recipient cell. Then, a passage (conjugation tube) is formed between the cells, and DNA moves from the donor to the recipient through this passage. In the final stage, which requires recombination if the donor contains an integrated plasmid, a segment of the transferred DNA becomes a part of the genetic complement of the recipient. If the donor contains a free plasmid, only the plasmid will be transferred and it will reside in the recipient in the free-plasmid form.

3.2.1 Transfer Genes

In the conjugation process certain strains designated as F+ (fertility plus) always acted as donors (males) and others designated as F– (fertility minus) always acted as recipients (females). Later it was discovered that all F+ strains contain a plasmid (termed the F plasmid, F factor, sex plasmid) that carries all the genes that encode conjugative genetic transfer. In fact, the F plasmid is not known to encode any additional function other than this one and its own replication (Fig. 3.1).

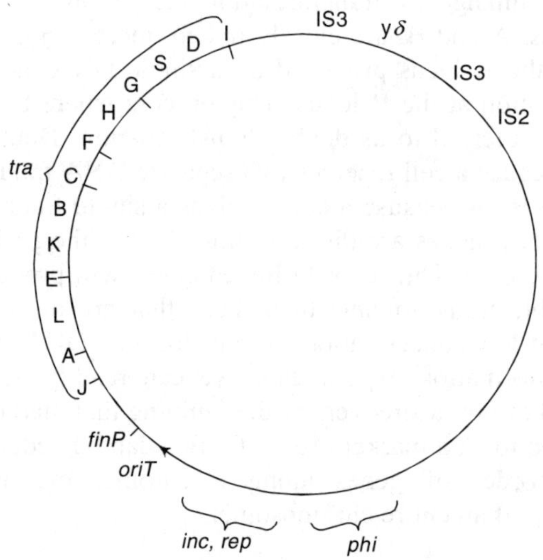

Figure 3.1

Genetic map of the F plasmid showing the relative position of genes encoding transfer functions (*tra*), fertility inhibition (*finP*), origin of transfer replication (*oriT*), incompatibility (*inc*), replication (*rep*) and phage inhibiting (*phi*). The positions of insertion sequences 1S2, 1S3, and y are also shown. The length of the genome is 94.5 kilobases.
(***Source:*** *Stanier, R. Y.; Ingraham, J.L.; Wheelis, M.L.; Painter, P.R. General Microbiology. © 1988 New Jersey, Prentice Hall Intl.*)

3.2.1.1 F Plasmid

A bacterial cell may contain one or more plasmids. Plasmids are circular DNA molecules, capable of replicating independently of the chromosome. There is a detailed discussion on plasmids in Chapter Two (2.3.1). F plasmids contain transfer genes that mediate conjugation in *E. coli.* The F plasmid encodes transfer of itself to other cells that lack an F plasmid. Thus, if F– cells are added to an F+ culture, all of them rapidly become F+. The F plasmid carries certain genes (*rep*) that allow it to be replicated by the host cell and, as directed by the genetic region *inc,* it exhibits the phenomenon of incompatibility; i.e. if a certain plasmid is present in a cell, replication of closely related plasmids is inhibited. Thus closely related plasmids are said to be incompatible; only one member of such a group of plasmids (termed an incompatibility group) can be replicated in a stable way in the same cell. The F plasmid belongs to an incompatibility group termed *Inc F1.*

The F plasmid is a double-stranded DNA with about 1,00,000 nucleotide base pairs. (The bacterial chromosome is about 40 times longer). One specialized segment for DNA transfer *Ori T* enters the recipient cell first and the rest follows sequentially in a linear order. In F+ strains the F factor is circular, and only one such F factor is usually present in each bacterial cell. This factor replicates once during each bacterial chromosome replication cycle, and one copy is distributed to each daughter cell.

In the case of F plasmid, transfer is encoded by 13 genes, *tra A* through *tra L* and *tra S*, that form an operon. 9 genes encode the synthesis of special pili, termed F pili or sex pili. Others encode a special type of replication termed transfer replication of the F plasmid, that occurs during transfer and mediates it. The *tra* genes of F plasmids are always derepressed. Thus, F+ cells always have F pili on their outer surface unless they have been subjected to vigorous shaking, an action that breaks off these long brittle appendages. An F pilus binds specifically to a protein in the outer membrane (*omp A*) of F-cells, thereby initiating transfer replication and the process of gene transfer by conjugation (Fig. 3.2.). A nick (the cutting of a single strand of DNA) is made in the F plasmid at the site termed *ori T* (origin of transfer); then a type of replication sometimes termed rolling circle mechanism, in which the intact strand is used as template for its own replication occurs and the 3′ end generated by the nick is used as the primer; the 5′ end of the nicked single strand is displaced and is transferred into the F-cell, where it is copied in the 5′ $\rightarrow$ 3′ direction (Fig. 3.3.).

It is not clear how this transfer occurs. The singlestranded molecule might pass through the hollow core of the F pilus or it might pass from the F+ cell to the F– at some other point of contact between them. If the latter case is true, the function of the F pilus would only be to hold the two cells together so that another direct conjugative bridge can form. Within the F-cell, the single stranded molecule of DNA is duplicated by a chromosomally encoded DNA polymerase

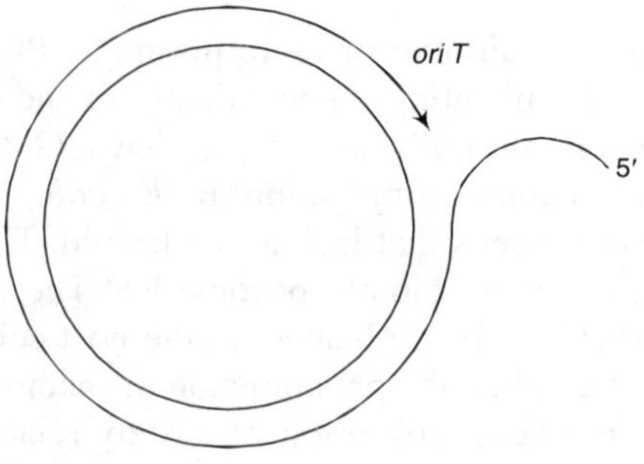

Figure 3.2

Transfer replication of an F plasmid. An F-encoded nuclease cleaves one strand of the plasmid at *oriT*. Then replication at arrow head occurs by a rolling *circle* mechanism whereby the newly synthesized DNA displaces a pre-existing single strand the 5′ end of which enters the F cell.

(***Source****: Stanier, R. Y.; Ingraham, J.L.; Wheelis, M.L.; Painter, P.R. General Microbiology. © 1988 New Jersey, Prentice Hall Intl.*)

and recircularized. By some unknown mechanism, the transferred linear F strand becomes recircularized in the recipient cell. Possibly the ends of the transferred piece of DNA become attached to a protein located in the cytoplasmic membrane, thereby holding the ends in appropriate *juxtaposition* to be joined by the action of DNA ligase. Once circularized, the transferred F plasmid can be replicated in the recipient cell. The genes it carries are expressed, and the cell then becomes F+.

3.2.1.2 Hfr cells

High frequency recombination cells are referred to as Hfr cells, in which the F plasmid and the bacterial chromosome become integrated into a single large circular molecule (Fig. 3.4.). Because of this, the recipients acquire the donor alleles with a high frequency. The integrated F element is ordinarily replicated passively along with the bacterial chromosome, and it is transmitted in this way from one cell generation to the next. But when conjugation is initiated, the replication apparatus of the F element is activated. The F element's DNA is nicked in one strand and the 5′ end of the nicked strand is drawn into the conjugation tube, apparently by the impetus of a rolling circle type of DNA replication (Fig. 3.5). The stages of transfer are much like those by which F+ is transferred to F– cells—namely, pairing of donor and recipient, rolling-circle replication in the donor, and conversion of the single stranded DNA to double stranded DNA by replication in the recipient. A portion of F is the first DNA transferred and the chromosomal genes are transferred next. (The replicative transfer begins with the F plasmid region at *ori* T and continues into the chromosomal region of the large circular molecule). Usually the entering chromosome breaks at some intermediate position due to the spontaneous breaking apart of the fragile conjugation bridge, thereby interrupting the genetic transfer.

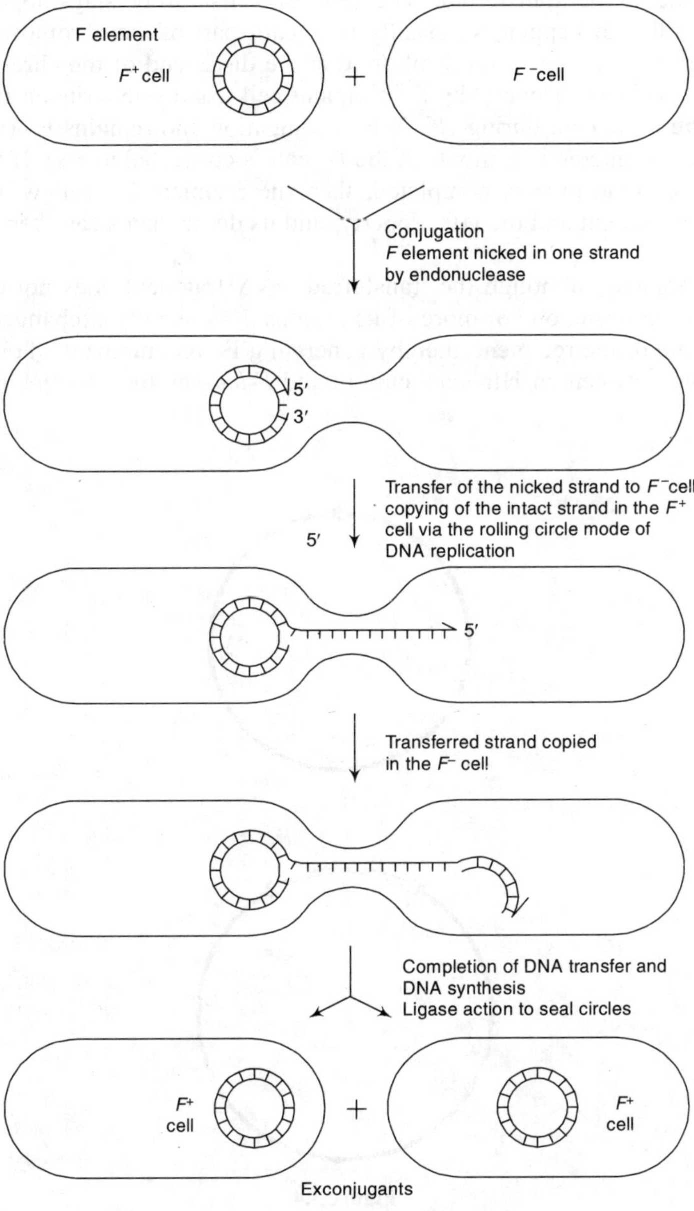

Figure 3.3

Transfer of the f element from an F+ to an F– cell during conjugation in *E. coli*.

(***Source:*** *Goodenough, U. Genetics. © 1986 New York, Holt, Rinehart and Winston Inc. Reprinted by permission.*)

A considerable time (about 100 minutes at 37°C) is required for the entire chromosome to be transferred. The pair of cells rarely stays together long enough for this to happen; so usually the major part of the chromosome is not transferred; the portion of the F plasmid at the distal end of the chromosome is also not transferred. Hence, the F– recipient cell usually inherits an incomplete copy of the F element during Hfr X F– conjugation and remains F– (in contrast to an F+ X F– interaction, in which the F– cell is converted to F+). If transfer of the entire chromosome is completed, then the recipient F– cell will inherit a complete F element and the Hfr property, and its descendants can then act as Hfr cells.

In Hfr transfer, although the transferred DNA fragment does not circularize and cannot replicate, one or more of its regions is frequently exchanged with the chromosome of the recipient, thereby generating F– recombinants. For example, in a mating between an Hfr *leu+* culture and *F-leu–* culture, F-*leu+* cells arise.

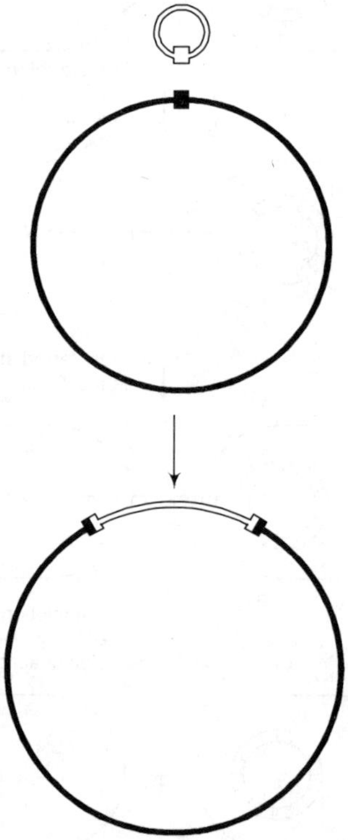

Figure 3.4

Integration of F+ by a reciprocal exchange between a base sequence in F and a homologous sequence in the bacterial chromosome.

(***Source:*** *Hartl, D.L.; Freifelder, D.; Snyder, L.A. Basic G enetics. © 1988 Boston: Jones and Bartlett Publishers. Reprinted by permission.*)

The genotype of the donor is unchanged. Genes can also be mapped by Hfr x F- matings. Sometimes a cross over occurs between two non-homologous regions, one at one of the two boundaries between the integrated F and the chromosome and the other in the adjacent chromosomal DNA. When such aberrant excision occurs, a plasmid containing chromosomal DNA, an F′ plasmid is formed. This replicates autonomously and has a circular structure.

This is also called substituted F factor. Because F′ carries a portion of the bacterial chromosome, it can act as an infective particle that 'F-duces' or 'sex-duces' F-recipients for the specific gene or genes that are carried. That is, male donor cells which are *F′ lac+,* for example, will preferentially transmit this gene to F– lac- recipients, converting them to *lac*+. This process, known as sexduction or F-duction, can be defined as the transmission of bacterial genes to a recipient cell through their incorporation into an autonomous conjugative plasmid. Sexduction by F′ is one of the examples of the use of a small particle as a vector for gene transfer.

Occasionally the F factor will leave its chromosomal position in an Hfr cell and reconvert the cell to an F+ cell. The sites at which integration between the F factor and the bacterial chromosome occurs are specific sections of DNA known as insertion sequences (IS). There are four such sequences on the F factor and more than twenty on the E. *coli* chromosome.

3.3 Transduction

Transduction is the transmission of DNA from a donor cell to a recipient by the incorporation of a fragment of donor DNA into a viral particle. Such a particle is called *transducing particle.* It contains DNA of the bacterial genome replacing part, or all of the normal complement of phage DNA. The protein capsid of such transducing particles does not differ from the capsid of a normal phage virion. Since it is the capsid that determines a phage's ability to attach to a sensitive bacterial cell and to inject its complement of DNA into the cell, the transducing particle can introduce bacterial DNA derived from the cell in which it developed with another sensitive cell. The result is the transfer of genetic material between these two cells. Two types of transducing particles and therefore two types of transduction exist. One of these is termed generalized or non-specialized transduction, because it mediates the exchange of any bacterial gene. The other is termed restricted or specialized transduction because it mediates the exchange of only a limited number of specific genes.

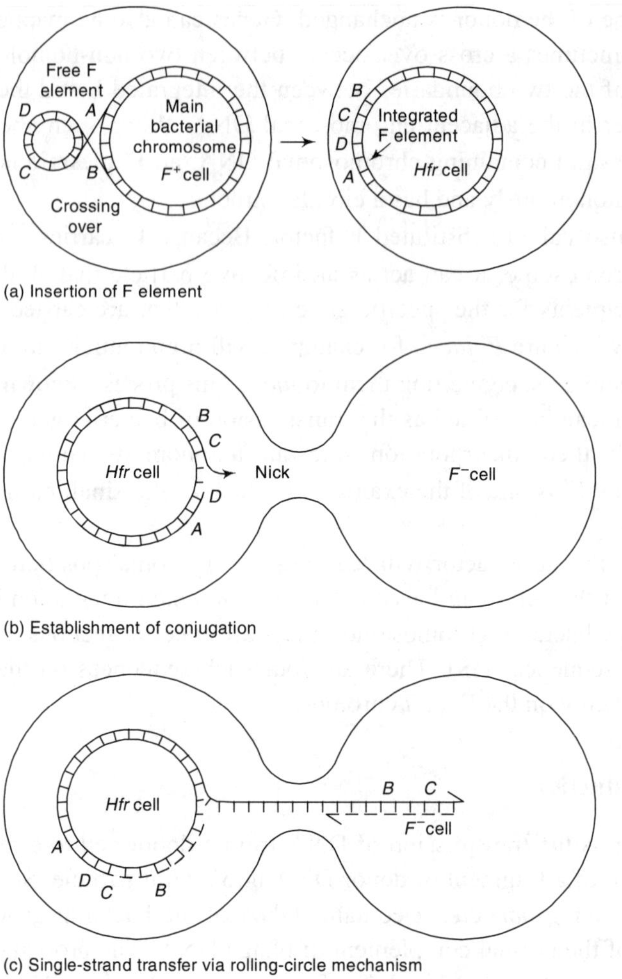

Figure 3.5

Integration of F+ element to form an Hfr cell and transfer of Hfr chromosome to an F– cell during conjugation in *E. coli.*

(***Source:*** *Goodenough, U. Genetics. © 1986 New York, Holt, Rinebart and Winston Inc. Reprinted by permission.*)

3.3.1 Generalized Transduction

During generalized transduction, a piece of a donor bacterial chromosome becomes incorporated into a phage head and is transduced (carried over) to a recipient bacterium, where it may insert into the recipient genome. In almost all cases of generalized transduction, very little or none of the phage DNA is carried in the transducing particle, which consists primarily of donor DNA surrounded by a phage envelope. Generalized transduction is performed by phages such as P1 of *E. coli,* P22 of *Salmonella,* and SPO1 and PBS1 of *Bacillus subtilis*.

3.3.1.1 Generalized Transduction Mediated by Phage PI

During infection by P1, the phage makes a nuclease that causes fragmentation of bacterial DNA (a common event in the life of many phage species). A single fragment of bacterial DNA comparable in size to P1 DNA is occasionally packaged into a phage particle instead of P1 DNA. The positions of the nuclease cuts in the host chromosome are random, so a transducing particle may contain a fragment derived from any region of the host DNA, and a large population of P1 phage will contain a particle consisting of each host gene. About one particle per 10^3 progeny is a transducing particle. On the average, any particular gene is present in roughly one transducing particle per 10^6 viable P1 phage. The bacterial DNA in this transducing particle can be efficiently injected into a second bacterium, and, since it shares a homologous sequence with a portion of the host chromosome, it occasionally inserts into the host chromosome. When the inserted DNA carries donor genes that differ from recipient markers, recombinants will result.

Let us take a look at the events that follow infection of a bacterium by a generalized transducing particle obtained, for example, by the growth of P1 on wildtype *E. coli* containing a *leu+* gene. If such a particle adsorbs to a bacterium whose genotype is *leu–* and injects the DNA it contains into the bacterium, the cell will survive because the phage head contained only bacterial genes and no phage genes. A crossover event exchanging the *leu+* allele carried by the phage for the *leu–* allele carried by the host will convert the genotype of the host cell from *leu–* to *leu+*. In such an experiment, typically about one *leu–* cell in 10^6 will be converted to *leu+* (Fig. 3.6). Such frequencies are easily detected on selective growth medium; i.e., if the infected cell is placed on a solid medium, lacking leucine, it will be able to multiply and a *leu+* colony will be formed. A colony will not be formed if crossing over does not result in insertion of the *leu* allele.

3.3.1.2 Generalized Transduction Mediated by Phage P22

Within the infected cell, probably by a rolling circle mechanism, long stretches of phage DNA composed of randomly repeated phage genomes (*concatamers*) are synthesized. In preparation for packaging into the phage head, the concatamer is initially cleaved by the action of a phage-encoded endonuclease at a specific site termed as *pac* (packaging) site. Then starting from the point of cleavage, headful amounts of phage DNA are sequentially packaged into developing phage heads. Each virion receives a length of DNA that is a complete phage genome plus a small amount of additional DNA at one end. The packaged DNA is therefore *terminally redundant* since the additional amount of DNA has same sequence as that at the other end. Transducing particles are made when

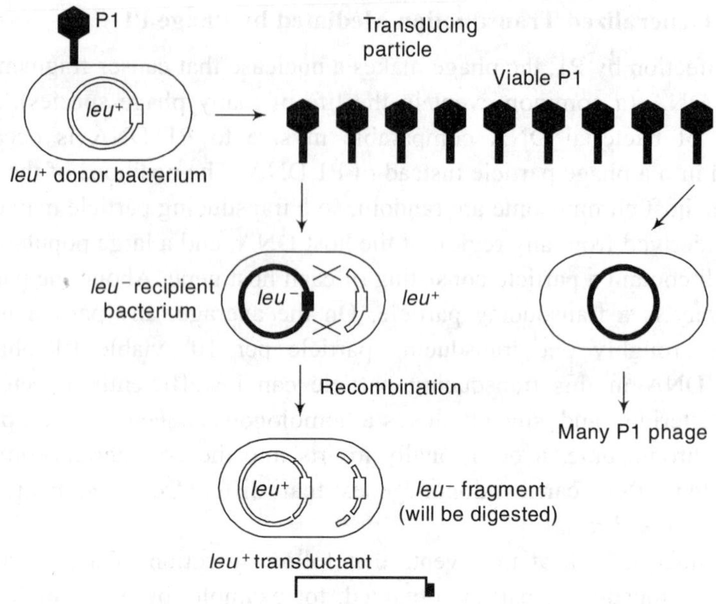

Figure 3.6

Transduction. Phage Pl infects a leu^+ donor, yielding predominately viable P1 phage with an occasional one carrying bacterial DNA instead of phage DNA. If the phage population infects a bacterial culture, the viable phage will produce progeny phage and the transducing particle will yield a transductant. Notice that the recombination step requires two crossovers. (***Source:*** *Hartl, D.L.; Freifelder, D.; Snyder, L.A. Basic Genetics. © 1988 Boston: Jones and Bartlett Publishers. Reprinted by permission.*)

cleavages occur in the bacterial genome at sites that resemble the *pac* site sufficiently to allow the phage-encoded endonuclease to act.

In P22, a phage specified protein, coded by gene 3 and most likely the endonuclease responsible for cutting P22 concatamers into headful lengths during virion maturation apparently recognizes particular signals in the *Salmonella* chromosome as well and cuts these into headful lengths. As a result, P22 will transduce certain *Salmonella* markers far more frequently than others. High-transducing (HT) mutants of P22 decrease the specificity of the endonuclease that *acts* at the *pac* site so that *pac*—like sites in the bacterial genome are cleaved with greater frequency. The small fragment of bacterial DNA contained in a transducing particle carries about 50 genes; so transduction provides a valuable tool for linkage analysis of short regions of the bacterial genome and mapping can be done. Simultaneous transduction of two genes is referred to as cotransduction. The frequency at which two genes are contransduced by a population of phages can be used to estimate their linkage, i.e. their relative distance from each other on the chromosome. Cotransduction frequency is inversely related to the distance between genes.

3.3.2 Specialized Transduction

Specialized transduction is a mode of gene transfer carried out by. temperate phages such as lambda. A specialized transducing phage produces particles containing both phage and bacterial genes linked in a single DNA molecule, and the bacterial genes are obtained from a particular region of the bacterial chromosome. Specialized transducing particles are formed by the inaccurate excision of prophages when they are induced to lytic growth. Rather than only the phage genome being excised by a recombinant event between the ends of the prophage region, a segment of DNA is excised that includes a portion of the bacterial chromosome and a portion of the prophage. If a significant portion of the bacterial chromosome is excised, the entire prophage cannot be included in the specialized transducing phage, because the phages are viable only if they contain an amount of DNA greater than 73 percent and less than 10 percent of the phage genome.

In a way, a specialized transducing phage is a new organism having gained certain genes from the bacterial chromosome and lost others from its own genome. These phages are designated by the bacterial genes that they carry and by the degree of deficiency caused by the loss of phage genes. For example lambda *d,gal* designates a specialized transducing lambda phage that carries *gal* genes (encoding the dissimilation of the hexose *gal*actose) and is defective because it has lost phage genes rendering it incapable of development except in a cell that contains another lambda phage (termed as *helper phage*) that contains the missing genes and thereby complements the lost phage functions of the specialized transducing phage. The phage harvest with increased transducing efficiency is called *Hft* (high frequency transduction *lysate*). Specialized transducing phages contain only those genes that are immediately adjacent to the site of integration of the prophage. Phage lambda usually integrates at a site, *att* lambda, located between two operons, *bio* (encoding the biosynthesis of the vitamin, *biotin*) and *gal* (encoding the catabolism of the sugar, *galactose*); so specialized transducing phages carrying either *gal* or *bio* genes can be generated inducing a normal lambda lysogen.

The lambda chromosome is a double-stranded DNA molecule, 47,000 base pairs long with a single-stranded projection of 12 nucleotides at each 5′ end. These projections are complementary to each other ('cohesive'), so that when injected into an *E. coli* cell as a linear molecule, the chromosome rapidly circularizes because of its cohesive ends. Circularity protects the lambda chromosome against degradation by host exonuclease enzymes and also offers advantages in replication, since non-circular lambda DNA cannot replicate vegetatively. Figure 3.7 gives details of the mechanism of the formation of specialized transducing particles by phage lambda. If a lambda phage lysate containing lambda *d,gal*+ phages is used to infect *gal*– bacteria, transductants are produced that are able to ferment galactose. They are almost invariably lysogenic for lambda. The entering lambda *d,gal*+ DNA first circularizes as in a normal phage infection (Fig.3.7a.) Its *gal*+ region then pairs with homologous *gal*– region in the recipient chromosome (Fig.3.7b), but the donor genes do not

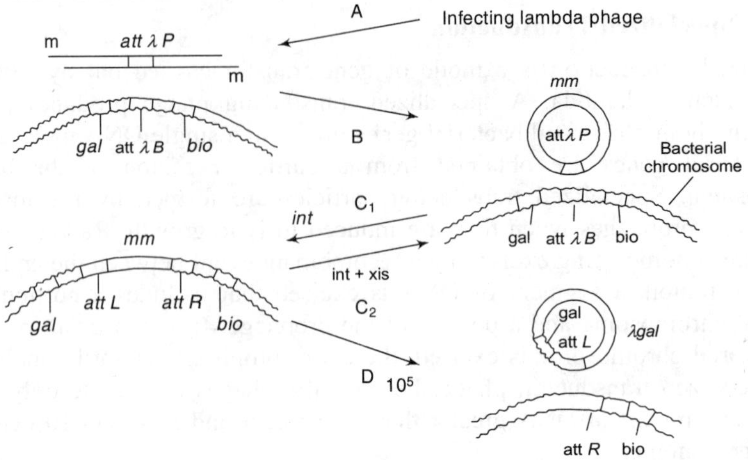

Figure 3.7

Mechanism of formation of specialized transducing particles by phage lambda. (A) On infection phage lambda DNA enters the cell as a linear molecule. (B) Its complementary single-stranded ends (m and m′) anneal circularizing the molecule. (C) A crossover mediated by a phage gene (*int*) *occurs between complementary regions on the phage (att p) and the chromosome (att B) integrating the* two *molecules and creating attL and attR* (C_1). By the action of *int* and *xis* this process can be reversed (C_2). (D) But sometimes at a lower frequency (10^{-5}) the crossover occurs between a region within the prophage and the chromosome creating a transducing particle (*dgal*) that carries a chromosomal gene (gal).
(***Source:*** *Goodenough, U. Genetics. © 1986 New York, Holt, Rinehart and Winston Inc. Reprinted by permission.*)

displace the recipient genes (in contrast to the situation in transformation or in generalised transduction). Instead, recombination occurs so that the lambda *d,gal+* DNA is inserted into the site where pairing took place (Fig.3.7c).

Meanwhile, the usual lambda attachment site (*att* lambda) in the *E. coli* chromosome remains unoccupied, and it is ordinarily filled by a second, normal lambda phage that infects the cell at the same time as the lambda *d,gal+* particle (Fig 3.7d). Thus the resulting transducing bacterium carries two copies of most (but not all) lambda genes and two copies of one or several bacterial genes (Fig. 3.7d).

The total length of the DNA that is packaged into a specialized transducing particle is roughly the same as that of a normal phage chromosome. A specialized transducing particle carrying a sizable piece of the bacterial genome will therefore usually (but not always) lack a corresponding length of phage genome. The missing phage genes are taken away from the end of the prophage chromosome opposite the one to which the bacterial genes are added. For this reason, such specialized transducing particles are denoted as *defective* in phage genes so that, for example, lambda *d,gal* is defective and *gal* is transducing, whereas lambda *dbio* is defective and *bio* is transducing. Specialized transduction provides an important method for mapping the bacterial chromosome. Bacterial genes transduced by a specialized transducing phage are identified as closely linked to the bacterial *att* site for that phage. So by placing the genes of interest next to known *att* sites, bacterial genes can be mapped.

Study Outline

Transformation

Transfer of genetic information into recipient cells in the form of exogenous DNA extracted from donor cells.

Conjugation

Gene transfer by means of cell-to-cell contact, promoted by genetic factor that can be incorporated into the bacterial donor chromosome.

Transduction

Transfer of donor gene into recipient bacteria by bacterial viruses that act as intermediary carriers.

Stages in Transformation Process

There are three general stages depending upon the bacterial cell wall structures. Cells that can take up DNA through changes on the cell wall is the first stage. This involves the formation or activation of special DNA receptor proteins that can be induced by polypeptide competence factors. DNA binding and uptake involves direct interaction between the cell wall receptors and donor DNA. This sequence is at first reversible but as more cell membrane proteins become involved DNA attachment is considerably increased. The third stage begins with intracellular transport of the transforming DNA to the recipient chromosome in some protected form.

Types of Transformation Mechanism

Natural transformation where entry into the competent state is signaled by certain environmental conditions.

Artificial transformation, where competence is induced by exposure of cells to high concentrations of divalent cations.

Role of the Donor Cell

Its role is passive. Donation of DNA depends on the occasional and random lysis of certain cells in the population.

Gene Linkage

It is brought about by transformation. In the case of closely linked genes, transformation at two loci may be produced. This is referred to as double transformation. Based on transformation experiments, we can define whether two markers are linked or not.

Conjugation

A bacterial cell may contain one or more plasmids. They are circular DNA molecules, capable of replicating independently. F plasmids contain transfer genes that mediate conjugation in *E. coli.* They encode transfer of themselves to other cells that lack an F plasmid. Thus if F cells are added to an F culture all of them rapidly become F.

Hfr Cells

High frequency recombination cells are referred to as Hfr cells. In this the F plasmid and bacterial chromosome become integrated into single larger circular molecule. Because of this, the recipients acquire the donor alleles with a high frequency. The integrated F element is ordinarily replicated passively along with the bacterial chromosome and it is transmitted from one cell generation to the next.

Generalized Transduction and Specialized Transduction

(a) *Generalized transduction:* During this any portion of a donor bacterial chromosome becomes incorporated into a phage head and it is carried over to the recipient genome. In this only very little or none of the phage DNA is carried into the transducing particle which consists primarily of donor DNA surrounded by a phage envelope.

(b) *Specialized transduction:* It is a mode of transfer carried out by temperate phages such as lambda. A specialised transducing phage produces particles along with phage and bacterial genes linked in a single DNA molecule and the bacterial genes are obtained from a particular region of the bacterial chromosome.

Questions

(1) Define transformation.
(2) What are the various stages in transformation?
(3) What is transduction? Describe the mechanisms of transduction.
(4) What is the significance of specialized transduction?
(5) Explain the method of conjugation in bacteria.
(6) Describe F plasmid, Hfr strains and F′ plasmids.
(7) What do you mean by cotransduction?

4
Transferring Genes into Plant and Animal Cells

Introduction

In 1976, Jaenisch who was working at the Salk Institute, California, first introduced foreign genes and integrated them into the genome of mice and their offspring. He infected morula stage mouse embryos with mouse leukaemia virus (M-MuLV) and then implanted them into foster mothers. He observed that about 10 to 40 per cent of the adults contracted the disease after a few months. He also showed that the disease which resembled leukaemia induced in mice by inoculation of the virus resulted from the integration of the virus genome into all cells of the embryo, including the germ line. In a high proportion of the embryos that grew into adult males, the virus was integrated into the cells of the germ line, since on mating with normal females they produced male offspring which transmitted the virus to 50 per cent of the next generation. Although the males which developed from infected embryos showed a variable and declining transmission of the virus, all somatic cells of the second generation of males contained viral DNA that was transmitted as a normal and dominant gene to 50 per cent of their offspring.

The work of Jaenisch and his collaborators, for the first time, gave the evidence that foreign genetic material could be integrated into the genome of mammalian cells in a stable way and that it could be expressed and transmitted to their offspring. These experiments also paved the way for the study of the cell-specific expression of a gene.

Molecular cloning of genes allows the investigation of gene structure and the sequences which control gene expression. Gene cloning technology can be manipulated in plants and animals for the benefit of human beings. This technology provides an additional tool for the breeder, to improve yield, nutritional quality and many other characters. In addition, plants and animals can be viewed as a genetic resource, genes being cloned into, and expressed in, bacteria. These bacteria can then be used to produce desirable products on an industrial scale using fermenters.

4.1 Vectors For Plants

The term plant gene vector applies to potential vectors both for the transfer of genetic information between plants, and also the transfer of genetic information from other organisms such as bacteria, fungi and animals to plants. Thus a vector is a 'go-between', transferring genetic information from one organism—the donor, to another—the recipient, and in the case of plants the equivalent of bacterial vectors are bacteriophage lambda, cosmids and plasmids. Several plant DNA viruses have been proposed as candidates for such a role but they are too complicated and limited with regard to the host range. The use of natural vectors such as viruses, tumour-inducing (Ti) plasmids and transposable elements is being explored. A subgroup of Ti plasmids inducing the hairy-root tumours are often referred to as Ri plasmids.

4.1.1 Agrobacterium Tumefaciens

The most promising method of transforming plant cells makes use of a plasmid called the Ti plasmid which is found within the bacterium *Agrobacterium tumefaciens.* This gram negative, rod-shaped, motile bacterium lives in the soil and invades many dicotyledonous plants and some gymnosperms when they are damaged at the soil level. The bacterium enters the fresh wound and attaches itself to the wall of an intact cell, after which it transfers a relatively small part of its Ti plasmid into the nucleus of the plant cell. This plasmid integrates some of its DNA into the chromosomes of its host plant cells (Fig. 4.1). This is a unique morphogenetic phenomenon where a permanent incorporation of a portion of bacterial genome completely diverts the host cell from its pre-determined path of development.

Because of this infection it causes a crown gall, a lump or callus of tumour tissue that grows in an undifferentiated way at the site of infection. The cells of the crown gall acquire the properties of independent, unregulated growth. When the crown gall cells are put into culture, they grow to form a callus even in media devoid of the plant hormones that must be added to induce normal plant cells to grow in culture.

4.1.1.1 Tumour—inducing (Ti) Plasmids

Ti plasmids have evolved solely for the benefit of the bacterium. The potential of the *Agrobacterium* Ti plasmid as a vector arises from the ability of the bacterium to somehow transfer, and stably integrate a piece of the plasmid DNA into the plant nuclear genome, a natural vector system. The transferred DNA is known as T DNA, and carries several genes which are expressed within the plants and which have dramatic effects on their metabolism. One gene codes for an enzyme which catalyzes the synthesis of an opine from amino acids and other common metabolites found within the plant cell. Opines are never found in normal plants and cannot be metabolized by them; but they can and are used as a source of carbon and nitrogen. The ability to induce and metabolize opines is encoded by plasmids in the bacteria. Host plant cells cannot use these new amino acids, so the bacterial infection not only causes cells to become tumorous but also subverts the plant's metabolism to making amino acids that only the bacteria can use as food.

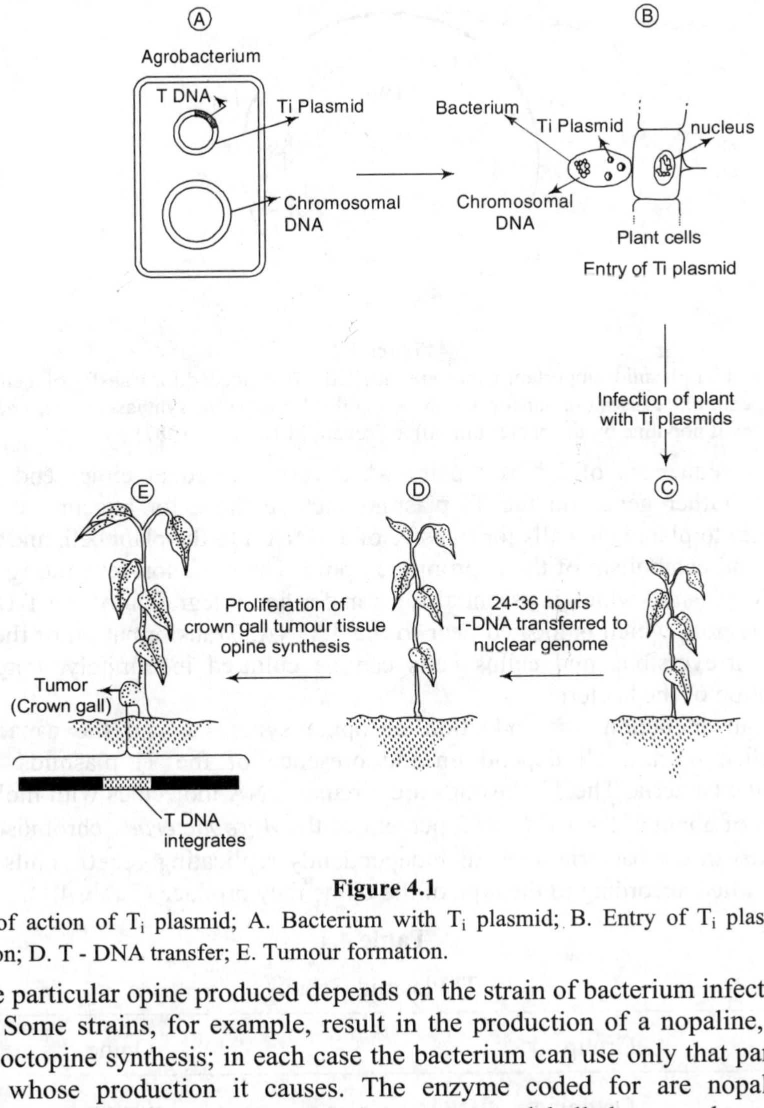

Figure 4.1

Mode of action of T_i plasmid; A. Bacterium with T_i plasmid; B. Entry of T_i plasmid; C. Infection; D. T - DNA transfer; E. Tumour formation.

The particular opine produced depends on the strain of bacterium infecting the plant. Some strains, for example, result in the production of a nopaline, others cause octopine synthesis; in each case the bacterium can use only that particular opine whose production it causes. The enzyme coded for are nopaline or octopine synthases, and their respective genes are labelled *nos* and *ocs*. They produce octopine (N-a-(D-1-carboxyethyl)-L-arginine) and nopaline (N-a-(1,3-dicarboxypropyl)-L-arginine). Not only does the T DNA ensure a supply of nutrient for the bacterium, but it also induces the disorganized proliferation of cells around the wound to form a callus which can be further colonized by the bacteria. This disorganized growth is the result of excessive production of phytohormones, and is coded for by the *onc* gene of T DNA. (Fig.4.2).

An important property of the T DNA is that, once inside the plant cell, it does not remain as an independent plasmid, but becomes integrated into the plant chromosomal DNA. This integration seems to depend on the presence of two

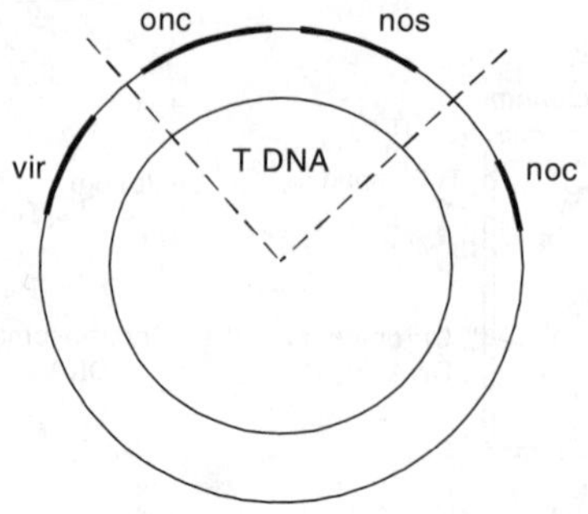

Figure 4.2

Structure of Ti plasmid: important genes are labelled: *vir* is needed for transfer of TDNA into the plant cell; *onc* causes tumour formation; *nos* codes for nopaline synthase; *noc* is needed for catabolism of nopaline by the bacterium (after Trevan, M.D. et *al.*, 1987)

repeated sequences of 25 base-pairs which are located at either end of the T DNA. Other genes on the Ti plasmid include those for attachment of the bacterium to plant cell walls for transfer of T DNA into the plant cell, and for the uptake and catabolism of the appropriate opine. The only non-integrating region of the Ti plasmid which is essential for transfer and integration of the T DNA is the *vir* region, which is located near to the T DNA. Transformation of the plant cells is irreversible, and callus cells can be cultured indefinitely, long after elimination of the bacteria.

Tumour induction, the induction of opine synthesis, and the capacity to metabolize opines, all depend on the presence of the Ti plasmids in the respective bacteria. The Ti plasmids are circular DNA molecules with molecular weights of about 1.2×10^8 (3 to 5 percent of the *Agrobacterium* chromosomes); they exist in the bacterial cells as independently replicating genetic units. They are classified according to the type of the opine they produce (Table 4.1).

Table 4.1

Ti Plasmid Groups

	Group	Opine
(a)	Octopine	Octopine
		Octopinic acid
		Lysopine
		Histopine
		Agropine
		Nopaline
(b)	Nopaline	Ornaline
		Agrocinopine

(***Source:*** *Mantell, S.H.; Mathews, J.A.; McKee, RA. Principles of Plant Biotechnology. © 1987 Oxford, Blackwell Scienttfic Publications. Reprinted by permission.*)

Most of these are either octopine or nopaline plasmids. *A. tumefaciens* cells harbour only one sort of Ti plasmid, either a nopaline or an octopine plasmid. The base sequences of the two plasmid DNAs are not closely related, except for four regions of extensive homology, one of which includes the genes responsible for crown gall transformation. This suggests that the nopaline and octopine plasmids may have diverse evolutionary histories. Ti plasmid encoded functions are listed in Table 4.2.

Table 4.2

Ti Plasmid Encoded Functions

—	Crown gall tumour induction
—	Specificity of opine synthesis in the transformed plant cell
—	Catabolism of specific opines
—	Agrocin sensitivity
—	Conjugative transfer of Ti plasmid
—	Catabolism of arginine and ornithine

(***Source:*** *Mantell, S.H.; Mathews, J.A.; Mckee, R.A. Principles of Plant Biotechnology.* © *1987 Oxford, Blackwell Scientific Publications. Reprinted by permission.*)

Avirulent bacteria (unable to elicit crown galls on susceptible plants) do not carry a Ti plasmid. Transfer of the plasmid from a virulent to an avirulent strain results in that strain becoming virulent; moreover, it can now utilize the specific opine produced in the crown gall tissue which it initiates. The ability of virulent strains to transfer the Ti plasmid is found to be dependent on the presence of the particular opine encoded by that plasmid.

Some Ti plasmid mutants have been reported. They fell into three major classes. One class failed to synthesize opines but could still induce crown galls; a second class could no longer induce tumours; a third class caused normal cells in the vicinity of the tumour cells to undergo abnormal differentiation, for example, excessive proliferation of roots or shoots.

4.1.1.2 TDNA

T DNA is the transferred DNA or transforming DNA of the Ti plasmid. When animal tumour viruses like SV40 and adenoviruses transform animal cells to malignancy, some or all of the viral DNA is integrated into the cell's chromosomes. The DNA of crown gall cells was therefore probed for plasmid DNA by using Southern blot hybridization techniques; as expected, copies of the T DNA segment (about 20,000 base pairs long) were found covalently integrated into the DNA of tumour cells. The T DNA segments of the octopine and nopaline Ti plasmids integrate at various places in the host chromosomes (but not in either of their mitochondrial or chloroplast DNA). The integrated T DNA induces and maintains the tumorous state as well as the synthesis of opines.

The T DNA in octopine tumour cells has seven genes that specify distinct RNA transcripts in the plant. Most, if not all, of these genes are controlled by separate promoters. Four or possibly five of the genes suppress shoot and root formation by tumour cells, and another gene specifies the enzyme that synthesizes the particular opine made by the tumour cells. The only DNA that moves from the Ti plasmid to host plant cell chromosomes is the T DNA. Is the T DNA a transposable element that has specifically evolved to enable *Agrobacterium* to thrive within the environment of a suitable host plant? DNA sequence analysis, however, does not reveal T DNA to have the structure of any previously analysed movable element. T DNA does not have the terminal inverted repeats of bacterial-type transposons or the long terminal repeats of the retroviral DNA. Once the T DNA is inserted in a chromosome, the T DNA behaves like a normal Mendelian plant gene.

4.1.1.3 A Useful Vector

Even though Ti plasmid DNA is an ideal vector, it poses several problems. Firstly, the plasmids are large and this does not allow easy manipulation of their DNA; also, they have a large number of restriction sites which are not usefully distributed. Secondly, the plasmids transfer functions on the T DNA which specify the production of substances which effectively convert the infected cells into tumour cells, and these cannot readily be regenerated into whole plants. Thirdly, only dicotyledonous plants are infected.

In spite of these problems, the potential of the Ti plasmid as a vector for the genetic manipulation of plants was quickly recognized. The genes in T DNA are eukaryotic in nature, even though derived from a bacterial plasmid, and are transcribed by the plant's RNA polymerase. They contain introns, which are excised correctly during maturation of the mRNA. Two properties of the T DNA of Ti plasmids make them virtually ideal vectors for introducing foreign genes into plants. First, the host range of *Agrobacterium* is quite broad; they are capable of transforming cells of virtually all dicotyledonous plants. Whether the range can eventually be broadened to include monocotyledons remains to be seen. Secondly, the integrated T DNA is inherited in a Mendelian way and its genes have their own promoters to which foreign genes can be coupled and expressed.

The simplest way to introduce T DNA into plant cells is to infect them with *A. tumefaciens* containing the appropriate Ti plasmid, and let nature do the rest. Therefore, we need to insert desired genes into the T regions of Ti plasmids. Since the Ti plasmid is very large (up to 235 kilobase pairs), it is not feasible to modify it directly, so it is useful to perform all manipulations on an excised piece of DNA including the T DNA, and then use *in vivo* recombination to swap the 'engineered' T DNA for its normal version in an intact Ti plasmid. Here is a strategy that has been developed (Fig. 4.3). First, the T region is cut out of a Ti plasmid with restriction enzymes and introduced into one of the standard cloning vector plasmids that are used in with *E. coli*. Large amounts of the vector carrying the T DNA can be grown in *E. coli* and then isolated. The next step is to use restriction enzymes and recombinant DNA techniques to insert a particular gene into the T DNA. This hybrid, containing the T DNA and the gene inserted into it, can be grown in large amounts in *E. coli* and then introduced into *A. tumefaciens* cells containing the corresponding entire Ti plasmid. Homologous genetic recombination between the T DNA segment of the native Ti plasmid and the cloned T DNA segment carrying the foreign gene results in transfer of engineered T DNA to the Ti plasmid and the displacement of its normal T DNA. The outcome is *A. tumefaciens* with a Ti plasmid whose T region carries the desired foreign gene. The last step is to infect plants with these engineered *A. tumefaciens* bacteria. The crown gall cells that result will be transformed by the T DNA carrying the foreign gene, and the goal of introducing a desired gene into plant cells is achieved.

The usual method to transform plant cells with T DNA is to paint agrobacteria that harbour Ti plasmids on a wound made in a plant shoot. However with improvements in techniques for plant cell and protoplast culture, a more convenient method that allows infection and transformation *in vitro* has been devised. Leaf cells are removed from plants, converted to protoplasts and put into culture. At this stage, when the protoplasts have just regenerated a cell wall and begun to divide, the culture is infected with agrobacterium and left for several hours. Antibiotics are then added to kill the bacteria, and the cells are grown in a medium containing plant hormones for a few weeks until they have formed small calli. At this stage, the medium is changed to one lacking plant hormones. Only the transformed cells will continue to survive and multiply. The transformed cells can then be tested for the presence of T DNA or its hallmark, the synthesis of opines. Sometimes cells from such cultures spontaneously regenerate into shoots or plants carrying T DNA and making opines.

A procedure for using the Ti plasmid as a vector. First the T DNA of the Ti plasmid is cut out with restriction enzymes and cloned into pBR 322. Next a foreign plant gene is inserted into the cloned T DNA region in the pBR322. The resulting hybrid plasmid is mixed with Agrobacteria colonies containing normal Ti plasmids; their T DNA recombines with that of the hybrid plasmids to form Ti plasmids carrying the foreign gene. The Agrobacteria carrying the foreign gene are used to infect plants, which incorporate the modified T DNA into their chromosomes.

With a much lower efficiency, it is also possible to transform protoplasts directly with Ti plasmid DNA. Freshly prepared protoplasts are exposed to plasmid DNA in a medium containing polyethylene glycol and Ca^{++} ions—essentially the same medium that is used to induce protoplast fusion. T DNA is taken up by the protoplasts, which are then cultured in a medium with plant hormones to allow regeneration of cell walls and cell division. After a few weeks, when calli have developed, the medium is replaced with the one lacking plant hormones. Only the transformed cells will survive and continue to multiply. The fact that protoplasts can be transformed by pure Ti DNA above proves that agrobacteria are not essential for transformation. Their role is solely that of a vector to bring Ti DNA into plant cells.

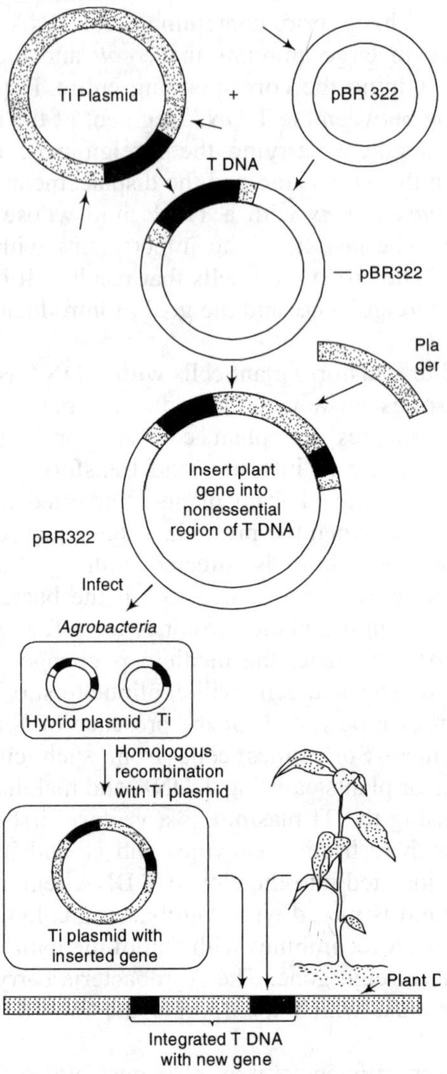

Figure 4.3

(***Source:*** *Watson, J.D.; Tooze, J.; Kurtz, D.T. Recombinant DNA—a short course. © 1983 New York, W.H. Freeman and company. Reprinted by permission.*)

Recent work has shown that all that is needed for agrobacteria to infect and transform plant cells is an intact T DNA region and another region of the Ti plasmid called *vir*. More important, from a practical standpoint, is that these two regions do not have to be on the same plasmid. If an agrobacterium harbours a Ti plasmid containing the *vir* region and another plasmid containing the T DNA, the bacteria can transform plant cells, and the T DNA (and whatever other genes have been inserted into it) will be incorporated into the plant genome.

The latest advance in the use of T DNA as a vector for introducing genes into plants is the use of specific plant promoters to express the transferred genes. The

Ti plasmid gene that codes for nopaline synthetase is isolated and sequenced, and its promoter region is identified. The structural genes for octopine synthetase is cloned downstream from this promoter and these hybrid genes are introduced into plant cells. These genes are found to be expressed in plant cells, under the control of the nopaline synthetase promoter.

A glimmer of hope has been provided by the discovery that *A. tumefaciens* can transfer its T DNA into certain monocots, resulting in the expression of the opine gene within the plant cells, but without inducing tumour formation. If the T DNA becomes integrated into the plant chromosomal DNA, and if similar results can be obtained using cereals, then the Ti plasmid will be even more suited to the transformation of monocots than dicots, since there seems to be no need to disarm the *onc* gene when infecting monocots.

4.1.2 Caulimoviruses

There are two groups of plant viruses which contain DNA—the caulimoviruses which have double stranded DNA, and the gemini viruses, which have single stranded DNA. Among the plant viruses the type virus of the caulimoviruses group, cauliflower mosaic virus (CaMV), is often cited as the most likely potential vector for introducing foreign genes into plants. This is mainly because caulimoviruses are unique among plant viruses in having a genome composed of double stranded DNA, which lends itself more readily to the manipulations involved in recombinant DNA technology.

4.1.2.1 Biological Properties

Only a small number of caulimoviruses are known and the most common ones are listed in Table 4.3.

Table 4.3

Host range of some caulimoviruses belonging to family caulimoviridae (sub family)

Virus	Host range	Serological relatedness
Carnation etched ring virus (CERV)	Caryophyllaceae	Related to CaMV and DaMV
Cauliflower mosaic virus (CaMV)	Several Cruciferae and two species of Solanaceae	
Dahlia mosaic virus (DaMV)	Several Asteraceae, some Amaranthaceae, Chenopodiaceae and Solanaceae	Related to CERV and CERV
Mirabilis mosaic virus	*Mirabilis* sp.	Unrelated to CaMV or DaMV
Strawberry vein banding virus	*Fragaria* sp.	

They all have similar particle size, *in vivo* behaviour and several are serologically related. Caulimoviruses have restricted host ranges and are confined to a few closely related plants in nature. There appears to be little, if any, overlap between the host ranges of the individual viruses within the group, in spite of some of the close serological affinities. Cauliflower mosaic virus, for example, infects only members of the Cruciferae in nature, although it is experimentally transmissible to a few plants outside this family. The Caulimoviruses are widely distributed throughout the temperate regions of the world and are responsible for a number of economically important diseases of cultivated crops.

The impetus for the development of CaMV as a vector stems from the study of the virus itself, as a consequence of its pathogenic activities on susceptible plants. Symptoms of infection vary, depending on the virus isolate, time of inoculation and condition of the plant, from mild vein clearing to more severe leaf stunting. The virus is transmitted by aphids in a non-persistent or style-borne manner. Successful transfer of CaMV by aphids requires the presence of a transmission factor in infected cells. This factor is not part of the virus particle but must be synthesized in response to infection since two non-transmissible isolates of GaMV have been identified. However, one of the main attractions is that both the virus and the isolated DNA are infectious, easily transmitted by abrasion of the leaves.

4.1.2.2 Structure and Properties of CaMV

The CaMV particles are spherical, isometric, about 50 mm in diameter and can be isolated from an inclusion body using urea and non-ionic detergents. There are probably four structural polypeptides but only two of these account for over 90 per cent of the viral protein. The major components have molecular weights of 37,000 and 64,000 and are present in a molar ratio of 5 to 1. From the proportion of these polypeptide species and the molecular weight of the virus particle, the most likely structure is an outer shell of 420 molecules of the 37,000 species surrounding a core of 60 molecules of the 64,000 species. The two remaining polypeptides have much higher molecular weights (96,000 and 88,000) and may be glycoproteins. Their function is not known.

The DNA molecule is about 8 kbp long and several varieties (totalling 50,000 bases) have been sequenced. The DNA exists in linear, open, circular and twisted or knotted forms; however, none of the circular forms is covalently closed due to the presence of site-specific single strand breaks (Fig. 4.4). These nuclease-sensitive single strand breaks are not true gaps but short oligonucleotide overlapping regions, having sequence complementarity, and thus forming short triple-stranded structures with a fixed 5′ end. There are three such sites, one (1) in the minus (coding or transcribed) strand yielding the large α fragment and overlapped by eight residues. The other two (2 and 3) are in the plus (non-coding or non-transcribed) strand yielding the β and γ fragments having 18 and 15.residue overlaps respectively. One of the plus strand discontinuities is dispensable and none is required for infection, as virus DNA previously cloned in bacteria and lacking the 'gaps' is as infectious as native DNA.

The sequence data obtained from CaMV have revealed six major and two minor, tightly packed, potential coding regions distributed between the three reading frames. Transcription of CaMV is found to be asymmetric, with only the α strand producing stable transcripts. The mechanism of replication seems to be as follows: The infecting CaMV DNA enters the plant nucleus, where the single-stranded overlaps are digested and the gaps ligated to give a supercoiled minichromosome. The function of this minichromosome is to act as a template for plant nuclear RNA polymerase II. The transcript thus formed is transported to the cytoplasm where it is either translated, or replicated by reverse transcription. A site 600 b downstream of the promoter of the large transcript binds the proposed primer of reverse transcription, methionine tRNA. The RNA transcript is then copied into minus strand DNA. Synthesis of the plus strand DNA starts at two primer binding sites near gaps 2 and 3. From gap 2 synthesis proceeds to the 5′ end of the minus strand DNA, whereas synthesis from gap 3 continues to gap 2. This DNA molecule gets packed into virus particles or re-enters the nucleus and undergoes another round of transcription and/or translation/replication.

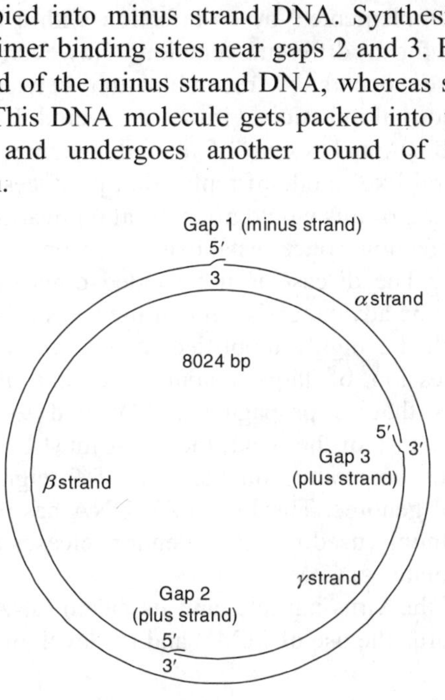

Figure 4.4

Cauliflower mosaic virus DNA
(***Source:*** *Mantell, S.H.; Mathews, J.A.; McKee, R.A. Principles of Plant Biotechnology. © 1987 Oxford, Blackwell Scientific Publications. Reprinted by permission.*)

4.1.2.3 Use of CaMV as a Vector

CaMV has several features which are in complete, contrast to those of Ti plasmid, some of which make it quite attractive as a vector. One useful feature is that the naked DNA being infective, is able to enter plant cells directly if rubbed onto a leaf with a mild abrasive. Once inside the cells, the DNA is replicated and encapsidated within virus particles, which then invade the rest of the plant. Although the CaMV DNA does not become integrated into the chromosomal DNA, and is therefore not certain to be handed on to all cells during cell division, its spread throughout the plant means that transformed plants can be effectively cloned by vegetative propagation.

But there are several problems associated with the use of CaMV as a gene cloning vector for plants. Firstly, the genome is so tightly packed with coding regions that there is little room to insert foreign DNA. Most deletions of any significant size destroy virus infectivity, except for small modifications in a specific region. Inserts up to 0.4 kbp long are tolerated, but those over 1.3 kbp destroy infectivity of the DNA. Attempts have been made to side-step this size limitation problem by using a helper virus system, where a substantial proportion of the viral genome is deleted and replaced with foreign DNA. The loss of function could be complemented' by co-infection with a normal viral DNA, or viral DNA deleted for a different function. However, the rescue of viral functions in all cases occurs by recombination between the inactive viral genomes, and only normal infectious virus is recovered. For this system to be of any use, the recombinational rescue of altered genomes must be suppressed, although the 'retroviral like' mode of replication produces a high recombination frequency and alteration of this would affect viral replication.

Secondly, the infection, once established, becomes, systemic, spreading throughout the plant. The disease is not handed down through the germ line cells. Hence this may be advantageous in that the CaMV DNA, and any inserted gene sequence, would be highly amplified in the host plant cells, potentially permitting the expression of large quantities of the foreign gene product. However, it appears that to propagate CaMV and to allow its movement throughout the vasculature of the plant, the DNA must be encapsidated and this would impose serious constraints on the size of foreign DNA which can be inserted into the viral genome. Thirdly CaMV DNA has multiple cleavage sites for most of the commonly used restriction endonucleases and this will limit the usefulness of wild isolates of CaMV.

The infectivity of the virus particle, and its naked DNA, are the most useful assets to date, as regards the use of CaMV and its development as a gene cloning vector for plants.

4.1.3 Gemini Viruses

As with the Ti plasmid *Agrobacterium,* and cauliflower mosaic virus, the potential of gemini viruses as gene cloning vectors for plants, stems from the work on several plant diseases now recognized as being caused by these agents. Both curly top virus (CTV) and maize streak disease virus (MSV) are gemini viruses which are characterized on the basis of their unique virion morphology and possession of single stranded DNA.

4.1.3.1 Structural Features

The most surprising features of this virus group are the small capsid size, 18-20 nm × 30 nm, their geminate (paired particles) morphology, which sets them apart from all other classes of viruses, and the unexpected covalently closed circular topography of the single stranded DNA which is in the molecular weight range of $7 \times 10^5 - 9 \times 10^5$. All gemini viruses recognized so far have a single major protein subunit in the range of $2.7 - 3.4 \times 10^4$ daltons.

Bean golden mosaic virus (BGMV) DNA was found to be 2510 nucleotides long, and if this was the complete genome it would be less than half the length of any other known autonomously replicating plant virus. By comparing the single stranded DNA of the virus particle with the viral double stranded DNA found in infected plants, it was found that the nucleotide sequence had a complexity twice that expected on the physical size of the viral DNA. This indicates that the BGMV DNA is heterogenous, has a divided genome consisting of two DNA molecules of approximately the same size, but different genetic content. It appears that gemini viruses consist of two populations of paired particles, differing only in the nucleotide sequence of the DNA molecules they contain. Transmission of the virus in nature occurs by leaf hoppers or the tropical white fly.

4.1.3.2 Use as a Cloning Vector

One advantage that this group of viruses has is that they contain DNA which, although single stranded, appears to replicate via a double stranded intermediate, which makes *in vivo* manipulation in bacterial plasmids more convenient. The virus group is known to infect a wide range of crop plants including monocots and dicots.

A potential disadvantage may relate to the observation that in infected plants BGMV particles are limited to phloem-associated elements. Also these viruses are not readily transferred by mechanical means from plant to plant, since they are transmitted in nature by insects in a persistent fashion. The small particle size may present packaging problems for modified DNA molecules.

4.1.4 Mitochondrial Elements

Studies of cytoplasmic male sterility (CMS) have revealed several of these extrachromosomal DNA elements. Unlike elements, these appear to replicate autonomously in mitochondria and may integrate into the mitochondrial genome. The cytoplasm of plants exhibiting CMS are classified into T, C and S, types based on their response to nuclear restorer genes, and this division correlates well with features of the mitochondrial DNA, and the presence of DNA elements. Wild type mitochondrial CMS cytoplasms contain a 1.95 kbp circular element, a small cryptic self-replicating plasmid; all except T-CMS contain in addition a 2.4 kbp linear element. Apart from these, C-CMS cytoplasm has two small circular elements of 1.55 and 1.42 kbp, and S-SMS cytoplasm contains two linear molecules of 6.2 kbp and 5.2 kbp called S1 and S2 respectively. These two elements have an inverted terminal repeat of 200 bp, sharing a region of homology of 1.3 kbp near to one end and, although they are linear and non-integrated, they appear to be capable of transposition within the mitochondrial genome. Indeed they may have been derived from this genome as regions of homology exist between S1 and S2 and normal mitochondrial DNA. These elements can be used as vectors.

4.1.5 Satellite RNAs

Satellite RNAs have perhaps the greatest potential being totally dispensable to the virus. They vary in size from 270 bases (tobacco ringspot virus satellite) to 1.5 kb (tomato black ring virus satellite). These satellites appear to share little homology with the viral genomic RNAs, have the templates for their own replication, and utilize the machinery for replication. They are not required for virus replication, but are capable of altering the pathogenicity of the viral infection. Satellite RNAs have a number of other unusual properties including the ability to code for proteins and stability in the plant in the absence of other viral components.

4.1.6 Viroids

The smallest and the simplest pathogenic agents known have also been proposed as plant gene vectors. They are small, 240-400 bases long, circular, single stranded although they undergo extensive base pairing, and consist of naked RNA. These non-protein coding viroids replicate in the host using host enzymes, probably host RNA polymerase II. They are mechanically transmissible, able to move through the sap and infect other parts of the plant; some may also be transmitted through the seed. They infect a wide variety of tropical (mainly) plants. They are certainly associated with the nucleus and may replicate in nucleus.

4.2 Vectors For Animals

The efficiency of transformation of animal cells can be greatly increased by using viral DNA as a vector, and allowing the viral particles to insert their DNA into the cells they infect. Viral DNA is an obvious for the introduction of foreign DNA into animal cells because so much is known about the life cycles of the viruses and their entry into and exit from animal cells. Also, depending on the cells they infect, they can either replicate to give progeny or integrate their DNA into host chromosomes. With virus infection it is possible to ensure that each recipient cell has many copies of the foreign gene. And since the viral genome includes strong promoters, it is possible to ensure efficient expression of foreign genes inserted into the viral DNA.

4.2.1 SV40 Vectors

SV40 is a papovavirus derived from simian virus 40. It has been the most commonly used vector for introducing foreign genes into animal cells for a number of reasons. These are:

(1) The genome consists of a single, small, covalently closed circular DNA molecule whose entire nucleotide sequences have been determined.
(2) The viral DNA is obtainable in large quantities.
(3) The genomic regions responsible for the various viral functions have been accurately located with respect to a detailed physical map of the DNA.
(4) The viral genome can multiply vegetatively or as an integral part of cellular chromosomes.
(5) A wealth of information exists on the replication and expression of the viral genome.

4.2.1.1 Basic Properties of SV40

SV40 viruses are spherical particles the capsomers of which are organised in icosahedral symmetry. The virus particle has a molecular weight of 28 megadaltons. It contains three polypeptides and one circular, double stranded DNA molecule that is associated with four histones, H2a, H2b, H3 and H4. Viral DNA which is about 5200 base pairs long contains the information coding for five or six viral proteins, three of which are part of the structural components of the capsid. The capsid is constructed from 420 subunits of the 47,000 dalton molecular weight polypeptide VP1. Two minor polypeptides VP2 and VP3, which consist largely of identical amino acid sequences are also present.

The DNA of SV40 is a covalently closed circle that can be divided into 'early' and 'late' regions (Fig. 4.5). The early region is expressed throughout the lytic cycle, whereas expression of the late genes occurs only after viral DNA replication has begun. Between the early and late regions there is a DNA sequence containing the origin of viral DNA replication.

Cells in which a papovavirus multiplies are called permissive and cells in which viral growth does not occur are non permissive. Generally speaking, a permissive cell line is derived from an animal in which a given virus normally reproduces. Non-permissible cell lines usually originate from animals which are insusceptible to the virus.

4.2.1.2 Modification of SV40 as a Vector

Wild-type SV40 cannot be used as a vector since the addition of exogenous DNA would generate a DNA molecule too large to be packaged into viral particles. However, SV40 mutants lacking the entire late region can be propagated in mixed infections with a helper virus that can provide the missing function. To produce SV40 virus particles containing recombinant DNA, either the early or the late region of the Sv40 DNA is replaced with a segment of foreign DNA. The recombinant DNA molecules cannot synthesize essential viral functions (either the T antigens if the early region has been replaced, or the

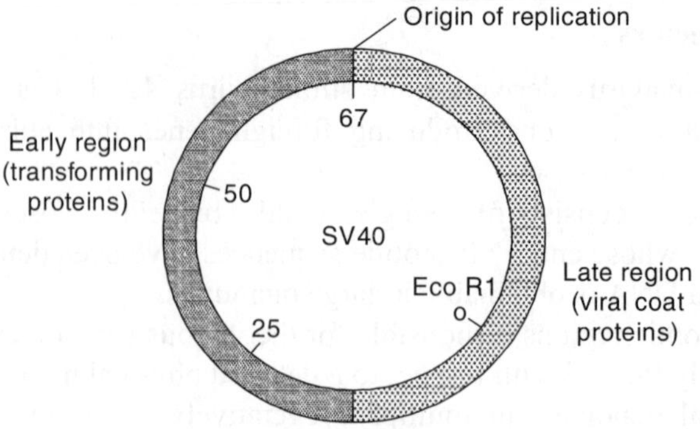

Figure 4.5

The SV40 chromosome. The early-region primary transcript codes for the transforming (large T and small t) proteins. The late primary transcript codes for the viral coat proteins (VP1, VP2, and VP3).

(***Source:*** *Watson, J.D.; Tooze, J.; Kurtz, D. T. Recombinant DNA—a short course. © 1983 New York, W.H. Freeman. and company. Reprinted by permission.*)

capsid proteins if the late region has been replaced). Therefore, in order to obtain virus particles containing the foreign DNA, the missing viral functions are frequently supplied by complementation using co-infection.

When the late region of SV40 is replaced with foreign DNA, a helper SV40 that has a deletion mutation in its early genes is used. Permissive cells are simultaneously transferred with the SV40 molecules containing the foreign gene and DNA extracted from the mutant helper virus particles. The SV40 recombinant produces the early gene products, while the co-infecting helper mutant provides the viral late proteins for new capsids. As a result, a mixed population of progeny virus particles is produced, some containing the foreign DNA, others the mutant viral genome.

When the early region of SV40 RNA is replaced by foreign DNA, production of recombinant virus particles depends on the supply of early gene proteins, the T antigens. One way to obtain T antigens while avoiding co-infection with a mutant helper virus is to introduce the recombinant DNA into a monkey cell line called COS. COS cells have been transformed by SV40 DNA that contains a functional early gene region but has a defective origin of viral DNA replication. As a result, the SV40 DNA integrated into the host chromosome specifies functional viral T antigens but the viral DNA, lacking an origin of replication, cannot replicate independently of the cell's chromosomes. When any SV40 molecule that lacks functional early genes but has an SV40 origin of DNA replication is introduced into these cells, it will replicate, because the T antigens provided by the cells will recognize the origin of replication in the incoming viral DNA. The advantage of replacing early genes by foreign DNA and propagating virions in COS cells is that all progeny virus particles will have the recombinant genome. There will be no contaminating helper virus. This overcomes the problem of separating recombination and helper viruses from each other after their recovery from cells.

In COS cells, any piece of DNA that includes an SV40 origin of replication will replicate because of the presence of SV40 T antigen in the cells. The foreign DNA will, at least transiently replicate independently of the cellular DNA.

4.2.2 Papilloma Virus DNA

Another DNA virus that is being used as a vector in eukaryotic cells is bovine papilloma virus (BPV). This virus which causes warts in cattle, has a genome of 8 kB (Fig. 4.6), The circular BPV DNA has the ability to transform certain mouse cell lines to the malignant phenotype. In these transformed cells, thc BPV

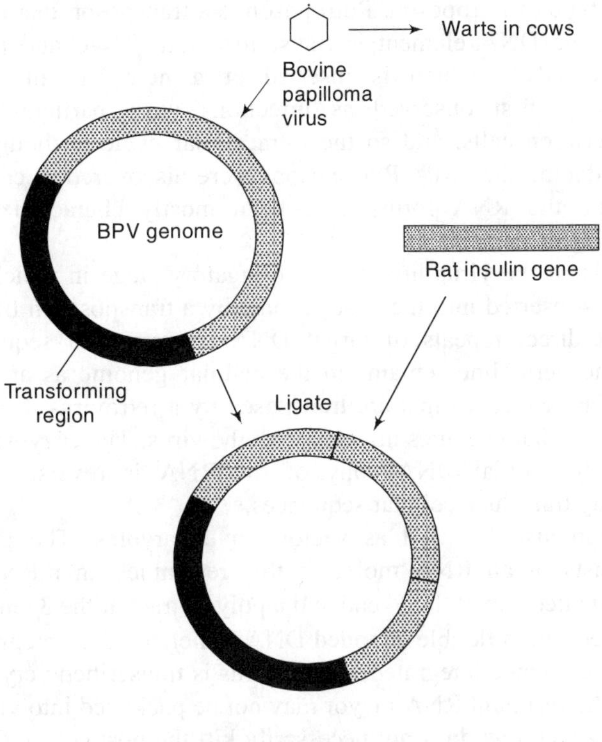

Figure 4.6
Bovine papilloma virus DNA replicates autonomously in mouse cells and remains stable at about 50 to 200 copies per cell. The rat insulin gene contained on such a replicating plasmid produces large amounts of insulin mRNA and protein.
(***Source:*** *Watson, J.D.; Tooze, J.; Kurtz, D.T. Recombinant DNA—a short course.* © *1983 New York, W.H. Freeman and company. Reprinted by permission.*)

DNA remains circular and extrachromosomal, at about 30 to 100 copies per cell. This is the only well-documented example of a plasmid being stably maintained in higher eukaryotes, Foreign DNA can be cloned into the BPV genome and introduced into mouse cells in this way. The recombinant molecules usually remain extrachromosomal. For example, rat insulin gene has been inserted into BPV DNA. In transformed mouse cells, 30 to 50 copies of the recombinant are maintained in a plasmid-like state, and high levels of insulin mRNA and protein are produced. If pBR322 sequences are also introduced into BPV DNA, the resulting recombinant can be shuttled back and forth between *E. coli* and mouse cells.

4.2.3 Retrovirus

Retrovirus is a single stranded RNA virus that propagates (replicates) through a double stranded DNA intermediate. It has the ability to insert DNA copies (proviruses) of an RNA viral genome into the chromosomes of a host cell. Retrovirus is a type of retroposon. Retroposon is a transposon that mobilizes via an RNA form; the DNA element is transcribed into RNA, and then reverse-transcribed into DNA, which is inserted at a new site in the genome. Retroviruses were first observed as infectious virus particles, capable of transmission between cells, and so the intracellular cycle is thought of as the means of reproducing the virus. Retroposons were discovered as components of the genome and the RNA forms have been mostly characterized for their functions as mRNAs.

The life cycle of the virus involves an obligatory stage in which the double stranded DNA is inserted into the host genome by a transposition like event that generates short direct repeats of target DNA. A retroviral sequence that is integrated in the germ line remains in the cellular genome as an endogenous provirus. Cellular sequences that are transposed by a retrovirus may change the properties of a cell that becomes infected with the virus. The enzyme responsible for generating the initial DNA copy of the RNA is reverse transcriptase. Retroviruses may transduce cellular sequences.

Retrovirus can also be used as vectors in eukaryotes. The genome of a retrovirus consists of an RNA molecule that resembles an mRNA in that it contains a methylated cap at the 5′ end and a poly-A tract at the 3′ end. The RNA genome is copied into a double stranded DNA molelcule that integrates into the genome of the cell. Once integrated, the provirus is transcribed very much like a cellular gene. The resultant RNA mayor may not be packaged into viral particles. The production of virions does not necessarily kill the host cell; the virions bud from the plasma membrane, and this is usually not cytopathic.

The integrated provirus contains the same DNA sequence at each end, the LTR sequence. The only known promoter for viral gene expression is contained in the L TR, and the production of the various RNAs coding for the different proteins is regulated at the level of RNA splicing. Cloned proviruses can therefore be used as vehicles for introducing genes into animal cells; this is done by replacing one of the viral genes with a foreign sequence. Cells infected with such a recombinant will produce large amounts of the new mRNA, with transcription initiating in the LTR. If a helper virus is included, the RNA copy of the recombinant virus will be packaged into viral particles.

4.3 Direct Transformations

Before the advent of genetic recombination techniques, somatic cell hybridization or the fusion of two somatic cells made it possible to transfer genes. When two cell lines are incubated with polyethylene glycol, fusion of cells of the two lines results in the fusion of nuclei that contain the chromosomes of the parent cells and express their characters. Such hybrid cells can be isolated in a selective medium; particular characters are thus associated with particular chromosomes and genes can be progressively mapped. In the course of multiplication a hybrid cell can lose chromosomes from one parent cell or both of them; a gene that has been repressed for several generations can also be expressed; sometimes a gene that is normally not expressed in a parent cell line is expressed in the hybrid cell.

4.3.1 In Plants

The development of gene cloning vectors for plants aims at introducing foreign DNA into the plant using some 'natural' system, viral or bacterial. When this is not possible, other methods are sought. It has been shown that plant protoplasts treated with polyethylene glycol, which is commonly used to induce protoplast fusion, will take up DNA from their surrounding medium. More importantly, this DNA can then be stably integrated into the plant chromosomal DNA. Using this technique, it has been possible to transform plant cells with a gene for kanamycin resistance linked to a strong plant promoter. The gene was expressed, and so transformed cells could be selected using a culture medium containing kanamycin. Plants regenerated from the transformed cells were resistant to kanamycin and this resistance was heritable. Apart from polyethylene glycol, other agents used to protect the nucleic acid from nuclease digestion are poly (L-ornithine), poly (L-lysine), protamine sulphate etc.

DEAE-dextran is a polycationic high molecular weight compound, which helps in the interaction between negatively charged DNA and the components of cell surface in endocytosis.

Pollen grains are soaked in DNA solution and are used in pollination. This helps in the transfer of DNA into the egg cell. But this method is not so successful. Another way is to inject DNA into the pollen tube and allow the pollen tube to carry this DNA into the egg.

The zygotic embryo is present in the seed. Grinding the seeds in chemicals like CCl_4 or cyclohexine can isolate the dry embryos of wheat, barley, pea or bean. When the dry embryos are immersed in a solution containing the desired gene they can take up DNA by imbibition. These embryos can be germinated and expression of the introduced gene can be assessed.

4.3.2 In Animals

The most straight-forward way of getting foreign DNA into a mammalian cell is to precipitate the DNA with Ca++ and mix this precipitate with the cells to be transformed. The DNA is taken up by the cells and once inside, the transforming fragments. are ligated to give a concatamer (a series of units linked together as in a chain) which is then integrated as one large block into the nuclear DNA. The integration occurs at random. The formation of concatamers is a particularly useful feature, since a selectable marker gene can be mixed with a gene to be cloned.

A great technical advance was the discovery that purified DNA from adenovirus, when precipitated with Ca++ and added to a monolayer of normal rat cells growing in culture, led to the appearance of many more transformed foci than when Ca++ was absent. The mechanism of the preferential uptake of Ca++ precipitated DNA by cells remains unclear, but apparently the cells actually phagocytosize the DNA granules, and a small fraction of the DNA molecules later stably integrates into the cell's chromosomal DNA. Since only a very small fraction of the added DNA finally becomes functionally integrated into cellular DNA, 'marker' techniques had to be developed to allow cells with integrated DNA to be selectively multiplied and easily identified against a background of much larger numbers of unmodified cells.

Several well-defined selectable genes (markers) have already been used in genetic studies in eukaryotic cells. The best characterized so far is the gene for thymidine kinase, an enzyme used in the salvage pathway of pyrimidine biosynthesis. The enzyme takes thymidine that has been formed by the degradation of DNA and phosphorylates it to dTMP, which by the addition of two or more phosphorylated groups becomes dTMP and gets reincorporated into DNA. Tk- cells will die in "HAT", a medium containing hypoxanthine, aminopterin (which blocks the normal dCDP—dTDP step), and thymidine. In this case the only source of dTTP for DNA biosynthesis is through thymidine kinase. In 1977, it was first found that exposure of tk- mouse cells to Ca++ precipitated DNA containing the thymidine kinase gene from herpes simplex virus resulted in the survival of resistant cell clones in HAT medium. Southern blotting confirmed that these survivors had indeed taken up and stably integrated the herpes tk gene. This meant that the tk gene could be used as a selectable marker for the integration of other genes linked to it.

The use of a cloned tk gene as a vector for gene transfer into eukaryotic cells obviously requires that the recipient cells be tk–. Though in principle it should be possible to render any eukaryotic cell tk–, in practice this is often very time consuming since both of the tk alleles of diploid cells must be inactivated; furthermore, the tk– cells used for gene transfer must have an extremely low frequency of reversion to tk+. Recently, much effort has been given to developing gene markers that work on normal cells as opposed to tk– mutant cells

Two such versatile vectors now exist (Fig. 4.7). Both use prokaryotic genes that have been linked to eukaryotic control signals. One contains a bacterial gene that lets bacteria utilize xanthine as a source of purine nucleosides by coding for the enzyme xanthine-guanine phosphoribosyl transferase (XGPRT). The corresponding mammalian enzyme HGPRT uses hypoxanthine; it can use xanthine only very inefficiently. This vector was made by inserting the cloned bacterial XGPRT gene between the promoter and poly-A addition sites of the SV40 large T antigen gene. Then SV40 promoter is extremely efficient, and consequently results in the expression of a large amount of bacterial XGPRT enzyme. This SV gpt vector not only transforms HGPRT–mammalian cells to the HGPRT+ phenotype, but, essentially, it can be used as a dominant-acting vector (that is, one that can transform wild-type cells) if the selection medium is a mixture of mycophenolic acid and xanthine. Mycophenolic acid blocks the HGPRT enzyme, making xanthine the sole source of purine nucleosides. So only cells that have taken up the SV gpt vector with the bacterial gene can survive, by using the xanthine in the medium and the acquired bacterial gene to metabolize it.

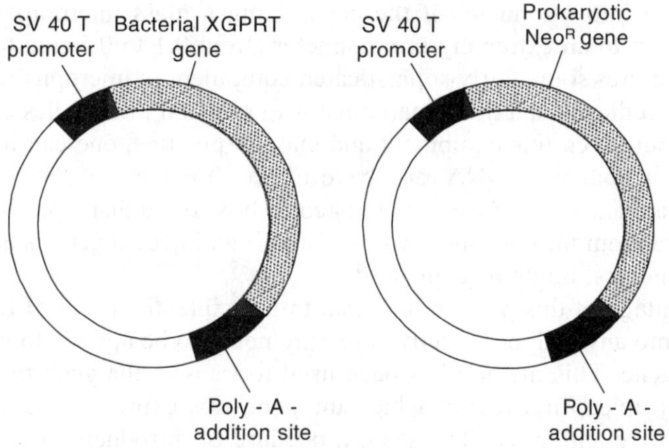

Figure 4.7

Dominant-acting vectors for gene transfer in eukaryotes. Both vectors use prokaryotic structural genes under the control of eukaryotic promoters.
(***Source:*** *Watson, J.D. Tooze, J.; Kurtz, D. T. Recombinant DNA—a short course. © 1983 New York, W.H. Freeman and company. Reprinted by permission.*)

The second dominant-acting vector consists of the prokaryotic neomycin-resistance gene (NeoR gene) ligated into the SV40 early region. This gene codes for an enzyme that phosphorylates and thus inactivates neomycin, which is toxic to ribosomes. Eukaryotic cells are sensitive to a neomycin analog called G418, which is also inactivated by the product of the NeoR gene. The SV neo vector can thus be used to transform mammalian cells to G418 resistant cells.

The existence of selectable markers led to the idea that it should be possible to introduce any gene into mammalian cells by ligating that gene to the cloned selectable marker. Analysis of mouse cells that had taken up the tk gene revealed that they had also incorporated other DNA sequences that were included with the tk gene in forming the Ca++ precipitate. (In gene transfer experiments, a large excess of carrier DNA is usually added to the cloned tk gene to form the precipitate). It was found that within the mouse cells, the exogenously added DNA is actually ligated into a large concatamer that can contain up to 800 to

1000 kb. Apparently this large structure is integrated randomly as a unit into a chromosome. Thus the DNA added with the tk gene (cotransformed DNA) is physically linked to the tk gene in the mouse cell. Using this technique of cotransformation, virtually any cloned segment of DNA can be easily introduced into eukaryotic tissue culture cells, if they are competent for transformation and if an appropriate selection is available, simply by including the cloned DNA along with the selectable marker when forming the Ca++ precipitate.

4.4 Other Methods

Microinjection

DNA can also be stably introduced into tissue culture cells by its direct microinjection into the nuclei of the cells, using a glass micropipette that has been drawn out to an extremely thin diameter (from 0.1 to 0.5 microns). Such a procedure requires some fairly sophisticated equipment (a micropipette puller for making the needles, and a micromanipulator to position the needles correctly for injections); but given this equipment and enough practice, one can inject 500 to 1000 cells per hour with DNA, and have up to 50 percent of the injected cells stably integrate and express the injected genes. It is found that injected DNA will integrate at random into the nuclear DNA, and if an injected gene is attached to a suitable promoter it might be expressed.

The advantage of this procedure is that in principle any piece of DNA can be introduced into any cell; no selective pressure needs to be applied to maintain the transferred gene. This method has been used to transfer the gene for rat growth hormone into mice, in a few of which the gene was expressed, resulting in the production of "giant" mice. The same procedure of introducing pieces of DNA into plant cells is also followed. The disadvantage of microinjection is the expensive equipment that is required, the extensive practice needed to master this tedious technique, and the relatively small number of cells that can be treated in one experiment. Also after microinjection, the egg must be re-implanted in a surrogate mother, and only after gestation can the progeny be screened for expression and correct regulation of the foreign DNA. This is therefore a slow, labour-intensive method of genetic manipulation, and the small size of population which can be produced for screening inevitably reduces the chances of success.

Macroinjection

This technique involves the injection of plasmid DNA using hypodermic syringe. Since the needles used for injecting DNA have greater diameter than the diameter of the cells this is called macroinjection

Liposomes

Liposomes can be preloaded with DNA and then are fused with protoplast to deliver their content into cytoplasm. Using this technique, it was easy to transfer DNA into animal cells, protoplasts of plants, yeasts and bacteria.

The system currently receiving most attention, and considered to be the most promising involves the use of liposomes. These are small artificial lipid vesicles prepared from phosphatidyl choline and stearylamine by a process known as reverse-phase evaporation. Nucleic acid entrapped in such liposomes renders it highly tolerant to attack by nucleases.

Direct Fusion

A further technique which would be useful when transferring DNA present in bacteria to higher plant cells involves the direct fusion of bacterial and plant cells. Transfer of Ti plasmid from *Agrobacterium tumefaciens* to tobacco cells in tissue culture has been achieved. *E. coli* cells and sphaeroplasts have been introduced into protoplasts of *Vinca rosea* using polyvinyl alcohol to mediate fusion.

Biolistic or Particle Gun

1-2μm tungsten or gold particles are coated with the DNA and using high pressurized helium gas, the DNA is delivered into the tissue.

Electroporation

This technique involves the introduction of DNA into cells by exposing them to very brief high voltage electric pulses.

Fibre-mediated DNA delivery

In this method DNA is delivered into the cell cytoplasm and nucleus by silicon carbide fibres.

Laser-induced DNA transfer

In this method laser is used to puncture the plasma membrane through which DNA may enter into the cell cytoplasm

Sonication assisted DNA transfer

In this method sonication is used to produce pores on plasma membrane through which DNA can enter the cell.

4.5 Nuclear Transplantation

To "clone" an animal, it is necessary to remove surgically, or totally inactivate with radiation, the nucleus in a fertilized egg, and replace it with a nucleus taken from another individual. It requires transplantation of a whole intact and developmentally competent nucleus (Fig. 4.8). Experiments of this sort were first done with frogs' eggs, large cells that are easy to obtain and relatively easy to manipulate. The results showed that as the donor cells from which nuclei are taken become progressively more committed to particular developmental pathways, their nuclei lose the capacity to replace the fertilized egg nucleus. Thus, nuclei transplanted from cells of very early frog embryos that are still totipotent can give rise to adult frogs. On the other hand, nuclei transplanted from the cells of adult frogs have so far never promoted the development of an adult animal; the developmental process always fails at some embryonic or larval stage.

Nuclear transplantation with frogs' eggs was first achieved in 1952. The technical problems of mammal reproduction by nuclear transplantation are much greater simply because it is extremely difficult to manipulate mammalian eggs without damaging them. In the immediate future there is little likelihood of nuclear transplantations being attempted with any other mammalian species. In theory, it could be attempted with human eggs and embryonic cells but has no practical application.

4.6 Isolation And Cloning Plastid and Mitochondrial Genes

Cloning organellar genes presents a rather different prospect to nuclear genes. Most mRNA molecules transcribed from organellar genes are non-polyadenylated; so conventional oligo-dT primed cDNA synthesis is not possible. However, the genomes are small, approximately 150 kbp for chloroplasts; therefore cloning of the genes directly from purified organellar DNA is relatively straightforward when compared with nuclear DNA.

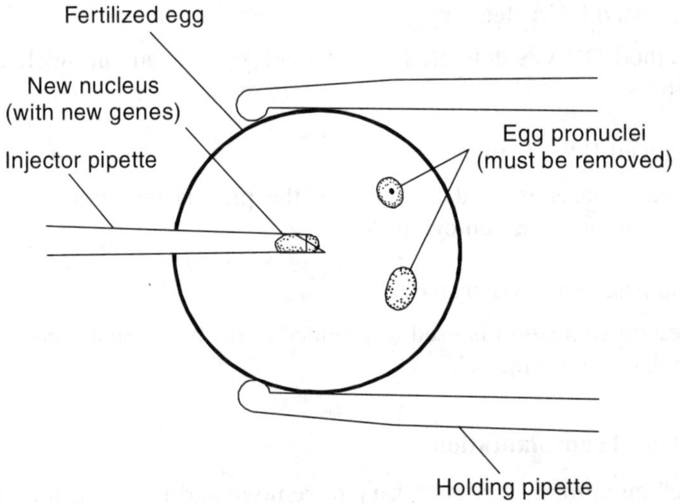

Figure 4.8
Transplanting nuclei to clone a frog. A fertilized egg is obtained and its two pronuclei are removed surgically or are inactivated with x-rays. A nucleus from another frog is then inserted into the egg.
(***Source:*** *Watson,J.D.; Tooze,J.; Kurtz, D.T. Recombinant DNA—a short course. © 1983 New York, W.H. Freeman and company. Reprinted by permission.*)

Chloroplast DNA, free from nuclear contamination, has been prepared reliably from intact, purified chloroplasts, which are treated with DNase prior to DNA isolation. If it differs in buoyant density from nuclear DNA sufficiently, chloroplast DNA can be isolated by $CsCl_2$ density gradient centrifugation. The differences in buoyant density is too small in higher plants. A number of chloroplast genes have now been cloned and it is apparent that some homology exists between species. A method often used now is to take cloned sequences from one species and use these to probe for genes from different species. This homology greatly facilitates organellar gene cloning and analysis of the structure of the genome.

Mitochondrial DNA has been studied less extensively compared to that of the chloroplast but interest in it is increasing. Quantitatively it is the smallest genetic component of a plant cell, often contributing less than 1 per cent of the total cellular DNA. In spite of the small amount present, mitochondrial DNA has been successfully prepared from purified, DNase-treated, mitochondria.

Until 1980, very few plant genes had been cloned but since 1980 the number has increased dramatically.

One of the biggest groups to be investigated is the seed storage proteins of a number of major crop plants. These storage proteins are synthesized rapidly over a short period during seed development, their expression is both tissue-and time-specific. The rapid synthesis correlates with high levels of mRNA, up to 50 per cent of the mRNA in the cells; so cDNA cloning of these genes is an attractive proposition. The gene for phaseolin, from french beans was the first, plant gene to have the presence of intervening sequences demonstrated. The protein sequence of the maize storage protein, zein, has a repeating unit. Leghaemoglobin genes from soybean have been cloned and extensively anlaysed. Many other plant proteins are being studied for their own sake and some of these may turn out to have biotechnological applications. One example is the sweet-tasting plant protein, thaumatin. This protein is considerably sweeter than sucrose on a weight for weight basis. A thaumatin gene has been cloned and expressed in *E. coli* demonstrating the presence of an amino acid extension at both the N and C termini.

Cloning of plant genes requires three basic approaches;

(i) the removal of genes from the plant and their return to the same or a different species after modification;
(ii) the use of plant genes in a unicellular organism to produce desirable plant products using fermenter technology and
(iii) the introduction of desirable genes into plants from other organisms. (eg. *nif* genes, salinity tolerance genes).

Study Outline

Vectors for Gene Cloning

A vector is a 'go between', transferring genetic information from donor to the recepient—e.g. bacteriophages, cosmids and plasmids. Ti plasmid from

Agrobacterium tumefaciens is considered to be the most promising vector used to transform plant cells.

Tumour Inducing (Ti) Plasmid

Tumour induction is a process during which a piece of plasmid DNA is transferred into plant nuclear genome. The transferred DNA is known as T-DNA which carries several genes. One gene from T-DNA codes for an enzyme which catalyzes the synthesis of opine from amino acids. Opines are never found in normal plants and cannot be metabolized by them. But it is used by the bacteria and also metabolized by them. The bacterium produces tumour and subverts the plant metabolism to make amino acids that only the bacteria can use as food. The plants are made to produce either nopaline or octopine depending upon the strains of bacteria.

TDNA

It is the transferred DNA or transforming DNA of the Ti plasmid. T DNA in tumour cells has seven genes that contain octopine and they specify distinct RNA transcripts in the plant.

Ti plasmid DNA as a Vector

Two properties that make TDNA of Ti plasmid as ideal vectors for introducing foreign genes are:

(a) the host range of Agrobacterium,
(b) inheritance is in a Mendalian way, and,
(c) its genes have their own promoter to which foreign genes can be coupled and expressed.

Caulimoviruses

There are two groups of plant viruses that contain DNA. (a) caulimoviruses: they have double stranded DNA, and have a restricted host range. They infect the members of the family Cruciferae only and cause economically important diseases of cultivated crops. (b) Gemini viruses: Curly top viruses (CTV) and maize streak disease viruses (MSV) are gemini viruses. They are single stranded DNA plant viruses. They have a small capsid which sets them apart from other viruses.

Viroids

Viroids are the smallest and the simplest pathogenic agents used as vector.

Viral vectors

The efficiency of transformation is increased using viral DNA as a vector. It is used to introduce. foreign DNA into animal cells. With virus infection it is possible to ensure that, each recipient cell has many copies of the foreign gene.

SV40 Vectors

It is derived from Simian Virus 40. It has been the most commonly used vector for introducing foreign genes into animal cells. SV40 viruses are spherical particles. They have a molecular weight of 28 megadaltons. They have 3 polypeptides and one circular double stranded DNA molecule.

Papilloma Virus DNA

Another DNA virus that is being used as a vector in eukaryotic cells is bovine papilloma virus (BPV). The circular BPV DNA has the ability to transform certain mouse cell lines to the malignant phenotype. Foreign DNA can be cloned into the BPV genome and introduced into mouse cells in this way.

Retrovirus

Retrovirus can also be used as vectors in eukaryotes. It is an RNA virus that propagates via conversion into duplex DNA. The genome of the retrovirus resembles the mRNA.

Direct Transformation

It is achieved through protoplasmic fusion which will take up DNA from their surrounding medium. It is strongly integrated into the plant chromosomal DNA. Another aspect of direct transformation is achieved through the micro-injection of nucleic acid into plant cells. Yet another technique is the direct fusion of bacterial and plant cells.

It is a straight forward way of getting foreign DNA into the mammalian cells. For this the DNA is precipitated with Ca++ and mixed with the cells to be transformed. DNA is taken up by the cells and once inside, the transforming fragments are ligated to give a concatamer (a series of units linked together as in a chain). The integration occurs at random.

Ca++ stimulates the uptake of DNA

The mechanism of preferential uptake of Ca++ precipitated DNA remains unclear, but the cells apparently phagocytosize the DNA granules and a small portion of the DNA molecule is integrated into the cell's chromosomal DNA.

Cotransformation

In mouse cells, the exogenously added DNA is ligated into a large concatamer. Apparently this large structure is integrated randomly as a unit into the chromosome. By using this technique of cotransformation, any cloned segment of DNA can be easily introduced into eukaryotic tissue culture cells if they are competent for transformation.

Microinjection

The transformation of cloned animal cells cannot be used for breeding purpose because it is impossible to regenerate whole animals from such cells. But DNA can be stably introduced into tissue culture cells by direct microinjection into nuclei of the cells using a glass micropipette. The advantage of this procedure is that in principle any piece of DNA can be introduced into any cell. The disadvantage of microinjection is the expensive equipment and extensive practice needed to master this technique.

Nuclear transplantation

It means the removal of the nucleus in a fertilized egg and replacing it with a nucleus from another individual. Nuclear transplantation with frog's eggs was first achieved in 1952.

Isolation and Cloning Plastid and Mitochondrial Genes

Cloning of the genes directly from purified organellar DNA is relatively straight forward compared with nuclear DNA. Chloroplast DNA, free from nuclear contamination has been prepared reliably from intact purified chloroplast. Chloroplast DNA can be isolated by CsCl density gradient centrifugation method. Mitochondrial DNA has been studied extensively as compared to the chloroplast DNA.

Questions

(1) What are the vectors used for gene cloning in plants?
(2) What is a Ti plasmid?
(3) Name the aminoacids synthesized by T DNA.
(4. Explain the structure and properties of CaMV viruses.
(5) What are gemini viruses?
(6) What is co-infection?
(7) Explain the uses of various cloning vehicles.
(8) What are viroids?
(9) Write about SV40 virus and its uses.
(10) What is a papilloma virus?
(11) What do you understand by direct transformation?
(12) How does Ca++ stimulate the uptake of DNA?
(13) What is the role of Tk genes as a selective marker?
(14) What is meant by cotransformation?
(15) What is microinjection? Critically comment on its application?
(16) Explain the discovery and the technique of nuclear transplantation.
(17) What are the advantages of cloning plastid and mitochondrial genes?
(18) What are liposomes?

5
Plant Cell and Tissue Culture

Introduction

In developing countries the most important challenges are to produce sufficient food, fibre and fuel for the continuously growing population from inelastic land area. Plant tissue culture offers excellent opportunities of mass propagation of plants in test tubes. Cell culture techniques are increasingly used for cloning purposes because a single cell can be induced to regenerate a complex individual. This idea of totipotency has been the foundation for tissue cultures of several species, and later, for somatic and sexual cells isolated from a large number of plants.

Plant cell and tissue culture is fundamental to most aspects of plant biotechnology. One of the significant contributions to the manipulative powers of modern biologists has been the development of cell and tissue culture technique. Tissue culture is the process whereby small pieces of living tissue (explants) are isolated from an organism and grown aseptically for indefinite periods on a semi-defined or defined nutrient medium. Explants range from large seedlings and organs (as in ovule and embryo culture) to small, single cells and protoplasts. With the discovery of auxin and cytokinin and their effects on cell growth and division, along with the advantageous inclusion of natural substances in media such as coconut milk (which in vivo supports growth and development of embryos in certain plants), it was shown that plant tissue explants could proliferate by repeated cell divisions. When appropriate cultural conditions are provided, cell masses could then proceed along various developmental pathways, to regenerate shoot and root organs and eventually whole plants.

Development of single cells into complex multicellular organs and tissues is a natural progression common to all higher forms of life. It constitutes that spectrum of development known as differentiation and is a series of highly coordinated and genetically determined processes, through which single or fused gametes (spores and zygotes) and somatic initials derived ultimately from a single cell primordium develop into whole plants. Patterns of plant development are reasonably consistent within definable ranges of genotype, i.e. taxonomic groups, so that the genetic constituents of the original germ cell in theory contain all the critical determinates of patterns of differentiation. This is the basis for the concept of totipotency. Totipotency is the capacity of a single cell to regenerate the phenotype of the complete and differentiated organism from which it is derived. The activity of meristems—regions of concentrated, most coordinated cell division—can be activated or suppressed according to patterns of differentiation dictated by genetic and/or environmental control mechanisms.

Cells at a relatively early stage of development, such as quiescent (non-dividing) types of parenchyma and the cells in meristems, such as vascular cambial tissues and embryonic tissues are in an undetermined condition. By definition, undetermined cells are capable of switching to different pathways of development depending on the environment imposed on them. Undetermined cells can also rapidly proliferate (dedifferentiate) and produce cell masses known as calluses. Undetermined plant cells can exhibit totipotency in addition to a high degree of plasticity in their response to physiological and environmental stimuli.

5.1 Historical Events

In 1839, Schwann proposed the cell theory which envisaged that each living cell of an organism, if provided with proper environment, would be capable of independent development. This theory gave birth to the concept of totipotency. Vochting in 1878, inspired by Schwann's cell theory, performed some basic experiments and stated that in every plant fragment, even the smallest ones rest the elements from which, the whole body can be built up by isolating the fragments under proper external conditions. In 1902, Haberlandt predicted that one could successfully cultivate artificial embryos from vegetative cells'. Thereafter the course of history reveals some dramatic advances in tissue culture techniques. Table 5.1 summarizes some of the major advances.

5.2 Media

Plants in nature can synthesize their own food material. In contrast, plants growing *in vitro* are heterotrophic, i,e. they cannot synthesize their own food material. Plant tissue culture media, therefore, require all essential minerals plus a carbohydrate source, usually added in the form of sucrose, and other growth hormones (regulators and vitamins). A significant contribution to the formulation of a defined growth medium suitable for a wide range of applications was made by Murashige and Skoog (1962). In their work to adapt tobacco callus cultures for use as a hormone bioassay system they evaluated many medium constituents to achieve optimal growth of calluses. By doing so, they improved upon existing types of plant tissue culture media to such an extent that their medium (the MS medium) has since proved to be one of the most widely used in plant tissue culture work. Table 5.2 gives the composition of MS medium.

Components of media for the growth of plant callus and suspension cultures can be classified into six groups, and this division is usually reflected in the way in which stock solutions are prepared and stored. These groups are:

Table 5.1

Major advances in the development of plant cell and tissue culture technique.

Period		Advances
1900	—	First attempts to culture plant cells and tissues in non-aseptic conditions.
	—	Formulation of problems (Haberlandt)
1920	—	Limited culture of excised pea and maize roots (Kotte)
1934	—	Discovery that auxin IAA promotes cell growth (Went)
	—	Indefinite culture of tomato roots (White)
	—	Indefinite callus cultures of tree species (Gautheret)
1935	—	Use of IAA in media (carrot cultures) (Gautheret)
1940	—	Use of tumour hybrid *Nicotiana glauca, N.langsdorffii* to produce callus cultures (White).
	—	Recognition of role of Vitamin B1 (Gautheret)
1941	—	Use of coconut milk to support embryoids of *Datura* hybrids
1950	—	(Van Overbeck *et al*).
	—	Discovery that adenine derived from nucleic acids enhances cell proliferation and bud formation in callus cultures (Skoog)
	—	Endosperm cultures established (La Rue)
	—	Culture of monocotyledons establised using coconut milk additive to media (Morel).
1951–	—	Discovery that the cytokinin, kinetin, promote cell division
1960	—	(Miller *et al*)
	—	Effects of graft transmissible growth regulatory substances on differentiation.
	—	Roles of auxin and cytokinin on shoot and root induction in tobacco callus cultures established (Skoog and Miller)
	—	Discovery of somatic embryogenesis in carrot callus cultures (Reinert)
1960–	—	(Shoot) micropropagation
1970	—	Effect of cytokinins on apical dominance
	—	Genetic stability - clonal propagation
	—	Pathogen (virus) elimination
		— systemic infection
		— isolation and regeneration of non-vascularised meristematic part
	—	Pathogen indexing
		— immunological tests
	—	Germplasm conservation

Contd...

Table 5.1 Contd...

Period		Advances
	—	Anther culture
		— Pollen embryogenesis
		— Haploid callus and plant regeneration
	—	Isolated microspore culture
	—	Ovule culture
	—	Interspecific hybridization and embryo culture
	—	*In vitro* pollination
	—	Isolated ovule and placenta culture
1971–980	—	Protoplast isolation — enzymatic digestion of cell wall, pectinase, cellulase
		— osmolarity of media
	—	Protoplast culture
		— cell wall regeneration
		— cell division
	—	Plant Regeneration from protoplast
		— cell and callus culture
		— organogenesis and/or somatic embryogenesis
	—	Protoplast fusion
		— PEG, electrofusion
		— Homo-heterokaryotic fusion
		— Hybrid cytoplasm
	—	Somatic hybrids
		— Selection of fusion products
		— New hybrid combinations
1981	—	—Somaclonal variation
		—isolation of auxotrophs by cell colony screening in haploid protoplasts
1982	—	—Naked DNA transformation of protoplasts — Electrofusion of protoplasts
1983	—	Industrial production of secondary metabolite by suspension culture
		—Cointegrate type of vectors designed for *Agrobacterium transformation*
1984	—	Transformation of *Nicotiana* protoplasts with plasmid DNA
1985	—	Transformation of leaf discs with *Agrobacterium tumefaciens*
		— Development of binary vector system
		— Gene transfer by electroporation
1987	—	Use of microprojectile gun form genetic transformation

Contd…

Period		Advances
1993	—	*In vitro* fertilization in maize plants
		—Green hairy roots showing photoautotrophy
1994	—	Marketing of genetically engineered tomato 'Flavr-Savr'
		—Improved plant transformation through electrophoresis
1996	—	Development of agrolistic method for plant transformation
1997	—	Sonication assisted *Agrobacterium* mediated transformation
		Contd...
2000	—	Sequence of *Arabidopsis thaliana* released
2002	—	sequence of rice genome released.
2004	—	Centrifugation assisted *Agrobacterium* mediated transformation
2005	—	*in vivo* transformation in pea plant

Table 5.2

Murashige and Skoog Medium composition and preparation.

Constituent	Molarity in Medium	Concentration of stock solution (mg/litre)	Volume of Stock per Litre of Medium (ml)	Storage of stock solution
Major inorganic Nutrients				
NH_4NO_3	2.06×10^{-2}	33000		
KNO_3	1.88×10^{-2}	38000		
$CaCl_2\ 2H_2O$	3.00×10^{-3}	8800	50	+ 4°C
$MgSO_4\ 7H_2O$	1.50×10^{-3}	7400		
KH_2PO_4	1.25×10^{-3}			
Trace Elements				
KI	5.00×10^{-6}	166		
H_3BO_3	1.00×10^{-4}	1240		
$MnSO_4\ 4H_2O$	9.99×10^{-5}	4460		
$ZnSO_4\ 7H_2O$	2.99×10^{-5}	1720	5	+ 4°C
$Na_2MoO_4\ 2H_2O$	1.00×10^{-6}	50		
$CUSO_4\ 5H_2O$	1.00×10^{-7}	5		
$CoCl_2\ 6H_2O$	1.00×10^{-7}			
Iron Source				
$FeSO_4\ 7H_2O$	1.00×10^{-4}	5560	5	+ 4°C
$Na_2\ EDTA\ 2H_2O$	1.00×10^{-4}	7460		
Organic				

Contd...

Table 5.2 Contd...

Constituent	Molarity in Medium	Concentration of stock solution (mg/litre)	Volume of Stock per Litre of Medium (ml)	Storage of stock solution
Supplement				
Myo-Inositol	4.90×10^{-6}	20000		
Nicotinic Acid	4.66×10^{-6}	100		
Pyridoxine - HCI	2.40×10^{-6}	100	5	+ 4°C
Thiamine – HCI	3.10×10^{-7}	100		+ 4°C
Glycine	3.00×10^{-5}	400		
Carbon Source				
Sucrose	8.80×10^{-2}	—	add as solid 30g/litre)	

(i) major inorganic nutrients,
(ii) trace elements,
(iii) iron source,
(iv) organic supplement (vitamins),
(v) carbon source,
(vi) organic supplement (plant growth regulators).

As plant growth regulator levels are usually the most critical factor for successful dedifferentiated growth of cultured plant cells, and since the optimum concentrations of auxins and cytokinins, for such growth, may differ from one species to another, they are usually modified for each medium.

Other plant tissue culture media proposed by Gamborg *et al* (1968), White (1963), Heller (1953) and Smith (1967) are also used in tissue culture work.

5.3 Culture Techniques

Establishment of any plant tissue culture follows standard procedures similar to the one outlined in Fig. 5.1. The general techniques used in the isolation and growth of cultures are described as follows.

5.3.1 Cleaning of Glassware

Cleanliness of glassware is a very important factor for the successful growth of a culture. There are different procedures used for cleaning of glassware, but the following method is very suitable. It is first boiled in 10% sodium carbonate solution for two hours followed by thorough rinsing with tap water. The glassware is soaked in 30 per cent nitric acid overnight, washed, cleaned and rinsed with distilled water and finally drained, dried and stored in a clean place. This operation can now be avoided by the use of disposable sterile culture vessels that are available commercially.

5.3.2 Sterilization of Glassware and Media

The cleaned glassware is sterilized using the following methods. Wet heat method requires an autoclave which helps to produce heat in the form of saturated steam under increased pressure and is responsible for killing microbes.

In case of media, the use of pressure allows exposure at a higher temperature without the liquid boiling over. Empty glassware is generally sterilized at 15 lb/sq.inch for one hour whereas for media, the time is reduced to 15 to 20 minutes. Glassware can also be sterilized in an oven at 160 °C for at least half an hour by dry heat sterilization using an oven. This cannot be used to sterilize culture media as the liquid would evaporate to dryness. Certain thermolabile solutions cannot be sterilized by heat and hence specific bacterial filters which have a pore size smaller than the microbial cells are used. This method is called filter sterilization method.

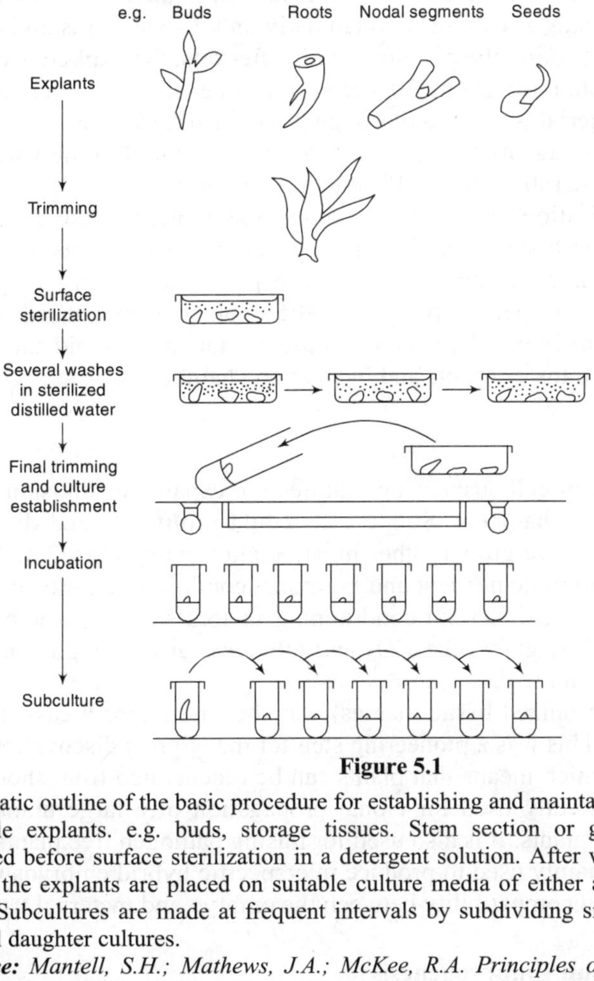

Figure 5.1

Schematic outline of the basic procedure for establishing and maintaining plant tissue cultures. Suitable explants. e.g. buds, storage tissues. Stem section or germinated seedlings, are trimmed before surface sterilization in a detergent solution. After washing in sterile distilled water, the explants are placed on suitable culture media of either a semi-solidified or liquid form. Subcultures are made at frequent intervals by subdividing single mother cultures into several daughter cultures.

***(Source:** Mantell, S.H.; Mathews, J.A.; McKee, R.A. Principles of Plant Biotechnology. © 1987 Oxford, Blackwell Scientific Publications. Reprinted by permission)*

5.3.3 Sterilization of Plant Material

Growing plants are usually contaminated with microorganisms present in the surrounding environment. Hence it is necessary to sterilize the plant material;

otherwise microbes will also grow in the medium and suppress the growth of the explant, ultimately causing death. Unlike the glassware and media, sterilization of plant material requires greater care, since both microbes and plant tissues are living cells. The microbes present on the surface area of the plant tissue have to be killed without killing the tissue. The method used is therefore also known as surface sterilization. The conditions for surface sterilization vary for each tissue and requires standardization both with regard to the concentration of the sterilizing agent and the time for the treatment.

The first step in the process involves cleaning of the plant material by thorough washing, often under running water. It is then treated with a detergent solution, which as a result of its ability to emulsify and dispense oils and dirt in the solutions helps in cleaning the plant material. After this, the explant is treated with 70 per cent alcohol for about 30 seconds to one minute. After alcohol treatment the plant material is washed thoroughly with distilled water.

The chemical sterilizing agents mainly used are 20 per cent chlorine water, 10 per cent bleaching powder, 0.01% or 0.1% mercuric chloride.

After surface sterilization, the flask containing the explant in the sterilizing solution is transferred to a sterile laminar airflow cabinet. The surface sterilized explants are removed and transferred to a sterile petridish with the help of a sterile pair of forceps. A specific portion of the explant is inoculated on the previously sterilized medium. Great care should be taken to avoid air borne contamination into the transfer rooms and incubation chambers.

5.3.4 Culture

Isolated single cells from cell suspension cultures are capable of division when they are placed in microchambers. Single cells could proliferate and divide to form calluses when they are grown either in association with "nurse" or feeder callus cells. When appropriate nutrient and hormonal conditions are met, calluses could regenerate new plants. Certain conditioning factors such as, amino acids like glutamine and serine, gases like CO_2 and ethylene, growth regulators like cytokinins are required in media.

Callus culture (unorganized tissue masses) was the first major break-through in plant tissue culture. This was a pioneering step for many great discoveries.

Meristem culture, which means that plants can be regenerated from shoot and root apices has been greatly used for clonal propagation of a large number of herbaceous and woody plants. It is also used for raising pathogen free plants.

Embryo culture is mainly used to produce interspecific hybrid embryos which otherwise abort due to incompatibility between the embryo and maternal tissue.

5.4 Organogenesis and Embryogenesis

Organogenesis refers to the induction of morphologically well defined organs like shoot, root etc. from callus cultures. Skoog and Miller, in 1957, pointed out that a balance between the relative levels of auxin and cytokinin played a great role in the initiation of shoot and root. Embryogenesis refers to the development of somatic bipolar adventive embryoids from callus cultures under certain nutritional and hormonal conditions. This development follows a sequence through pro-embryoid, globular and torpedo stages.

5.4.1 Organogenesis

Plant regeneration through adventitious bud formation can either be directly from the initial explant or through a callus phase. A callus can be increased substantially by subculture. But it is often subject to genetic aberrations resulting in variability and loss of totipotency. Root fragments, rhizomes, tubers, bulb scales, stem fragments, petioles, pedicels, flower parts etc. have direct adventive organogenetic capacity. Shoot mer!stems may arise from single cells of the epidermis and also from many cells in subepidermal layers. This technique is used extensively for vegetative propagation of tubers, vegetables, trees, ornamentals etc. mostly in vegetatively propagated plants.

Organogenesis has been studied in a number of plants and these studies shed light on several factors responsible for plant regeneration. The enhancement of regeneration by wounding and temperature is thought to be related to ethylene biosynthesis. By changing the carbon dioxide concentration in culture vessels, a better organogenetic response could be obtained.

5.4.2 Embryogenesis

Somatic embryogenesis offers many advantages over organogenesis but this is still a relatively rare phenomenon in many important crop plants. Plant regeneration through somatic embryogenesis has several advantages and appears to be most promising for future large scale, rapid plant propagation. The totipotency of cells is best expressed in the formation of somatic embryos from single cells and their growth and development to form a complete plant. Somatic embryogenesis has great implications in tissue culture technology. Firstly, because somatic embryos have formed root and shoot meristems, thereby reducing several of the labour intensive steps involved in the subculture and separation and rooting of individual shoots. Secondly, if the single cell origin of somatic embryos is universal, then potentially all single cells in cell suspensions could be induced to form embryoids.

The single cell origin of somatic embryos is also beneficial for the plants produced. They can be used for mutation breeding, genetic analysis and maintenance of germ plasm, where as plants obtained through the other routes are of multicellular origin and are consequently chimeras, not ideal for mutation breeding and genetic analysis. Somatic embryogenesis has now been observed in a wide range of plants including some of the major crops. In cereals and legumes it has only recently been achieved. Direct regeneration from protoplasts through somatic embryogenesis has also been achieved.

A few methods of enhancing somatic embryogenesis have been reported recently. Visual identification of highly embryogenic calli and media optimization has been used to achieve a rate of embryogenesis upto 33 times higher in cereal cultures. Such calli appear white, smooth and knobby in contrast to the yellow, transluscent, non embryogenic calli. Plasmolysis using 1M solution of sucrose is reported to enhance embryogenesis presumably by isolating cells from each other and creating a situation similar to the egg cell. Ultrastructural differences in embryogenic and non-embryogenic cells have also been identified. Regular arrangements of endoplasmic reticulum, accumulation of starch, sugars, lipids and proteins indicate competence of cells for somatic embryogenesis. A synergistic interaction of ammonium ions with amino acids especially proline has also been reported. Glutamine can substitute ammonium ions. Other reports indicate that polyamines play an important role in somatic embryogenesis, probably by controlling ethylene biosynthesis. Glycerol and GA_3 stimulate embryogenesis.

Somatic embryos are perfectly suited for large scale plant production since they can be made to simulate seeds and hence are amenable to mechanised sowing. Artificial seeds are prepared in the laboratory by encapsulating somatic embryos with various polymers such as calcium alginate. For example, it has been estimated that three grams of celery tissue per litre produces 7,50,000 embryos in three weeks, enough to plant 70 acres. A prototype machine to produce 5000 capsules per hour has been developed. The present procedure involves mixing the embryos in a solution of sodium alginate and dropping the individual embryos into a 50 mm solution of CaClz to get a coating of calcium alginate. Artificial seeds could be a part of future genetic engineering procedures where genetically modified plants are regenerated from protoplasts through somatic embryogenesis.

5.4.3 DNA Amplification and Tissue Culture

DNA sequences in eukaryotes can be resolved into three distinct classes differing in the degree of redundancy: highly repetitive, intermediate, and unique. Highly repetitive sequences are not transcribed. The unique sequences belong to structural genes in a strict sense. The intermediate group comprises interspersed short sequences and "reiterated" clusters of genes (eg. ribosomal RNA, 5s RNA, t-RNA, histone messenger RNA). Several hypotheses have been put forward with regard to the function of different kind of sequences. However, no unifying theory has been proposed till now, which might explain in teleological terms the reason for the large differences in multiplicity at the inter and intraspecific levels and their influence, if any, on plant developmental processes. In this context, plant tissue cultures have been exploited very recently to shed light on the problem of the function of amplification and its relation to redundancy.

The difference between these two phenomena seems to be that the first is considered as a transient process directly connected with specific developmental stages, whereas all the differences in multiplicity at the inter and intraspecific level which are heritable fall under the second category.

5.4.3.1 Transient Amplification

All those phenomena which directly or indirectly suggest the selective replication of specific DNA portions, concomitant with specific changes in developmental patterns and limited in time are referred to as transient amplification. Table 5.3. gives the names of some plants where transient amplification has been noted.

Table 5.3

Direct and indirect indications of transient DNA amplification in some plants

	Material	Evidence
(i)	*Helianthus* tuber slices	Inhibition of expansion growth by DNA synthesis inhibitors
(ii)	*Vicia faba* primary root	Loss of labelled DNA in aging stems
(iii)	*Lycopersicon esculentum collenchymna tissue*	*DNA turnover*
(iv)	Allium *cepa* roots	rDNA amplification associated with metaxylem differentiation
(v)	Germinating wheat embryos	Loss of ribosomal genes during germination
(vi)	Wounded *Vicia faba* stems	DNA synthesis without cell division after wounding
(vii)	*Cucurbita melo* seeds	Synthesis of a DNA satellite during cold stress
(viii)	*Phaseolus* suspensor	Cytological and biochemical evidence of amplification
(ix)	*Solanum tuberosum* tuber	DNA synthesis without mitosis tissue in vitro
(x)	*Cymbidium* maturing parenchyma *in vitro*	Cytological and biochemical evidence of DNA amplification and extrusion into the cytoplasm.
(xi)	*Ginkgo biloba* female gametophyte	Cytological evidence of localized DNA Systhesis

5.4.3.2 Amplification in Differentiating and Differentiated Systems

Many experiments have been conducted which merely give indirect proof of DNA amplification, mainly based on the need of non-mitotic DNA synthesis for specific growth and differentiation patterns, eg. cell elongation and expansion. Series of experiments on elongation have shown the need of an early DNA replication preferentially localized in chromocenters. Another cell differentiation process where an important role for gene amplification has been suggested is xylem differentiation. During the sequence of events leading to xylogenesis, an extra replication of DNA sequences coding, at least in part, for ribosomal RNA has been reported. A similar temporal sequence has been found for cell maturation. Nuclei in root hair and parenchyma cell were found to show disproportionately large chromocentres and DNA values exceeding those expected from a normal endopolyploidization process.

Besides transient DNA amplification occurring during a dynamic differentiation process, there are some cases of extra DNA synthesis in highly specialized cells such as suspensor, gametophytes, cells of quiescent centre. In general we can conclude that, differential replication may be a common, though complex phenomenon associated with the differentiation of non-dividing cells.

5.4.3.3 Amplification in Dedifferentiating Cells

The first results on DNA amplification during dedifferentiation are derived from the knowledge obtained from wound healing experiments mainly carried out to gain insight into the problem of *Agrobacterium tumefaciens* induced tumorogenesis. These studies are particularly related to the so called "conditioning" phase i.e. a period between the wound and infection with the bacterium. A sharp increase in DNA has been reported after wounding which was not connected with mitosis. This DNA plays an important role in tumour induction, which suggests the need of a specific extra DNA synthesis for cell proliferation after wounding. Following the wounding (cutting) of tissue portion during culture DNA synthesis without mitosis has been reported. Presence of gene amplification processes essential for further proliferation and differentiation have also been reported. Amplification capacity and proliferation capacity are under genetic control or hormonal control.

5.4.3.4 General Nature of Transient Amplification

The widespread occurrence of dynamic DNA amplification phenomena in different phases of plant development allow us to formulate a working hypothesis that selective replication might be one of the, main control mechanisms in plant growth and morphogenesis. Since this process is often found to be under hormonal control, genotypes may also exert an important influence on it. The amplified DNA is labile in nature.

5.4.3.5 Semipermanent Amplification

If amplification of specific portions of plant genomes increases rates of growth and protein synthesis, the permanence of these situations over longer periods of time could be of importance in altering developmental behaviours. Processes like gene compensation and magnification have been reported in plants. Gene compensation refers to developmental increases in the multiplicity of genes in one chromosome, in the presence of a deletion in its homologue. Gene magnification refers to the increase in rRNA cistrons which can be inherited. Although both these phenomena seem to provide an answer to artificially altered genetic situations, they nevertheless represent well-studied instances of semipermanent gene amplification. But the various experiments carried out so far do not throw clear light on semipermanent amplification. The biochemical nature of amplified portions is not yet established.

5.4.3.6 Differential Redundancy

A wide variation in the relative proportions. of different DNA species both at the inter and intraspecific levels have
been reported. Nothing is known as yet about the real mechanism of induction of the observed variability, which could occur either through amplification and integration of new DNA copies or through processes like unequal crossing over.

5.5 Androgenic Haploids

Haploid plants are sporophytes possessing the gametic rather than the somatic chromsome number. They may be obtained spontaneously or produced by a number of techniques during different stages of the plant life cycle. The usefulness of haploid plants is based on the assumption that homozygous inbred lines can be rapidly and readily achieved through them; also it is easier to detect mutations in haploids because of the presence of a single set of chromosomes. Yamada *et al*(1963) were the first to report the isolation of a haploid angiosperm tissue from anther cultures of *Tradescantia reflexa*. Soon Guha and Maheshwari (1964) reported the formation of embryo-like structures in *Datura innoxia*, and later confirmed the haploid nature of the embryoids and their origin from immature pollen grains. The embryo ids recapitulate various stages of zygotic embryogeny within the locule before they emerge from the anther. It is the potential use of androgenic haploids in the production of inbred lines, genetic analysis, selection and mutation research that has stimulated much interest and has led to extensive studies.

There are three major approaches in the culture of anthers and pollens (Fig. 5.2).

(1) Culture of anthers on semi-solid media and the proliferation of pollen derived embryos and plantlets through the dehiscence of mature anthers;

(2) Culture of anthers on liquid media and the release of their pollen leading to the formation of embryos and plantlets directly from released pollen;

(3) *ab initio* (from the beginning) culture of immature pollen extracted from developing anthers.

The physiological condition of the donor plants, the type of pre-culture treatment applied to excised flower buds, the stage of pollen development reached when anthers are cultured, and the presence or absence of growth regulator supplements in media are some of the critical determinants of successful culture and production of plants.

Pollen dimorphism in an anther or pollen refers to the presence of two different morphologies which have the potential to develop into two different types of generations—gametophyte and sporophyte. and is affected by the genotypic differences among the donors.

Pollen grains in cultured anthers give rise to androgenic haploids through a marked shift in the pattern of their normal development. Following the first microspore mitosis, which may or may not be normal, a haploid callus tissue or embryoid is formed instead of the normal male gametophyte. One of the most critical requirements for the successful induction of androgenesis *in vitro* is the stage of microspores at the time of anther excision and culture. Experience has shown that in most species, the maximum response is obtained when anthers are excised just before, during or immediately after the mitosis of the microspore nucleus. Several methods of culture are used to induce the formation of androgenic haploids. These include the culture of excised anthers on agar nutrient media, floating anthers on a liquid medium, culture of isolated microspore and the culture of whole inflorescence in liquid media.

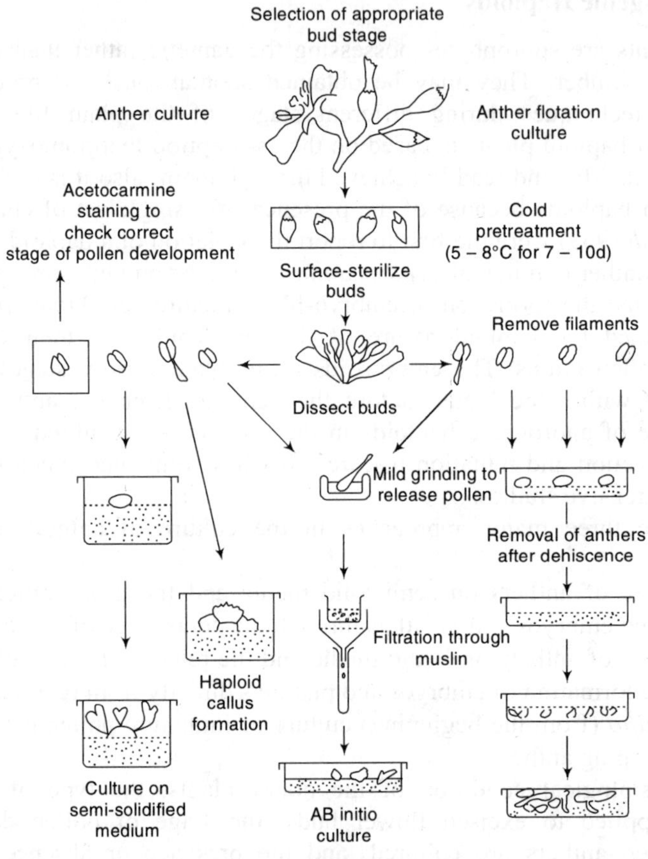

Figure 5.2

Different cultural procedures that can be followed to establish anther and pollen cultures and from which embryoids and plantlets can be produced.

(***Source:*** *Mantell, S.H.; Mathews, J.A.; McKee, R.A. Principles of Plant Biotechnology. © 1987 Oxford, Blackwell Scientific Publications. Reprinted by permission)*

Excised anthers are placed in culture so as to be in direct contact with the nutrient medium. The nutrient requirements for inducing a switch from the gametophytic phase to androgenic development are quite simple. Plant growth substances, particularly auxins and cytokinins, have been successfully used for the induction of androgenic development. The appearance of haploids in nature, as well as the ability of microspores to form embryoids or callus *in vitro*, is under genetic control.

5.5.1 Uses

Anther culture eliminates many cycles of selection and back-crossing required to produce homozygous plants. Genetic stabilization, homozygosity, and the development of pure lines can be achieved in a matter of months by anther or microspore culture. Even in self-incompatible species homozygosity could be achieved through haploids. Because mutagenesis and selection can occur in the vegetative, state, even those mutants which cannot pass through the sexual cycle can be obtained. The high purity of lines obtainable through androgenesis also makes it possible to achieve maximum heterosis. Haploids can be used to transfer the genotypes of inbred lines into cytoplasm that caused male sterility. Haploids are useful in the induction and isolation of auxotrophic mutants. They are of importance in selection and parasexual hybridization. Haploids can also be of use in cytogenetic investigations, e.g. in the study of pairing relationships between chromosome sets, in genetic analysis to establish inheritance patterns, as an aid to stabilizing chromosomes in those instances where there is a high degree of nonhomology, and in the production of monosomics, nullisomics etc.

Haploids offer the following advantages:

(a) In principle, plants of haploid origin are, homozygous. Even if they were to diploidize spontaneously, or through colchicine treatment, they would retain this quality, which is an essential pre-requisite for meaningful breeding trials.

(b) Homozygotes induced in tissue culture following meiotic segregation could reveal a number of valuable recessive characters which have accumulated and remained unexpressed in natural heterozygous populations. Many valuable genotypes, such as those governing low nutritive requirements and resistance to cold, drought or heavy metals, are of this type, and their expresssion in spontaneous or induced mutants will be promptly detected.

(c) In favourable cases, the number of androgenetic progeny can be phenomenally large and the time taken to obtain plants is considerably shortened when compared to that involving hand-pollination, fruiting, seedset and germination required to produce inbreds by conventional methods.

(d) Widespread self-incompatibility in trees can be overcome through androgenesis.

(e) Haploid cells and protoplasts are ideal material for gene transfer.

5.5.2 Monoploid Production by Chromosome Elimination

Here monoploids are defined as sporophytes with the basic gemetic chromosome number. They have a single genome or chromosome set ($2n = X = 7$ in *Hordeum vulgare*). Monoploids are generally sterile but by doubling the chromosomes, homozygous diploid fertile plants are produced (Fig. 5.3). Monoploids can be produced by interspecific hybridization followed by chromosome elimination. The hybridization method consists of crossing cultivated barley, *Hordeum vulgare* L ($2n = 2X = 14$), with the wild, diploid cross-pollinating and perennial *H. bulbosum* L ($2n = 2X = 14$). This technique, the Bulbosum method, consists of the following steps: the female gamete of barley is fertilized by the *H. bulbosum* gamete. During the formation of the embryos, the chromosomes of *H. bulbosum* are eliminated; only the barley genome is in the embryos. These are cultured *in vitro* as immature embryos. Plantlets from these monoploid embryos can be made to give fertile flowers bearing homozygous offspring, following an efficient chromosome doubling technique.

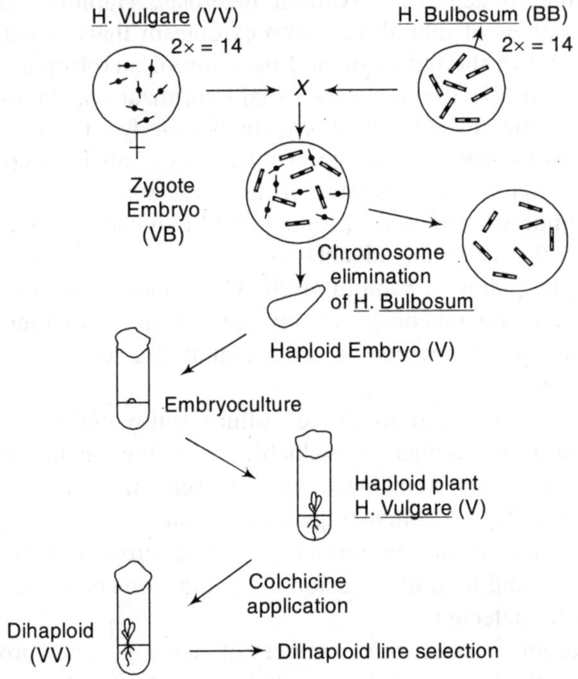

Figure 5.3
Schematic representation of chromosome elimination; principles of Bulbosum method.

There are two routes by which monoploids can be induced artificially (Fig. 5.4). One route is based on the male gamete (microspore) and the other is based on the female gamete (megaspore). Potentially, the first route, via anther or microspore culture, has an advantage because there are far more potential monoploids per spike in the form of male gametophytes than there are female gametophytes. Both methods are based on embryogenesis and the development of plants from monoploid embryos followed by chromosome doubling to obtain homozygous diploids.

The advantages of monoploids as tools in plant breeding or genetics become more apparent when their direct applications are visualized. 1. They provide the quickest possible way towards complete homozygosis. 2. They may serve to recover recessives. 3. Linkage data can be obtained directly by sampling gametes as monoploids. 4. Doubled monoploids give an immediate product of stable recombinants from species crosses. 5. Monoploids can be used up to determine homology within a genome and between genomes. 6. They are ideal for the

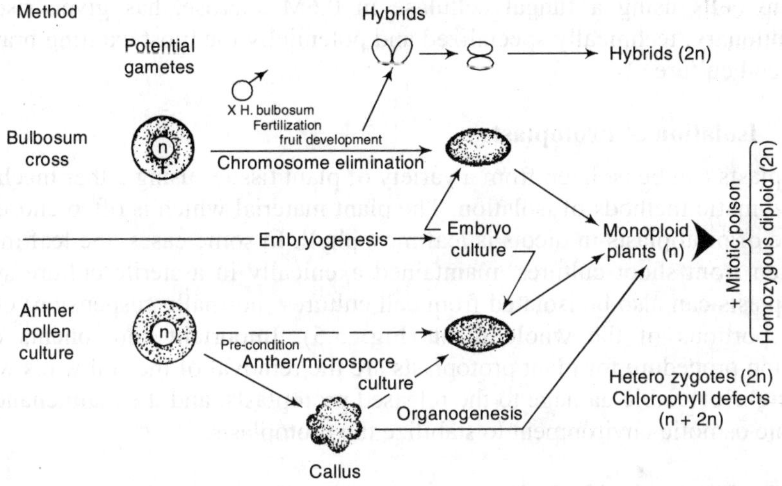

Figure 5.4

Schematic representation showing possible routes of monoploid and doubled monoploid production

study of mutation frequencies and spectra. 7. They provide an ideal system for fundamental cell biological problems (i.e. biosynthesis) in cell and protoplast culture. 8. Monoploid cells as protoplast provide a unique material for gene transfer, host pathogen reactions, and cytoplasmic and/or chromosomal incompatibility. 9. For breeding purposes, one of the main advantages of using monoploids is that completely homozygous lines are produced directly from gametes of F1 hybrids or from later (advanced) selections, This allows for a direct fixation of quantitative characters. 10. For practical plant breeders, these save time and the desired product is recognized easily. 11. Monoploid protoplasts are a powerful tool in plant modification and somatic hybridization.

5.6 Isolation and Transformation of Protoplasts

By definition, plant protoplasts are cells without a cell wall but bound by a plasma membrane. They are naked cells which are potentially capable of cell wall regeneration, growth and division. The absence of a cell wall makes the protoplasts suitable for a variety of experimental manipulations that are not possible with intact cells. Plant protoplasts have a great potential in securing genetic recombinations through somatic hybridization in sexually incompatible crosses and also for plant modification studies. Somatic hybridization involves the fusion of two distantly related or closely related plant protoplasts at intraspecific, interspecific and intergeneric levels with subsequent regeneration of hybrid cells into hybrid plants, while plant modification studies involve the uptake of DNA and organelles and uptake of single cells of bacteria and algae into protoplasts or selective transfer of beneficial gene or genes into protoplasts.

Protoplasts are most useful for plant cell manipulations. The initial observation by Cocking (1960) that plant protoplasts could be released from root-tip cells using a fungal cellulase in 0.6M sucrose, has given rise to a revolutionary, technically specialized and potentially the most exciting branch of plant cell culture.

5.6.1 Isolation of Protoplasts

Protoplasts can be isolated from a variety of plant tissues using either mechanical or enzymatic methods of isolation. The plant material which is often chosen as a source of protoplasts in dicots is leaf mesophyll. In some cases, the leaf material is taken from shoot cultures, maintained axenically in a sterile culture system. Protoplasts can also be isolated from cell cultures (normally suspension) or from other portions of the whole plant (Fig. 5.5). Important components of the isolation procedure for plant protoplasts are the removal of the cell walls without causing irreversible damage to the released protoplasts, and the maintenance of a suitable osmotic environment to stabilize the protoplasts.

5.6.1.1 Mechanical Isolation

All early attempts to isolate plant protoplasts relied entirely on mechanical methods. The mechanical method is dependent on preliminary plasmolysis of cells within tissues and the subsequent dissection of the tissue and deplasmolysis to release the preformed protoplasts. Large vacuolated cells or elongated cells were plasmolysed to cause the plasmalemma to retract away from the cell wall, resulting in the formation of a rounded protoplast in the centre of the cell. Tissues containing such plasmolysed cells were cut into thin strips, and often the end walls were removed without damaging the protoplasts. Protoplasts from such cut cells can be easily released by osmotic swelling when the tissue is placed in solutions causing rapid uptake of water. This method generally produces relatively low yields of viable protoplasts after a tedious procedure. This method is not universally applicable and is restricted to certain tissues.

5.6.1.2 Enzymatic Isolation

The disadvantages of mechanical methods are overcome by enzymatic method which is more gentle and less injurious. After peeling the epidermis the tissue is immersed in a cell wall digesting enzyme mixture in an osmoticum such as mannitol, sorbitol etc. The enzymes used in the preparation of protoplasts are mostly derived from fungi (e.g. crude cellulase from *Myrothecium verrucaria;* a mixture of cellulase and pectinase from *Trichoderma viride;* macerozyme from *Rhizopus* sp.). The preparations are crude and contain a mixture of many enzymes, but some of the commercially available enzymes like "pectolyase Y-

23", "Onozuka R-10", "Meicelase", "Rhozyme" and "Macerozyme R-10", are of sufficiently high quality to give rapid release and high yields of protoplasts. Some other enzymes like Macerase, Pectinase, Cellulase R-10, Cellulysin and Driselase are also used.

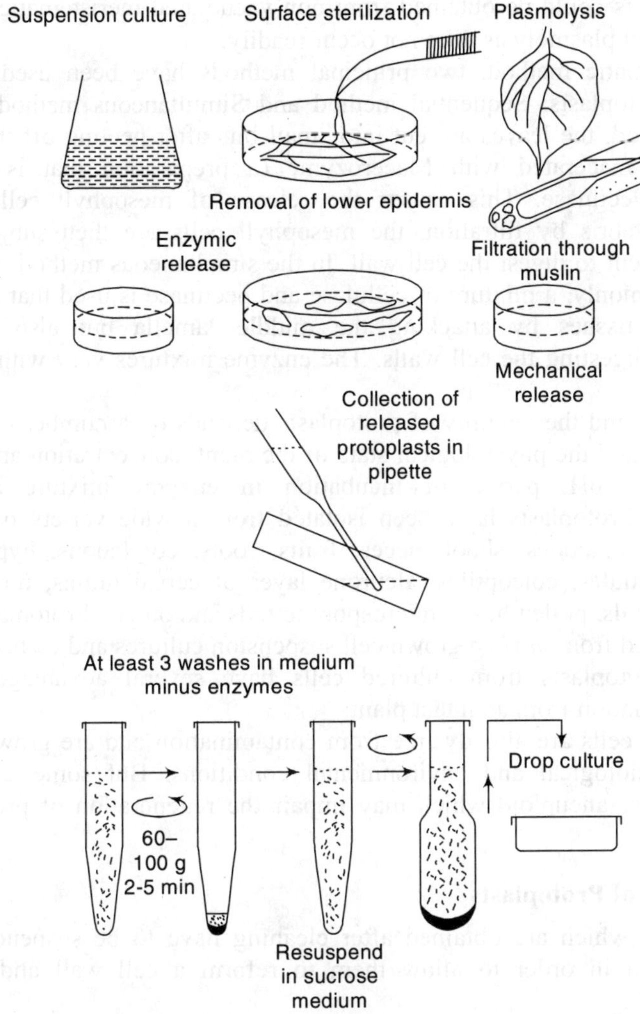

Figure 5.5

Schematic representation of the major methods used to isolate plant protoplasts. (***Source:*** *Mantell, S.H.; Mathews, J.A.; McKee, R.A. Principles of Plant Biotechnology.* © 1987 *Oxford, Blackwell Scientific Publications. Reprinted by permission.*)

The advantages of using enzymatic method of isolation of protoplasts are as follows:

(1) Large scale reproducible isolation of protoplasts from various tissues is possible and the method is more or less universal in application.

(2) Osmotic shrinkage is minimum and the deleterious effects of excessive plasmolysis are minimized.
(3) The cells are intact and are not injured as in the case of mechanical methods of isolation.
(4) Protoplasts could be obtained from non-vacuolated meristematic cells in which cell plasmolysis does not occur readily.

In the enzymatic method, two principal methods have been used for the isolation of protoplasts: Sequential method and Simultaneous method. In the sequential method, the leaves are cut into small bits after peeling off the lower epidermis and macerated with Macerozyme (a preparation that is rich in pectinase) or Pectinase. This causes the release of mesophyll cells. After removing the debris by filtration, the mesophyll cells are then subjected to cellulase treatment to digest the cell wall. In the simultaneous method, which is used more commonly, a mixture of cellulase and pectinase is used that not only macerates the tissues by attacking the middle lamella but also releases protoplasts by digesting the cell walls. The enzyme mixtures vary with species and materials.

The isolation and the viability of protoplasts depends on a number of factors such as the age and the physiological state of the plant, concentration and purity of the enzyme, pH, period of incubation in enzyme mixture and the plasmolyticum. Protoplasts have been isolated from a wide variety of tissues such as leaves, cladodes, shoot pieces, fruits, roots, cotyledons, hypocotyls, legume root nodules, coleoptiles, aleurone layer of cereal grains, microspore mother cells, petals, pollen tubes, microspore tetrads and others. Protoplasts have also been isolated from *in vitro* grown cell suspension cultures and callus tissues. Isolation of protoplasts from cultured cells have several advantages when compared to isolation from an intact plant.

The cultured cells are already free from contamination and are grown under controlled physiological and environmental conditions. But some times the cultured cells are aneuploid which may impair the regeneration of protoplasts into plants.

5.6.2 Culture of Protoplasts

The protoplasts which are obtained after cleaning have to be suspended in a suitable medium in order to allow them to reform a cell wall and initiate divisions

5.6.2.1 Nutrient Media

The nutrient requirements of isolated protoplasts are very similar to those of cultured cells and tissues. Since protoplasts lack the cell wall, they tend to be very efficient in the uptake of nutrients from the medium. Hence, the nutrient media used for the culture of protoplasts are generally modified to contain reduced levels of inorganic substances. Due to the absence of the cell wall, leakage of some metabolites may also take place from protoplasts. This also necessitates modification of the nutrient medium. The Murashige and Skoog's medium is modified by reducing the levels of inorganic substances, especially ammonium which is detrimental to protoplast survival. Calcium concentrations are increased 2-4 times as it is important for protoplast membrane stability. Concentrations of iron and zinc can also be lowered. Similarly, organic growth factors of MS and Gamborg media need to be carefully controlled in the modified media. Compared to these simple media, Kao and Michayluk in 1975 and Kao in 1977 used rather complex media for the culture of a single protoplast or *Vicia bajastana.* Their medium contains, in addition to the normal complement of inorganic substance, 14 vitamins, auxins and cytokinins, various organic acids 10 sugars and sugar alcohols, 21 amino acids, 6 nucleic acid bases, casein hydrolysate and coconut water.

Osmotic stabilizers and plant growth substances are two important ingredients in the protoplast culture medium. Proper osmolarity is achieved through the inclusion of mannitol. glucose, sorbitol, sucrose or xylose either alone or in combination. The most commonly used growth substances are the synthetic auxins such as 2,4-D, NAA, IAA and Cytokinins such as BA and Kinetin.

5.6.2.2 Methods of Culture

The methods employed in protoplast culture are the modifications of the methods used for the culture of plant cells.

(a) *Suspension or Droplet Cultures* Protoplasts are suspended in a liquid medium at a density of about 10^5/ml either in conical flasks or plastic petridishes. The droplet culture technique consists in placing approximately 50 ml of droplets containing protoplasts previously adjusted to 1×10^4 or 1×10^5 /ml in plastic petridishes. The plastic petrtidishes are sealed with parafilm and incubated at 25° C to 30° C at low light intensities or in the dark.

(b) *Plating Method* Protoplasts are suspended in a liquid medium in a petridish at double the concentration that is planned for the experiment and mixed gently but quickly with an equal volume of the medium containing double the agar concentration than is used for culture of cells and tissues. The petridishes are sealed with parafilm and incubated upside down in continuous light (1000–2000 lux) at 23° to 25° C.

(c) *Microculture Chambers* This method requires the eulturing of 30-50 µl of medium containing one or more protoplasts on a microsopic slide, which is enclosed by a cover glass resting on two other cover-glasses placed on either side of the drop. The cultures are sealed with sterile paraffin oil and incubated in light at 23° to 25° C.

(d) *Feeder Layers and Nurse Cultures* Non-dividing but metabolically active, X-irradiated protoplasts embedded in nutrient agar support the growth of protoplasts plated at very low densities (5 to 50 protoplasts per millilitre) above them. Nurse cultures are also used, where the fast growing protoplasts aid the recalcitrant (slow growing) species.

(e) *Micro-drop Array Technique or MPA Screening Technique* This method consists of hanging droplets of 40 *ml* representing one combination of regeneration factors to be tested. The droplets are arranged in a regular array of 7 × 7 drops on the lid of a 9 or 10 cm petridish.

5.6.2.3 Cell Wall Regeneration

Protoplasts which are cultured in an appropriate medium show rapid cytoplasmic streaming, respiration, synthesis of RNA protein and polysaccharides, increase in size, formation of numerous cytoplasmic strands; and most of the cell organelles particularly the chloroplasts aggregate conspicuously around the nucleus. The rate and the regularity of cell wall formation depends on the state of differentiation of the donor tissue/cells, conditions of isolation of protoplasts and the plant species. Usually cell wall formation occurs within 24 to 48 hours of culturing of protoplasts. Exceptions to this are protoplasts of legumes and cereals which may require about four days for cell wall regeneration. The newly synthesized cell wall can be observed under a fluorescence microscope using calcoflour white. Cell wall regeneration takes place by the deposition of cellulose microfibrils on the surface of the plasma membrane. The newly deposited cell wall is composed of loosely organized cellulose microfibrils, which later become more organized to form a typical plant cell wall.

The first cell division after the formation of a new cell wall usually occurs between two to seven days after the culture. However, the protoplasts isolated from actively dividing cell cultures undergo the first division much earlier than the protoplasts isolated from differentiated cells such as mesophyll tissue. Successive sustained cell division of the daughter cells leads to the formation of multicellular colonies after one to three weeks of culture, which can be transferred to an appropriate nutrient media for further growth and multiplication of the protoplast-derived cell colonies. The formation of a protoplast-derived callus depends on the kind, the concentration and the ratio of growth regulators, such as auxins and cytokinins used in the medium and the composition of medium, genotype of the donor tissue and environmental culture conditions.

5.6.2.4 Regeneration of Plants

The regeneration of protoplast-derived calli into whole plants is either through embryogenesis or through organogenesis. Cell colonies formed from protoplasts can be transferred to fresh nutrient media for further growth and multiplication. In many species, shoot and root differentiation and plantlet formation can be induced in protoplast-derived callus tissues with the help of auxins and cytokinins. In some species embryoids are formed from protoplast-derived colonies. Regeneration of whole plants through callus development and organogenesis has been achieved in a wide variety of plants. In general, organogenesis consists of the transfer of protoplast-derived callus to a cytokinin free medium for the induction of shoots and to a medium containing an auxin for root formation. More than 38 species of Solanaceae were regenerated from cultured protoplasts. More recently more than 28 non-Solanaceae members from dicots and monocots (e.g. *Pennisetum sp., Vigna aconitifolia, Trigonella foenumgraecum, Santalum album)* have been regenerated. Plant regeneration from protoplasts is a pre-requisite for the utilization of protoplast technology in somatic hybridization and genetic manipulation.

5.6.2.5 Samaclanal Variation

Somaclonal variation is a term coined by Larkin and Scowcroft to cover all those types of variations which occur in plants regenerated from cultured cells or tissues. Although cell culture techniques are being used to propagate plants clonally and thereby maintain desired characteristics in the progeny, the culture procedures often elicit genetic variability in the plants produced from the cultured cells. This variability may provide a way of producing desirable new characteristics in established varieties of crop species. All the somatic cells of an individual plant should have the same genetic composition, and the plants regenerated from those cells are expected to be identical. Instead they often show a great deal of diversity in their characteristics.

Several mechanisms may be responsible for the induction of somaclonal variation. These include the gross karyotypic changes which accompany *in vitro* culture via calluses, cryptic chromosomal rearrangements, somatic crossingover with sister chromatid exchange, transposable elements, gene amplification or diminution, or perhaps various combinations of these processes. Although the majority of somatic cells in a plant contain a representative somatic chromosome number, one consequence of natural developmental processes is altered ploidy levels induced in certain tissues through endoreduplication and endomitosis or even mutagenesis induced by solar sources of radiation. These processes yield cells with increased ploidy level. If such cells are inadvertently present in high numbers in the original explants, this will lead to culture products which differ from the somatic type. Some of the observed variations in tissue cultures are undoubtedly due to the *in vitro* development of totipotent aneuploid and polyploid cells present in the original explants. These variations are associated with changes in karyotype and chromosome number occurring in the nuclear genomes of dedifferentiated cells and of cells in adventitious meristems derived from dedifferentiated tells with changes in cytoplasmic genomes and alterations in the expression of genomes (so called epigenetic changes).

Observed nuclear changes include polyploidy, aneuploidy Le. the presence of cells containing chromosomal numbers other than those in the polyploid series, structural changes such as the frequency and occurrence of chromosomal bridges at anaphase and mitotic aberrations such as multipolar spindles, lagging chromosomes, fragments and unequal separation of chromatids. Both polyploidy and aneuploidy may also arise as a direct result of the use of synthetic auxins like NAA and 2,4-D in culture media. These compounds are known toinduce spindle failure and other abnormalities of mitosis in intact plants.

Different types of cryptic chromosomal arrangements are reciprocal translocations, deletions, inversions, non-homologous translocations and acentric and centric fragment formations. Such rearrangements probably cause losses of genetic material or at least a realignment and transportation of chromosomal material. This can lead to the expression of previously silent genes, especially where loss or switching off of a dominant allele has occurred.

The tissue culture environment may enhance the frequency of somatic crossing-over, and if a proportion of such an exchange is asymmetric or between non-homologous chromosomes, then genetic variants could be generated as a consequence. It is known that the frequency of sister chromatid exchange in plants is quite high.

Transposable elements may be responsible for certain types of genetic instability in cell cultures and it may well be that such elements contribute significantly to somaclonal variation. The conditions used for plant tissue culture apparently stimulate the movements of transposable elements, thereby leading to the high frequency of somaclonal variation in plants derived from the cultured cells. With increased study of the cytoplasmic genomes of plants, evidence on the variation of these genomes in cultured cells, tissues and in the plants regenerated from tissue cultures is accumulating.

Somaclonal variations encountered in plants regenerated from cultured cells is higher than the frequency of variations enountered in conventional breeding experiments, or by chemical or physical mutagenesis. The regeneration step seems to have a 'cleansing' effect that helps to eliminate deleterious changes because plants do not readily regenerate from cultured cells that have undergone harmful changes.

The plants that display somaclonal variation may have the potential for improving crop species (Table 5.4).

Table 5.4

Examples of somaclonal variation in crop plants

Plants	Somaclonal variant characters
Oats	Plant height, heading date, leaf, striping, twin culms awn morphology, heteromorphic bivalents, ring chromosomes.
Maize	Pollen fertility
Barley	Plant height, tillering, fertility
Sorghum	Fertility, leaf morphology, growth habit.
Onion	Bulb size and shape, clove number, aerial bulbil germination
Rape	Flowering time, glucosinolate content, growth habit.
Lettuce	Leaf weight, length, width, flatness and colour, bud number.
Pelargonium	Leaf shape, size and form, flower morphology, plant height fasciation, pubescence, anthocyanin pigmentation, essential oil composition.

(*Source: Scowcroft, W.R.; Larkin, P J. Plant Improvement and Somatic Cell Genetics*.. © 1982 *New York, Academic Prrlss. Reprinted by permission*.)

For example, strains that have traits such as the increased resistance to downy mildew and mosaic virus and increased yield can be used in conventional breeding programmes that aim to produce better varieties. The early-flowering trait could also prove useful in this regard by shortening generation times. Because somaclonal variation is basically simple and easy to achieve, it is assuming an important role in the biotechnological applications of plant cell and tissue culture.

5.6.3 Somatic Hybridization or Protoplast Fusion and Cybrid

Protoplast fusion facilitates mixing of two whole genomes and may be exploited in crosses which are not possible by conventional technique due to incompatibility. This technique helps in the extension of the range of hybrid plants. Mixing of two genomes opens the door to gene transfer and to study gene expression and stability of several traits. When two protoplast plasma membranes come into intimate contact and if they are given an appropriate stimulus, they will fuse together forming one cell. Protoplast fusion could be spontaneous during isolation of protoplasts or it can be induced by mechanical, chemical and physical means.

By mixing protoplasts of two different origins, fusions may be accomplished between protoplasts of the same plant population—homokaryon (synkaryon), —between protoplasts of the same plant species (different populations), intraspecific heterokaryon,—between protoplasts of the different species or genera—interspecific, intergeneric heterokaryon,—between protplasts of the same or different species, one of which is enucleated by irradiation—cybrid.

5.6.3.1 Spontaneous Fusion

When the callus cultures or cells grown in suspension are subjected to enzymatic degradation of the cell wall, the plasmodesmata of adjoining cells expand instead of breaking down. This facilitates spontaneous fusion of protoplasts. This type of fusion is usually observed when protoplasts are isolated from tissue cultures grown *in vitro* and is rare when protoplasts are isolated from mesophyll tissue. However, spontaneous fusion products do not regenerate into whole plants except undergoing a few divisions. Similar spontaneous fusion is also common during the preparation of protoplasts from meiocytes. In general, spontaneous fusion is non-reproducible and very rare.

5.6.3.2 Induced Fusion

Compared to uncontrolled, random, very rare occurrence of fusion of protoplasts spontaneously, techniques developed for 'induced fusion' of protoplasts are reproducible and efficient. There are three major types namely, (a) Fusion through mechnical means, (b) Fusion through chemical means, and (c) Fusion through an electric charge.

(a) *Fusion through Mechanical Means* In this method, the protoplasts of two different species or of the same species are passed through a micropipette, the tip of which is blocked partially. During this, the protoplasts come into intimate contact and are retained and remain compressed by the flow of the liquid. This method is not used very commonly even though fusion products have been obtained in *Glycine max, Arachis hypogaea and Vinca rosea.*

(b) *Fusion through Chemical Means* Protoplasts with similar osmotic properties can be fused in the presence of salts like sodium nitrate which is the fusogen (Fig. 5.6). This fusogen produces at least 25 per cent fusions. Even though sodium nitrate induced fusion of protoplasts is reproducible, it promotes a very low incidence of fusion. This could be due to the requirements of nearly identical osmotic characteristics of the protoplasts under fusion and the poor effect on the protoplast viability. High alkaline medium containing high Ca++ ions (pH-10.5) at high temperature (37°C) induces more fusion. It is believed that under these conditions the negative charge present on the protoplast membrane is lost facilitating agglutination and subsequent fusion of protoplasts. More than 25 per cent fusion has been reported with this modified method.

Some chemicals like antisera, and lectins, high molecular weight polyvinyl alcohol, dextran sulphate, poly-L-ornithine or polyethylene glycol (PEG), in the presence of high Ca++ and high pH induce a wide range of levels of fusion such as 1 to 100 per cent depending on the operator and the material used. The method most frequently used today is the PEG method as put forward by Kao and Michayluk in 1974. This method envisages the incubation of protoplasts in a high molecular weight PEG and Ca++ ions in lower concentrations. In PEG the protoplasts agglutinate and during elution of the PEG with a medium containing high amounts of Ca++ at pH 10.5, the agglutinated protoplasts fuse. For inducing fusion, high molecular weight PEG 1540 to 6000 is generally used at 25 to 30 per cent concentrations; the PEG induced fusion is non-specific and therefore useful for intra, interspecific, intergeneric or interkingdom fusion involving plant and animal cells. The mechanism of action of PEG is not known clearly. However, it has been suggested that PEG acts as a molecular bridge thereby dissociating the plasmalemma. The other view attributes the PEG function to its high polar nature as well as to its weak ionic charge which facilitates the integration of groupings on the proteins and lipids of opposite membranes.

Some modifications to Kao and Michayluk method, such as addition of concanavalin A to the PEG solution to increase the incidence of fusion and addition of dimethyl sulphoxide ($DMSO_4$) to make protoplasts more susceptible to PEG treatment, have been proposed.

(c) *Fusion through Electric Charge* Surface charges on plasmalemma membranes of protoplasts are altered with short pulses of direct current which, unlike chemical fusogens, have relatively little effect on protoplast viability.

In this method, the protoplasts are brought in close contact by applying a non-uniform AC field of low intensity to the suspension followed by a brief intense DC pulse. The DC pulse induces remarkable breakdown of cell membranes in the contact areas of the adjacent cells resulting in fusion. This technique is also referred to as electrofusion or electrical depolarization. This method was developed by Zimmermann and the electrofusion apparatus is named as "Zimmermann cell fusion TM system".

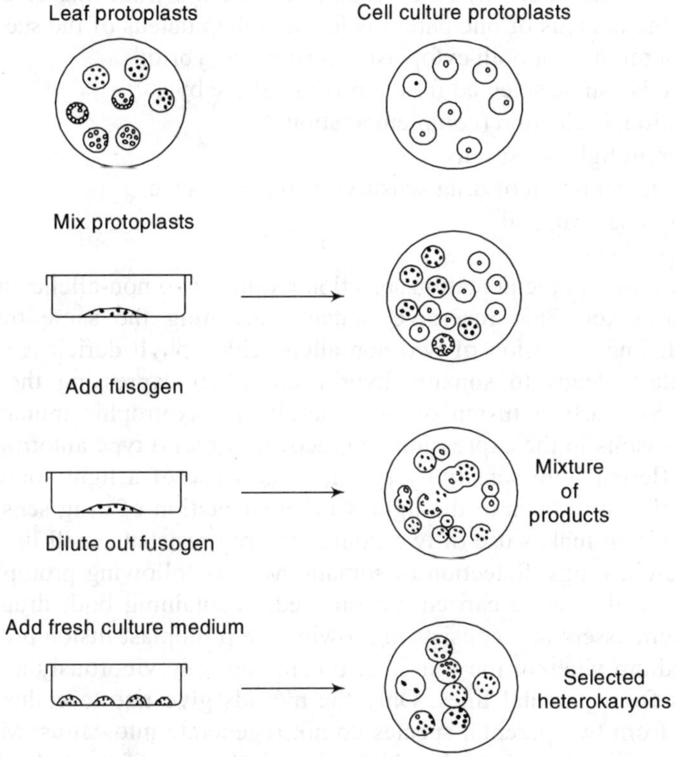

Figure 5.6

The basic protocol for achieving protoplast fusions through the use of chemical fusogens. (***Source:*** *Mantell, SH.; Mathews, J.A.; McKee, R.A. Principles of Plant Biotechnology.* © 1987 *Oxford, Blackwell Scientific Publications. Reprinted by permission.*)

5.6.3.3 Identification and Selection of Hybrid Cells

The fusion of protoplasts results in a coalescence of the cytoplasm. When protoplasts of two different species are induced to fuse, a variety of fusion products may be formed. If A and B are the protoplasts of two different species which are subjected to fusion, fusion products such as AA, AAA, BB, BBB, AAB, ABB, AB and unfused A and B protoplasts are formed. This is because, fusion induced by PEG or by other methods is random and uncontrolled. Even though in most cases the heterokaryotic fusions are in the range of 15 to 50 per cent, the true hybrid cell formation is not too common, as the nuclear fusion of the two parental protoplasts is a rare event. Also, the low number of true hybrid cells formed may get lost in the population of actively dividing homokaryotic fusion products and unfused parental protoplasts.

After protoplast fusion, several genome combinations are possible; (i) nuclei fuse forming a true hybrid, (ii) nuclei survive independently in mixed cytoplasm forming a heterokaryon, (iii) chromosome loss occurs from one or both of the nuclei, (iv) the nucleus of one parent is lost and the nucleus of the second parent survives in a mixture of both cytoplasms forming a cybrid.

Hybrid cells can be selected from a mixed culture by;

(i) nutritional selection (complementation);
(ii) different light sensitivity,
(iii) complementation of drug sensitivity and resistance,
(iv) growth pattern, and
(v) morphology.

Nutritional or complementation selection requires two non-allelic chlorophyll-deficient or auxotrophic recessive mutants, affecting the same trait, in the parental cell line. A fusion of two non-allelic chlorophyll deficient mutant cell line protoplasts leads to somatic hybrid formation expressing the wild-type phenotype. Similarly a fusion of two non-allelic auxotrophic mutant cell line protoplasts results in the expression and recovery of wild type autotroph somatic hybrids. Different light sensitivity system makes use of a light source and the sensitivity of hybrid cells to the light. Complementation of drug sensitivity and resistance system makes use of two dominant drug resistance cell lines resistant to two different drugs. Selection of somatic hybrids following protoplast fusion of such two cell lines is carried out on media containing both drugs. Growth pattern system essentially consists in growing the protoplast fusion products on a defined medium wherein the true hybrid cells multiply vigorously as compared to the cells from parental lines. Only the hybrids give rise to callus while the protoplasts from two parental species do not regenerate into callus. Morphology selection system is based on the abnormal morphology of the hybrid cells, the callus and the regenerated plants.

The selection systems described above have been based on complementation, selection and formation of media which selectively favour the growth of hybrid cells. Under such selection pressures which strongly favour the recovery of amphidiploid somatic hybrids, other potentially valuable cell components with complete genome of one patent and a few genes of the other parent are completely lost. Two selection methods have been developed to overcome this problem, namely

(i) mechanical isolation of fusion products ('fishing') and
(ii) flow sorting of fusion products.

The mechanical method 'fishing' for recovery of somatic fusion products using micro-manipulator and micro pipettes is based on the visual differences between the cell types involved in fusion. This method does not require the presence of mutants for selective recovery of somatic fusion products. Even though the mechanical method of isolation of somatic fusion products is the most tedious, it may be the probable method of recovery of somatic hybrids in a variety of different plants, especially legumes, cereals and tree species, in which mutants for complementation selection are very rare.

Another universally applicable method is to sort out electronically the heterokaryons formed by fusing protoplasts of two parents labelled with different vital fluoresecnt dyes. Vital dyes such as rhodomine isothiocyanate and fluoresceine isothiocyanate have been used for labelling the two parents. The fused and the unfused products can be sorted out in a "cell sorter" machine based on the presence or absence of fluorescence of both the dyes in the fusion products.

The majority of hybrid plants which have been produced through one or the other selection systems described above by somatic hybridization can also be obtained by sexual crossing.

5.6.3.4 Partial Genome Transfer

Production of full hybrids through the fusion of protoplasts of distantly related plants now appear unrealistic because of the widespread instability of the two dissimilar genomes in common cytoplasm (somatic incompatibility). Such hybrids would also be\undesirable as they are likely to exhibit structural and developmental abnormalities and it would require several generations of back-crossing and selection to eliminate undesirable genes from the hybrid. Therefore protoplast fusion is now being tried for partial genome transfer.

One of the ways by which partial genome transfer could be effected in higher plants is through cybridization or fusion of normal protoplasts of the recipient with enucleated (nucleus is removed) protoplasts of the donor. In cybridization, before protoplast fusion, the nuclear genome of one parent, "the donor" is inactivated either chemically or with irradiation. Fusion of untreated "recipient" protoplasts having a different plasmone and culturing under conditions that will prevent division of "recipient" protoplasts should result in cybrid plants having the "recipient" nuclei and "plasmone" traits of the "donor". The net effect is that the cybrids are similar to those obtained by sexual hybridization and subjected to extensive back-crossing. Since some agronomic important characters such as herbicide resistance, disease resistance or cytoplasmic male sterility are controlled by extra-nuclear genes; considerable interest has been shown in cybrids. The controlled and directional transfer of only cytoplasmic traits without interference with the nucleus of one of the parents has been successfully carried out in transferring cytoplasmic male sterility, streptomycin resistance, in correcting deficiencies, nitrate reductase and xanthium dehydrogenase activities.

An alternate method for controlled cybridization is the fusion of normal protoplasts of the recipient with the enucleated protoplasts of the donor. Enucleated protoplasts could be readily produced by centrifuging protoplast suspensions at a high speed. This method of production of cybrids is comparable and parallel to those methods involving ovum-transformation by highly irradiated compatible pollen, where parthenogenetically produced plants contain a few genes of the pollen parent. Cybridization studies have proved convincingly that male sterility is associated with mitochondrial DNA, while antibiotic resistance is encoded in chloroplasts.

5.6.3.5 Uses

Somatic hybridization has an important potential, in the following areas:

(a) Production of fertile amphidiploid somatic hybrids of sexually incompatible species.

(b) Production of heterozygous lines within a single species which normally could only be propagated by vegetative means, ego potato and other tuber and root crops.

(c) Transfer of limited parts of a genome from one species to another by the formation of heterokaryons in which unidirectional sorting of cytoplasmic elements occur. This enables hybrids with a mixed nuclear component to be obtained against a common cytoplasmic background. Conversely, the irradiation of one of the parents enables the selective loss of one nuclear genome and the combination of single nuclear genomes against a segregated cytoplasm,ic background as in cybrid formation (Fig. 5.7).

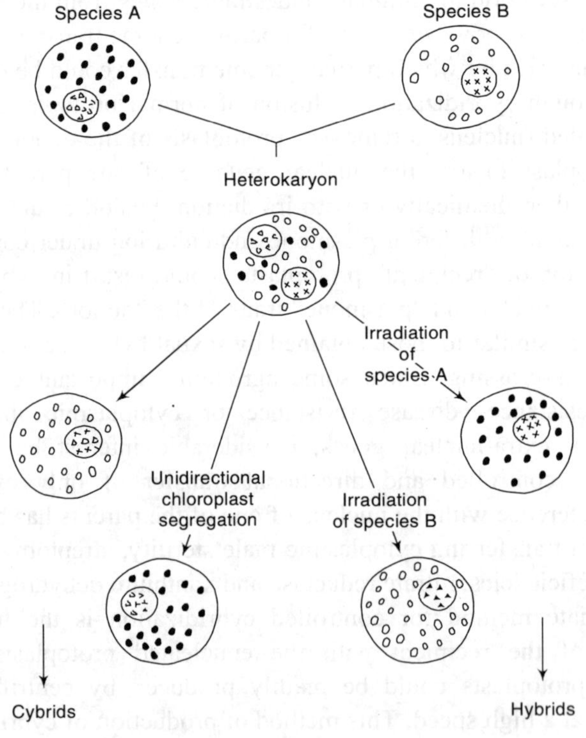

Figure 5.7

The various combinations of cell products which can be obtained through protoplast fusions particularly as far as the segregations of nuclear and chloroplast genomes are concerned. (***Source:*** *Mantell, SH.; Mathews, J.A.;* McKee, *R.A. Principles of Plant Biotechnology.* © 1987 *Oxford, Blackwell Scientific Publications. Reprinted by permission.*)

(d) Production of novel interspecific and intergeneric crosses between plants that are difficult or impossible to hybridize conventionally, e.g. hybrids of wheat and rye (triticale), of turnip and cabbage (raphanobrassica), of potato and tomato (pomato). There are limitations, however, to these types of somatic hybridizations since plants regenerated from some combinations are not always fertile and do not produce viable seeds.

(e) In rice, enhanced disease resistance and salt tolerance might be achieved by fusing the protoplasts of cultivated rice strains with those of wild species of rice.

(f) Direct transfer of cytoplasmic male sterility between strains.

5.7 Uptake of Dna By Plant Cells

Genetic modification of plants by scientists has long been centered around their activities to continually generate efficient agriculture for food and fibre. Boundaries set by natural genetic barriers have placed limits on extending the gene pool and new genetic variability to enhance agricultural efficiency. In recent times, attempts have been made to circumvent classical genetic technologies that are limited by natural genetic barriers. Technologies for efficient insertion of foreign genes into crop plants is one of these endeavours. The new technological advances in the insertion of foreign DNA into plant cells try to avoid the natural genetic barriers in plants. A common feature of all these new methods is that a DNA receptor has to be combined with a DNA donor (not the whole organism carrying the genetic material but the DNA carrier). For reasons of survival the DNA receptor must possess a certain level of organization, while in the case of the DNA donor, one could even use "pure" DNA, (Table 5.5).

The uptake of DNA by plants can be demonstrated in numerous ways. Typically the recipient is exposed to donor DNA that is tagged by some physical marker, such as radioactivity, density or both. After a period of incubation and washing or deoxyribonuclease (DNase) treatment to remove the external DNA, the recipient is ground, the DNA extracted and the presence of the donor DNA demonstrated. In the case of radioactivity this can be accomplished by counting the DNA preparation or by autoradiography of sections of the treated tissues.

In all these uptake experiments, the binding and uptake or exogenous genetic material must be proven. The expression of the introduced foreign genetic material must be demonstrated. Expression would involve transcription and translation. There should be integration of the exogenous genetic material into the genome or plastome of the DNA receptor. There should be replication of the exogenous genetic material-a prerequisite that must be fulfilled if the new genetic information is to be maintained through several generations.

Table 5.5

DNA donor-receptor systems used in genetic manipulations with higher plants

	DNA receptor	DNA donor
(i)	Cell organelles (nuclei)	Bacterial DNA
(ii)	Protoplasts	Plant DNA Bacterial DNA Plasmids Phages Cell organelles Protoplasts
(iii)	Cells and tissues in culture	Plant DNA Bacterial DNA Phages
(iv)	Cells in organisms (embryos, seedlings/plants)	Plant DNA Bacterial DNA Phages
(v)	Egg cell or early embryo (pollen as carrier)	Plant DNA Bacterial DNA Plasmids Phages

5.7.1 Isolated Cell Organelles as Receptors

If we intend to create whole plants with new characteristics by genetic manipulations, then isolated cell organelles are of no value as receptors of exogenous genetic material; but they offer the possibility of testing the utilization of the foreign gene material in an *in vitro* system. Whole organelles are easier to handle and allow more conclusions to be drawn regarding the behaviour of the whole cell and the nucleus. When isolated nuclei of *Petunia* were incubated with *Escherichia coli* DNA, the bacterial DNA was transcribed as revealed by DNA-RNA hybridization. Transcription took place either on the surface of the nuclei or in the surrounding medium. Part of the exogenous DNA may penetrate into the nuclei, but this is not yet conclusively proved. This system is easy to practise and shows that foreign DNA can be used by the plant system.

5.7.2 Protoplasts as Receptors

In most instances studied so far, higher cells, unlike microbial systems, do not seem to require a special state of competence for DNA uptake. Protoplasts of higher plants behave like mammalian cells in their uptake of DNA, presumably by pinocytosis or by cell fusion. Protoplasts apparently engulf what is brought in contact with them like TMV, TMV-RNA, proteins, polystyrene latex particles, plastids, nuclei and even other protoplasts. DNA, plasmids and phages could also be incorporated.

Protoplasts fed with labelled foreign DNA showed the presence of this foreign DNA when subjected to autoradiographic analysis. Some experiments have even shown that a significant portion of the exogenously added DNA was re-utilized. Many workers have confirmed exogenous DNA uptake by various pro top lasts and the association of significant portions of the DNA with protoplast nuclei. Scientists have demonstrated the uptake of plasmids; much of the plasmid was cleared in the protoplast's cytoplasm, but a significant portion did become associated with the nuclei. Protoplasts have been proved to take up phages, organelles, microorganisms. From what we have said so far it is clear that protoplasts can take up foreign DNA. There is substantial evidence that foreign DNA becomes associated with the nuclei of protoplasts. Data on the expression of exogenous genetic material in isolated protoplasts, or in cells derived from these protoplasts, have been rather rare and not always sufficiently substantiated.

5.7.3 Cells and Tissues in Culture as Receptors

Exogenously fed labelled DNA has been recovered from culture cells. In an experiment with *Allomyces* fungus, minor amount of exogenous labelled DNA was found incorporated into the recipient genome. Data on the expression of exogenous DNA in cultured cells are more convincing. For example, in the above mentioned *Allomyces* system the position of the gametangia could be changed. Normally, *Allomyces macrogynus* is epigynous; however following the treatment of its meiospores with DNA of the hypogynous *Allomyces arbusculus,* some hyphae showed the hypogynous character. Similarly in *Neurospora* mutants, which showed defective synthesis of inositol, pyridoxine and so on, revertants could be selected after treating with normal strain's DNA. Reports have shown that gene transfer into cells in culture helped in better growth of cells.

5.7.4 Cells in Plants, Seedlings and Embryos as Receptors

DNA uptake by vegetative parts of adult plants have only remote relation to genetic manipulations. There are several reports which state that exogenous labelled bacterial DNA when applied to the shoot was found inside the cell either in cytoplasm or adsorbed to the nuclei. Exogenous bacterial DNA was extracted from the seeds which were brought into contact with labelled solutions. Even partial breakdown and reutilization of foreign DNA has been reported. Translocation of bacterial DNA stored in the cotyledons to the flowers has been demonstrated. In some cases it has been shown that bacterial DNA covalently linked end to end to the plant DNA. Some reports show a weak phenotypic expression of the transferred gene material. Some data are also available in favour of a replication of the exogenous gene material.

5.7.5 Pollens as Receptors

When the pollen is incubated and germinated in exogenous gene material, this DNA is taken up or at least firmly fixed to the pollen. This pollen is used for pollination of plants of the same species. The exogenous genetic material, taken up or adhered, is transmitted with the growing pollen tubes through the stylar tissue. During fertilization it is brought into the egg cell or it is taken up later on from the surrounding tissues into the young developing embryos and later seeds could be obtained with exogenous DNA. The liquid culture medium offers the best conditions for DNA uptake. Experiments have shown that labelled DNA is found inside the pollen. Proteins and phages also have been taken up. Expression of the exogenous DNA that was taken up has also been established in some cases.

5.7.6 Chloroplast Uptake and Genetic Complementation

The ability of genetically dissimilar chloroplasts to survive in the same cell has been demonstrated in *Spirogyra.* It has been shown that protoplasts from mutant plants were capable of spontaneously pinocytosing normal green chrloroplasts, and under suitable culture would regenerate whole plants, with a normal complement of green functional plastids. Bonnett and Eriksson (1974) have succeeded in transferring chloroplasts of the alga *Vaucheria dichotoma* with a high frequency into the protoplasts of *Daucas carota.* Chloroplasts were seen in the cell cytoplasm after the transfer.

Complementation can occur if one partner lacks the ability to form a particular substrate or product, and the other partner is capable of stimulating the formation of that substrate or product. This is considered as true genetic complementation since the formation of new messenger RNAs and the subsequent synthesis of new proteins are involved.

To date there is no evidence of genetic complementation in the case of chloroplast uptake by plant protoplasts. There seems to be some evidence for the genetic complementation of chloroplasts by protoplast fusion. Giles (1973, 1974) showed that fusion of protoplasts containing green chloroplasts from the striped mutant of *Zea mays* with protoplasts of the white deficient mutant containing only white undeveloped plastids, caused the greening of the white deficient chloroplasts. A lack of genetic information in one nucleus of the heterokaryon is complemented by its presence in the other, allowing at least partial development of chloroplasts. Melchers and Labile (1974) reported complementation between certain chlorophyll deficient and light sensitive mutant varieties of tobacco.

5.8 Recent Advances

Since the dawn of the era of biotechnology, scientists have been trying to develop plants with higher yield, better resistance to pests and diseases, tolerance to various stress conditions and requiring less fertilizers. Plant tissue culture offers ways of circumventing these problems and several others.

5.8.1 Plant Propagation

Interest in plant tissue culture so far has been the greatest in the area of rapid clonal propagation of plants. A number of commercial laboratories now routinely use micropropagation for different foliage and ornamental plants. Three distinct routes to plant production are generally recognised. (a) through enhanced bud proliferation and multiple shoot formation, (b) organogenesis or adventitious bud formation, and (c) somatic embryogenesis.

In enhanced bud proliferation, which is similar to vegetative propagation through rooted cuttings, the normally dormant axillary buds are induced to grow into shoots by a judicious use of-hormones, especially cytokinins. The shoot number increases logarithmically with each subculture to give greatly enhanced multiplication rates. Plants obtained through this method, show minimum variability. The need for a separate rooting stage is, however, a disadvantage of this method. The use of a two stage culture technique, where the initial solid medium is overlaid with a liquid medium to avoid subculture, has been reported to improve multiplication rates and prevent vitrification.

The potential number of plants regenerated through adventitious bud formation either directly from the initial explant or through callus is very high. Sometimes the callus looses its regenerability. Somatic embryogenesis offers greater potential in plant propagation.

5.8.2 Plant Improvement

Several new varieties have been developed through anther culture. These include varieties for high yield, early maturity, low temperature tolerance, disease resistance etc. Anther culture eliminates the many cycles of selection and backcrossing required to produce homozygous plants.

The prospect of somatic hybridization and genetic manipulation has given an impetus to protoplast technology in recent years. The recently introduced electrofusion technique offers a simple and highly synchronous fusion procedure. Fusion products are viable and divide to form new cells. In the selection of protoplast fusion products, flow cytometry is employed. Dyes are also used as markers for cell sorting e.g. 3,4-B-benzpyrene, lucifer yellow etc. One technique of increasing plating efficiency is by the use of feeder cells on a solid medium overlaid by transparent cellophane. The protoplasts or cells plated on this sheet can be easily examined under a microscope or transferred without damage.

Plant genetic engineering is a very useful way of transferring selected genes to desired plants. Successful genetic engineering could mean transfer of useful genes from any plant, animal or microbe or even improved genes into an important crop plant and obtain proper expression. Efficient techniques for regenerating whole plants from single isolated protoplasts are thus a pre-requisite for most genetic engineering programmes. Naked or liposome encapsulated plasmid DNA is taken up by protoplasts in the presence of 15 per cent PEG 6000. Bacterial spheroplasts are attached to a plant protoplast. Co-cultivation of protoplasts with *agrobacterium* is being tried. Microinjection, electroporation, shot gun methods are also used to introduce foreign DNA into cells. In spite of these various techniques to introduce genes, the proper expression of the transferred genetic information remains a problem. There are some cases where introduced genes have expressed; e.g., phaseolin gene from beans and zein gene from maize have been expressed in sunflower.

5.8.3 Secondary Metabolite Production

Plant tissue culture is an important tool in the production of secondary metabolites. In recent years it has been shown that the spectrum of compounds that are produced in culture is even beyond the ability of whole plants, By feeding precursors not normally available to the plant cells, several novel compounds of biomedical importance have been obtained, One compound, a red dye and pharmaceutical shikonin is being produced as a cosmetic product for 4000 US dollars/Kg. High yields of secondary products are obtained with the use of a two-stage bioreactor where rapid cell division is achieved in the first stage and in the second, a late growth phase is stimulated by the reduction of nutrients and hormones. By immobilizing cells, the cell densities are increased and spectacular increases in metabolite production are achieved. Mechanical problems like clogging, flocculation and shear sensitivity of the plant cells are avoided,

5.8.4 Germplasm Conservation

One outcome of the development is the drastic narrowing down of the genetic diversity of our crop species. Our natural forests which house the wild races of most of our crops are being threatened. The result is the erosion of gene pool and germplasm. Maintenance of germplasm is usually in the form of seeds, with or without cold storage. This has its own problems ego loss of viability, space, labour, epidemics etc. *In vitro* techniques appear very promising. More attention is focussed on cryopreservation by which tissues can be preserved indefinitely. Apart from this, the cultures occupy very little space and *in vitro* conditions offer a controlled, sterile and protected environment. There are two methods for *in vitro* germplasm conservation;

(a) cold storage under minimal growth conditions and

(b) cryopreservation. By manipulating the culture conditons, minimum growth is achieved and frequent subcultures are avoided. This is helped by the use of growth retardants, higher osmotic levels, omission or reduction of some growth factors. Cryopreservation is done by storing the tissues at an extremely low temperature of liquid nitrogen at – 190°C. All biological functions cease at this temperature, hence growth and aging are suspended as long as the temperature is maintained. Pre-freezing treatments and cryoprotectants help in preventing the formation of ice crystals,

5.8.5 Trees

Trees have typically long reproductive cycles with a long juvenile phase. Many are cross-breeding. Most of the successful work on trees has been with juvenile explants like seedlings or embryos. Many problems are overcome by tissue culture. The growth conditions and pretreatment of species help to prevent contamination problems. The death of explants due to oxidation of exudates like phenolics is also prevented by the use of antioxidants. With an increase in subculture, increase in percentage of rooting is seen. Artificial seeds will be widely used in the future. Tissue culture is poised to revolutionize forestry by mass production of planting stock from 'elite' trees and also tree improvements by selection at *in vitro* levels.

Study Outline

Historical Events

Haberlandt in 1902, predicted the successful culturing of embryos from vegetative cells in artificial media.

Medium

Plants in nature can synthesize their own food materials but in *in vitro* conditions they are unable to synthesize them. So to culture tissues in an artificial condition, we have to supply the essential minerals, carbohydrates and growth regulators. There are several media prescribed by various tissue culturalists. They are being constantly renewed and updated. Of these MS medium is one of the most widely used.

Culture Techniques

Cleanliness of glassware is a very important factor in culture. Glassware is boiled in 10 per cent sodium carbonate solution for 2 hours followed by rinsing in tap water. The glassware is then soaked in 30 per cent nitric acid and rinsed, dried and sterilized using an autoclave at 16 lb/sq. inch for 1 hour and for the medium the time is reduced to 15 -20 minutes. Glassware can also be sterilized in an oven at 160°C by dry heat sterilization. It is not suitable for medium.

Sterilization of Plant Material

Unlike glassware and media, sterilization of plant material requires greater care since both microbes and the plant tissue are living cells. One has to kill the microbe on the plant material without killing the plant tissue. The method used is surface sterilisation. Plant materials are cleaned with water and detergent. After that the explant is treated with 70 per cent alcohol. Then it is washed with distilled water. The sterilizing agents used are 20% chlorine water, 10 per cent bleaching powder, 0.01 to 0.1 per cent mercuric chloride. Following sterilization the explant is transferred to the medium aseptically in a laminar flow chamber.

Culture

Isolated single cell proliferates to produce calluses. When an appropriate nutrient solution is given, the callus will regenerate to new plants. Meristem culture of shoot or root apex is generally used for herbaceous or woody plants. Embryo culture is done mainly to produce interspecific hybrid embryos. Callus culture was a major break- through in tissue culture.

Organogenesis and Embryogenesis

Organogenesis refers to the induction of morpologically well defined organs like shoot, root etc. from callus. Embryogenesis refers to the development of somatic bipolar adventive embryoids from a callus culture under certain nutritional and hormonal conditions. By changing the CO_2 concentration in culture vessels, a better embryogenesis response could be obtained. Somatic embryogenesis offers many advantages over organogenesis but this is still a rare phenomenon in many important crop plants. Direct regeneration from protoplasts through somatic embryogenesis has also been achieved. It has been reported that polyamine, glycerol and GA_3 stimulate embryogenesis. Somatic embryos are perfectly suited for large scale plant production in since they can be made to stimulate seeds. Artificial seeds are prepared in the laboratory by encapsulating somatic embryos with various polymers such as calcium alginate.

DNA Amplification and Tissue Culture

All those phenomenon that directly suggest the selective replication of specific DNA portions concomitant with specific changes in developmental patterns and limited in time are referred to as transient amplification. The other differentiation patterns e.g. cell elongation, xylem differentiation, cell maturation etc. also help in DNA amplification. There are some cases of extra DNA synthesis in highly specialized cells such as suspensor, gametophytes and cells of quiescent center. DNA amplification has been studied in dedifferentiating cells also. A sharp increase in DNA after wounding has been reported and this DNA played an important role in tumour induction. This amplified DNA is labile in nature.

Androgenic Haploid

Haploid plants are sporophytes possessing gametic chromosome number. Pollen grains in cultivated anthers give rise to androgenic haploids. Four principal sources of haploid formations are: (a) vegetative cell (b) generative cell, (c) generative and vegetative cell, (d) microspore. The uses of androgenic haploids are genetic stabilization, homozygosity, development of pure lines, induction and isolation of auxotrophic mutants.

Monoploid Production by Chromosome Elimination

Monoploids are defined as sporophytes with the basic gametic chromosome number. There are two ways by which monoploids can be induced artificially. One is based on the male gamete and the other is based on the female gamete. Monoploids provide the quickest possible way towards complete homozygosis; they serve to recover recessives; linkage data can be obtained directly; doubled monoploids give an immediate product of stable recombinants; monoploids can be used to determine homology within a genome; they are ideal for the study of mutation frequencies; they provide a unique material for gene transfer; the desired product is recognized easily.

Isolation and Transformation of Protoplasts

Protoplasts are the most useful materials for plant cell manipulations. They can be isolated from a variety of plant tissues using either mechanical or enzymatic isolation. The viability of pro top lasts depend on various factors such as the age and the physiological state of the plant, concentration and purity of the enzyme, pH, period of incubation in enzyme mixture, ete.

Culture of Protoplasts

The medium contains sugars, aminoacids and nucleic acid bases, casein hydrolysate and coconut water in addition to the inorganic acids. Osmotic stabilizers and plant growth substances are the important ingredients in the protoplast culture medium. The methods employed in protoplast cultures are suspension culture, or droplet culture, microculture, plating method, feeder layers, nurse cultures and micro drop array technique.

Somaclonal Variation

It is a term coined by Larkin and Scowcroft to cover all those types of variations which occur in plants regenerated from cultured cells or tissuses. Several mechanisms may be responsible for the induction of somaclonal variations. The important ones are gross karyotype changes, cryptic chromosomal rearrangements, somatic crossing over, gene amplification and transposable elements.

Somatic Hybridization or Protoplast Fusion and Cybrids

Protoplast fusion facilitates mixing of two whole genomes. This technique helps in the extension of the range of haploid plants. Protoplast fusion may be spontaneous or it could be induced by mechanical, chemical and physical means.

Partial Genome Transfer

One of the ways by which partial genome transfer could be effected in higher plants is through cybridization or fusion of normal protoplasts of the recipient with enucleated protoplast of the donor.

Uses

Somatic hybridization has important potentials: (a) production of fertile amphidiploid somatic hybrids of sexually incompatible species, (b) production of heterozygous lines within a single species, (c) transfer of limited parts of genome from one species to another, (d) production of novel interspecific and intergeneric plants, (e) enhanced disease resistance and salt tolerance and (f) direct transfer of cytoplasmic male sterility between strains.

Uptake of DNA by Plant Cells

New technological advances in the insertion of foreign DNA into plant cells try to avoid the natural genetic barriers in plants. A common feature of all these new methods is that a DNA receptor has to be combined with a DNA donor. Such DNA receptors are isolated cell organelles, protoplasts, cells and tissues in culture, cells in plants seedlings and embryos, pollens etc.

Recent Advances

Three distinct routes to plant production are generally recognized:

(a) through enhanced bud proliferation and multiple shoot formation;

(b) organogenesis or adventitious bud formation and

(c) somatic embryogenesis. Several new varieties have been developed through anther culture. These include varieties for high yield, early maturity, low temperature tolerance, disease resistance etc. Plant genetic engineering is another very useful way of transferring selected genes to desired plants. Plant tissue culture is an important tool in the production of secondary metabolites. Germplasm conservation and cryopreservation also help in preserving genetic diversity. Tissue culture is poised to revolutionize forestry by mass production of trees and also tree improvements by selection at *in vitro* level.

Questions

(1) What are the common media used for various cultures?
(2) What is the importance of sterilization?
(3) How are plant materials sterilized?
(4) What is callus induction?
(5) Define organogenesis and embryogenesis.
(6) What is DNA amplification?
(7) How are androgenic haploids produced? Enumerate their uses.
(8) What is a monoploid culture? Explain their uses.
(9) Describe the isolation and fusion of protoplasts.
(10) What are the advantages of protoplast culture?
(11) Explain callus induction and organ regeneration from protoplast culture.
(12) What do you mean by somaclonal variation?
(13) Explain in detail the prospects of somatic hybridization.
(14) What is a cybrid?
(15) Explain the various techniques by which DNA uptake of a plant cell is achieved.
(16) What is pollen dimorphism?
(17) Explain the technique of electroporation.
(18) What is microinjection?
(19) Enumerate the recent advances in plant tissue culture techniques.

6
Animal Cell and Tissue Culture

Introduction

A Cell is a biological unit, delimited by a semipermeable membrane which is capable of self-reproduction in a suitable medium. The organisms made up of only one cell are called unicellular organisms while those having many cells in their body are called multicellular organisms. The culturing of animal cells *in vitro* was first shown in 1907 but reproducible and reliable large-scale culture of mammalian cells has been achieved only from 1988 onwards. Originally large-scale culture was developed for the production of animal viruses to be used as vaccines. Recently the goal has been the production of human proteins of potential therapeutic value and monoclonal antibodies. Most animal cells can be grown *in vitro* using synthetic medium supplemented with serum or some other complex nutrient source. From the early 1950s, *Poliomyelitis* virus has been grown in cultures of mammalian tissues with a view to manufacture vaccines. Since then, human cell line cultures have become indispensable in the isolation and the growth of other viruses, in the production of highly specific proteins (such as antibodies and interferons), in cancer research and in antiviral chemotherapy.

History of animal biotechnology

1891 – First successful embryo transfer.
1900 – In vitro embryo culture development.
1951 – FDA approved antibiotics as feed additives for farm animals.
1961 – Mouse embryo aggregation to produce chimeras.
1966 – First report of microinjection of mouse embryos.
1970 – First chimeric mice were produced.
– Cytogenetic analysis using chromosome banding.
1973 – Foreign gene funcitn after cell transfection.
1974 – Development of teratocarcinoma cell transfer.
1977 – mRNA and DNA transferred to *Xenopus* eggs.
1980 – MRNA transferred into mammalian ova.
– The cloning technologies of embryo splitting (EMS) and embryonic nuclear transfer (NT) were introduced into dairy cattle breeding.
1980-81 – Transgenic mice first documented.
1981 – The term 'transgnic' was first used by J.W. Gordon and F.H. Ruddle.
– Transfer of ES cells derived from mouse embryos.

1982	– Transgenic mice and a growth hormone phenotype were produced.
1983	– Tissue-specific gene expression in transgenic mice.
1985	– Transgenic pig, sheep, rabbit, fish produced by microinjection.
1987	– Chimeric 'knowck-out' mice described.
	– Retrovirus – mediated transgenic chicken produced.
1989	– Targeted DNA integration and germ-line transgenic mice.
	– Microinjection for transgenic cattle.
	– First sperm-mediated reports in animals.
1990	– First clinical trial of gene therapy began.
1991	– Microinjection for transgenic goats.
1993	– Germ-line chimeric mice produced using co-culture.
	– FDA approved the use of bovine somatotropin (BST) to increase milk yield from dairy cows.
1996	– Embryonic Stem (ES) cells used for nuclear transfer.
1997	– The first cloned sheep 'Dolly' and the transgenic sheep 'Polly' were revealed.
2000	– Transgenic sheep carrying human gene for α, 1-antitrypsin was successfully produced.
2003	– A horse gave birth to Idaho Gem, a healthy mule.

6.1 Culture

Culture refers to growing of whole organism, organ, tissue, fragment or dispersed cells on a suitable nutrient medium. Freshly isolated cell cultures are called primary cultures. When this is subcultured, it gives rise to cell lines. Tissue culture strictly refers to tissues grown *in vitro* but is generally used to include the culture of dissociated cells. It is an art and an indispensable tool.

6.1.1 Isolation of Cells

The major problem associated with the isolation of free cells and cell aggregates from organs is that of releasing the cells from their supporting matrices without affecting the integrity of the cell membrane. Various methods have been employed to achieve this goal.

(1) *Mechanical technique* This includes forcing the tissue through cheese or silk cloth or shaking the tissue with glass beads in an appropriate buffer. There is considerable damage to the cell due to this technique. It also results in low cell yield.

(2) *Biochemical technique* This technique largely overcomes the problems caused by mechanical dissociation. Collagenase and hyaluronidase in a calcium free medium have been used for hepatocyte isolation. The liver is thinly sliced and then incubated with the enzymes.

Animal cells may be broadly subdivided into: (i) those which remain viable only when attached to a solid substrate (e.g. cells in primary cultures, normal diploid fibroblast cell strains), and (ii) those that will proliferate in a fine suspension (e.g. human tumour cells, HeLa cell lines and hybridomas). The material to which cells stick must be non-toxic, sterilizable and preferably transparent so that the cells may be observed microscopically. The surfaces which have been used successfully include plastic, glass, teflon tubing, DEAE-sephadex; cells may be detached from such surfaces by mild trypsin digestion.

6.1.2 Preparing Cells in Culture

A piece of tissue from the organism is usually quite complex and contains many types of cells. The cultivation of animal cells from a particular tissue begins with the dissociation of the tissue fragment into its component cells by treatment with a proteolytic enzyme, usually trypsin. After removal of trypsin, the cell suspension is placed in a flat-bottomed glass or plastic container together with a suitable liquid medium. After a lag period the cells attach themselves to the bottom' of the container and start dividing mitotically. A culture of this type, arising directly from differentiated tissue is referred to as a primary culture or primary cell line. Eventually the bottom of the culture vessel is covered with a continuous layer of cells, often one cell thick and hence referred to as a monolayer.

In clonal cultures a relatively small number of cells are added to the dish, each of which after settling and attaching to the surface, is at some distance from its neighbour. The proliferation of the cells generates individual colonies or clones of cell whose members are all derived from the same original cell. Thus cells derived from a single cell through mitosis constitute a clone.

Even though a variety of cells present in the tissue mass are taken for the preparation of primary culture, the cells that multiply best in culture are the fibroblasts. They migrate in a radial manner from the explant. The fates of various types of cells multiplying in a culture vary enormously. Many of them are quite short-lived, e.g. most of the blood cells die and disappear from the culture within two or three days. Other cells, such as neurons and muscle cells, frequently persist in culture, sometimes for months without dividing at all and then eventually die. Still other cells begin to divide rapidly and continue to do so for sometime. However, many of these also die after a period which varies from weeks to months. The shape of cells in culture is not invariable and can be affected by the composition of the medium and the presence of infectious agents.

Primary cultures can be used advantageously because:

(1) The expense and inconvenience of maintaining established cell stocks are avoided.

(2) They are particularly suitable for vaccine production since the probability of *in vitro* transformation of cells to malignancy is minimized.

(3) Massive quantities of tissue can be obtained conveniently for short term studies.

(4) They are hardy and can be well sustained in media of relatively simple composition.
(5) Their degree and range of sensitivity to viral infection may exceed that of the common established cell lines.

The use of primary cell cultures has its own Inherent disadvantages such as (i) they may get contaminated with latent viruses (e.g. foamy virus in monkey kidney tissues), (ii) long term experiments concerning the biological properties of cells cannot be carried out, and (iii) mixed populations of cells may confuse the interpretation of experimental findings.

The cells of primary cultures can be detached from the culture vessel by trypsin treatment or the addition of the chelating agent EDTA. These cells can be used to initiate secondary cultures by reseeding them in fresh media at high density. Cells from primary cultures can often be transferred serially a number of times. The cells multiply at a constant rate over successive transfers and such cells comprise a cell strain. Cell strains do not have infinite life and divide only a few times before their growth rate declines and they die; for example, human cells generally divide only 50-100 times before dying.

6.1.3 Established (Continuous) Cell Lines

Frequently, primary cell lines go on dividing at quite a high rate for a long time and can be passaged repeatedly. Sometimes, a few cells become altered in such a way that they acquire a different morphology, grow faster and multiply. They can be cultured for a long time and they seem to have developed the potential to be subcultured indefinitely *in vitro.* Such cell lines are called established cell lines. As a general rule, a line is not designated as established unless it has been subcultured at least 70 times at intervals of 3 days between subcultures. The transition from a primary cell line to an established cell line is smooth and gradual in some cases.

During repeated subculturing, cell lines can undergo extensive changes in their cultural properties; e.g., the density of division may' increase in such a way that the cells grow in clumps rather than in monolayers and the cells may be irregularly oriented with respect to each other. Such cell lines are said to be transformed; these type of cells are generally neoplastic, i.e. they produce cancer if transplanted into related animals. Lines of transformed cells can also be obtained by infecting them with oncogenic viruses or by treating them with carcinogenic chemicals. All primary cell lines at first have the normal number of chromosomes whereas established cell lines almost invariably have an unusual number.

Cancer cells, unlike those cells of cell lines derived from primary cultures, generally possess extra chromosomes, that is, they are aneuploid. The properties of a number of common cell lines are shown, in Table 6.1.

Table 6.1

Properties of some commonly used mammalian cell lines

Cell line	Species of origin	Tissue of origin	Morphology	Ploidy	Growth in suspension
3T3	Mouse	Connective tissue	Fibroblast	Aneuploid	No
L	Mouse	Connective tissue	Fibroblast	Aneuploid	Yes
CHO	Chinese hamster	Ovary	Epithelial	Quasidiploi d	Yes
BHK 21	Syrian hamster	Kidney	Fibroblast	Diploid	Yes
HeLa	Human	Cervical carcinoma	Epithelial	Aneuploid	Yes
WISH	Human	Amnion	Epithelial	Aneuploid	?
Hep-2	Human	Carcinoma of larynx	Epithelial	Aneuploid	?
KB	Human	Nasophary ngeal	Epithelial	Aneuploid	Yes

*(**Source:** Primrose, S.B. Modern Biotechnology. © 1987 Oxford, Blackwell Scientific Publications. Reprinted by permission.)*

Established cell lines behave in a remarkably similar manner irrespective of their origin.

1. They have short doubling timings, of the order of 12 to 20 hours.
2. They are invariably aneuploid.
3. They have similar nutritional requirements, whatever their origin.
4. They grow to much higher densities than primary cell lines.
5. They do not usually show much evidence of spatial orientation.
6. It is rare for them to show obvious specialized functions.
7. They will often grow from dilute inocula
8. Most of them can be established in suspension cultures, whereas it is exceptional for primary cell lines to grow in suspension.

The tendency of cell lines to change continuously on repeated cultivation necessitates that stocks of cells generally be maintained in the frozen state. Usually the cells are mixed with additives such as glycerol or dimethyl sulphoxide to minimise cellular damage by ice crystals. They are distributed in ampoules and stored in liquid nitrogen. Cells maintained in this way remain viable for years. New cultures can be initiated readily on thawing them.

6.1.4. Organ culture

Maintaining and growing small parts or pieces or organs *in vitro* is called organ culture. The aim of organ culture is to maintain the architecture of tissue and to direct it towards normal development. Different techniques are used which employ solid medium and fluid medium. In **plasma clot**, the explant is cultured on the surface of a clot consisting of chick plasma and chick embryo extract contained in a watch glass. In **Raft method**, the explant is placed onto a raft of lens paper or rayon acetate that is floated on serum in a watch glass. In **agar gel method**, the medium is gelled with 1% agar and the explant is placed on it. The agar gels are usually kept in embryological watch glasses and sealed with paraffin wax. In **grid method**, the tissues are placed on the grid made of suitable wire mesh or perforated stainless steel sheet whose edges are bent to form four legs of about 4 mm height. In **cyclic exposure**, the explants are rhythmically exposed to the fluid medium and gas phase. The explants are attached to the bottom of a plastic culture dish and are covered with fluid medium. The dishes are enclosed in a chamber containing a suitable gas mixture. The chamber is mounted on a rocker platform. The chamber is rocked at several cycles per minute to ensure intermittent exposure of the explants to medium and gas.

One of the important applications of organ culture has been the production of tissues for implantation in patients (tissue engineering). Human skin and cartilage have been successfully produced *in vitro* and used for transplantation.

It is now possible to grow skin by *in vitro* technique using the epidermis portion of skin. Keratinocytes derived from any type of stratified squamous epithelium (from epidermis, cornea, mouth, tongue etc.) will divide *in vitro* to form colonies and eventually a continuous epithelium. It involves addition of collagen matrix in a medium for the growth of the tissue. Regenerated skin is not completely normal since it lacks hair follicles and sweat glands.

Artificial cartilage developed in vitro by culturing the human chondrocytes has promising role in human implantation particularly in cases of injuries, arthritis, etc.

6.1.5 Animal Cell Fusion

Hybrid cells can be formed by the fusion of two different types of somatic cells. Cells can be fused with the help of inactivated Sendai virus and other agents that affect membrane structure, such as polyethylene glycol (PEG) and lysolecithin. By adhering to plasma membrane of cells, they help in fusion. Fusion of two cells produces a single hybrid cell with two nuclei (heterokaryon). Then both nuclei undergo mitosis synchronously, form a single metaphase plate, divide and produce a hybrid cell line. The cells of a hybrid cell line have single nucleus containing chromosomes from both parental nuclei.

Hybrid cells are useful in gene or chromosome mapping, to study the control of cell division and pattern of expression of gene, in hybridoma production etc.

6.2 Kinetics Of Cell Growth

The primary cell lines and the established cell lines have their own specific growth kinetics.

6.2.1 Primary Cell Lines

Primary cell lines do not behave in quite the same way as established cell lines. When established cell lines have become stationary, the medium in which they have been grown is usually inadequate for the maintenance of a fresh inoculum of cells. However, it can often be observed that cultures of primary cell lines stop growing before the medium is exhausted. This is due to a phenomenon called contact inhibition. This was first described by Abercrombie and Heaysman. They observed that when certain kinds of normal cells, mainly fibroblasts, come into contact with each other, they were immediately immobilized.

Along with cell movement, cell division, DNA synthesis, RNA and protein synthesis are much reduced or eliminated when a cell sheet becomes confluent. When primary cell lines become transformed, there is a great diminution of contact inhibition. This is why transformed cells grow to higher densities and pile upon each other. The primary cell lines exhibit ideal growth kinetics when there is no contact inhibition.

6.2.2 Established Cell Lines

Cells in culture display the same type of growth pattern as microorganisms. In particular, they show the classical growth kinetics as demonstrated by cultures of bacteria, yeast and protozoa. The culture exhibits the following phases:

(1) *Lag phase* During this period, practically no growth occurs and may last for some hours to a few days before growth begins.

(2) *Logarithmic (log) phase* During this phase, growth proceeds steadily with the population, doubling every 15 to 20 hours in the case of fast growing cells.

(3) *Stationary phase* At the end of the log phase, maximum population density is reached and the growth becomes stationary.

The growth rate of cultured cells is not necessarily always the same. It may vary to some extent from one cell strain to another, but in particular it varies considerably with environmental conditions such as pH, temperature and osmotic pressure.

6.2.3 Interaction Among Cells

Besides contact inhibition, the most interesting interaction is the ability of like-cells to recognize and adhere to each other. Holtfreter showed that when amphibian embryonic cells were disaggregated in calcium and magnesium free salt solution and the separated cells were then allowed to mix together, they first adhered in a random manner and then sorted themselves into groups of like-cells. Eventually the entire embryo was reconstructed. Moscona demonstrated the same phenomenon with mammalian and arian cells. One school of thought postulates that there is a kind of intercellular cement which sticks like-cells to each other; the other school of thought suggests that the adhesion phenomenon is an intrinsic property of the cell membranes themselves.

6.2.4 Genetics of Culture Cells

Primary cell lines usually retain their diploid karyotype. Transformed cell lines show a great variation in karyotype. Shortly after transformation, the incidence of tetraploid cells increases. Then the aneuploid cells make their appearance and stable established cell lines commonly have an aneuploid karyotype with a wide spread of chromosome numbers. The emergence of aneuploidy is due to non-disjunctive cell division. Later on, in the established cell lines the morphology of the individual chromosome also changes; it is because of chromosome breaks, fusion and translocations that mutant cells also arise in tissue culture.

6.2.5 Metabolism

Just as the cultural properties of cell lines may be different from those of normal cells, so is their metabolism; e.g., cells from liver-derived hepatomas fail to synthesize most of the normal liver enzymes but may continue to secrete the major liver product albumin. Similarly, cell lines from some tumours secrete hormones in an uncontrolled fashion, e.g. cells from tumours of the testes secrete androgen while pituitary tumour cell lines secrete adrenocorticotrophic hormone and growth hormones.

In cultured cells, the metabolism of glucose proceeds by way of glycolytic and Krebs pathways as in the tissues of the intact organism. However, many cells show a marked tendency to accumulate lactic acid and keto-acids in the medium.

Cultured cells have highly variable needs for oxygen and a considerable part of the energy requirements can be met by the breakdown of 6-carbon compounds such as glucose to 3-carbon compounds such as lactic acid and pyruvic acid, a process which requires no oxygen. Cells can be grown in the complete absence of oxygen for rather short periods of time.

Tissue culture cells can synthesize lipids from simple chemical substances such as acetate. It is not known whether fat can be taken up as such from the medium and stored. Some cells are capable of synthesizing cholestrol. Cultured cells can build nucleic acids readily from simple compounds in a medium (such as formate, glycine and bicarbonate).

6.2.6 Modes of Cell Growth

Under optimal conditions primary epithelial cells form layers one cell thick, while the layers formed by fibroblasts are usually two or three cells thick. Such cells generally grow only when attached to surfaces. The same principles apply for cell strains and cell lines derived from normal cells. Only rarely can cell lines be derived that multiply well in suspension and these usually arise from transformed cell lines. Cultures of cells which grow well in suspension produce many more cells than those whose growth is restricted to surfaces. Transformed cells and cells of some lines can grow and form colonies on semi-solid media, e.g. agarose, and this is particularly useful when cloning cells, as in hybridoma selection.

6.3 Culture Media For Animals

One of the most crucial factors in achieving the successful cultivation of animal cells *in vitro* is' the composition of the growth medium. To be a satisfactory medium, it must fulfil the following criteria.

(i) The medium must provide all requirements of the cell.
(ii) The medium must maintain a pH value of 7.0-7.3 despite the production of acid, i.e. it must be adequately buffered.
(iii) The medium must be isotonic with the cell cytoplasm.
(iv) The medium must be sterile.

The growth media in common use are complex and generally not completely defined because of the presence of serum, although this can sometimes be replaced simply with albumin. The base component of these media is a balanced salt solution whose functions are mainly to provide: (a) essential inorganic ions, (b) the correct osmolality, (c) the correct pH, (d) a source of energy in the form of glucose, and (e) phenol red as pH indicator. The compositions of two widely used balanced salt solutions are given in Table 6.2.

Table 6.2

Comparison of two balanced salt solutions

Ingredients	Amount (mg/l) in balanced salt solution of: Earle	Hanks
NaCl	6800	8000
KCl	400	400
$CaCl_2\ 2H_2O$	264	185
$MgSO_4\ 7H_2O$	200	200
$Na_2HPO_4H_2O$	140	—
Na_2HPO_4	—	47.5
KH_2PO_4	—	60
$NaHCO_3$	1680	350
Glucose	1000	1000
Phenol red	17	17

(***Source:*** *Primrose, S.B. Modern Biotechnology. © 1987 Oxford, Blackwell Scientific Publications. Reprinted by permission.*)

Although cells will remain alive for several hours in a balanced salt solution, many more ingredients must be included if proliferation of cells is to occur. These ingredients include most of the common amino acids, eight vitamins and 5-10 per cent of serum. The precise contribution made by the serum is not fully understood. Some components of serum like a-globulins and hormones, may exert a beneficial effect by promoting the attachment and spreading of the cells and by stimulating cell division. The most popular source of serum is from fetal calves since this maintains better growth of cultured cells than serum from adult animals.

6.3.1 Culture Media Containing Naturally Occurring Ingredients

In spite of the vast use of chemically defined media in tissue culture, it is still necessary to depend on naturally occurring substances derived from the organism. The various kinds of such media which are in use may be, (i) blood plasma, (ii) blood serum, (iii) tissue extract and (iv) complex natural media.

6.3.1.1 Blood Plasma

The first tissue cultures were made by Harrison (1907) in clotted frog lymph. Burrows (1910) substituted a coagulum prepared from chicken plasma. After many years, it was found that plasma provided a complete nutrient in which cells could survive and multiply slowly for extended periods under conditions that resembled those found in the body in many respects. Plasma is still being used to advantageously for the following purposes:

(1) To provide a nutritive substrate and a supporting structure for many types of cultures, just as it also provides a matrix for new cells during the repair of injury in the body.
(2) To provide a means of conditioning the surface of glass for better attachment of cells.
(3) To provide a means of protecting cells and tissues from excessive traumatic damage during subculture.
(4) To provide some degree of protection from sudden changes in the environment at times of fluid change.
(5) To provide localized pockets of conditioned medium around cells.

For culture work, plasma from the adult chicken is preferred to mammalian plasma because it forms a clear, solid coagulum even when diluted several times. Mammalian plasma is either too opaque for good optical work or else it fails to produce solid clots.

The plasma is obtained by centrifugation of whole blood before coagulation takes place. The tissue is then placed in a small quantity of the plasma and coagulation encouraged by the addition of a small amount of tissue extract or thrombin. This is done because the cells in culture require a solid support for continued growth and activity. In case of fowl, the blood is obtained from the wing, heart and carotid artery. In case of mammals it is obtained from the carotid artery and heart.

6.3.1.2 Blood Serum

Blood serum (plasma minus fibrinogen) with or without other nutritive substances may be used either as the entire culture medium or as the fluid phase of a medium consisting partly of a plasma coagulum. For many years it was assumed that whole serum was toxic, that plasma was useful only as a supportive structure and that the nutritive requirements of the cells were supplied by the embryo extract that was usually added to the medium. Eventually, however, it was found possible to cultivate tissues in serum alone without plasma or tissue extract.

The following Table 6.3 summarizes the advances in serum development.

As some of the more elaborate chemically defined solutions were developed, it was found that they had to be supplemented with 10 to 20 percent serum to provide a completely adequate medium for the continuous propagation of established cell lines and freshly explanted tissues for extended periods. Harris (1959) concluded that medium 199 and NCTC 109, as well as the simpler basal medium of Eagle (1955) are all deficient in one or more factors that occur in serum dialysate and are essential for the growth and maintenance of chick skeletal muscle fibroblasts. Thus serum does provide some of the growth factors or some of the physical conditions, or both, that are presently lacking in synthetic media.

Table 6.3

Advances in serum development

Year	Advances
1928	Successful cultivation of many mamalian tissues in diluted serum (*des* Ligneris).
1933-1936	Cultivation of chick tissues in serum (Parker).
1936-1942	Introduction of an ultra filtrate of serum that was used as basal medium for many purposes including the propagation of viruses (Simms; Simms and Sanders).
1946	Biotest-Serum-Institut GmbH was founded by Carl-Adolf Schleussner and Hans Schleussner. The family fim concentrated initially on research in the field of blood group serology.
1948	The anti-D test serum for the determination of the Rhesus factor was introduced as the only product of this type in the world
1949	Production of the first non group-specific conserved blood, 'Biseko'
1971	Production of the first immunoglobulins
1986	Biotest-Serum-Institut GmbH changed to Biotest AG, pursuing the further expansion of the pharmaceutical and diagnostics divisions
1987	Biotest was listed on the Frankfurt Stock Exchange as a global concern
1993	Production of the first doubly virus-inactivated Factor VIII preparation for haemophilia patients
2004	The comprehensively modernised pharmaceutical production facility was taken into service
2005	The TANGO fully automated blood group typing system and associated reagents were licensed on the US American market

6.3.1.3 Preparation of Chicken Serum

The fluid plasma from which the serum is prepared should be completely coagulated. The plasma is coagulated deliberately by adding a drop or two of embryo tissue extract to each tube or an equivalent amount of thrombin, and leaving the tubes to incubate for several hours at 37°C. The coagulated plasma is broken up into fragments and it is ground in a mortor with sterile quartz sand. After grinding, the serum is separated by centrifugation.

6.3.1.4 Preparation of Mammalian Serum

The mammalian blood is left at room temperature for an hour. The clot is removed by a glass rod and then centrifuged for 30 minutes at 3000 rpm and the serum is separated. Carrel (1912) discovered that the embryo tissue extract had remarkable powers of promoting cell growth and multiplication in cultures of connective tissue cells from chick embryo heart. Since Carrel's experiments, there have been many attempts to determine the chemical nature of the substances responsible for the stimulating effect of embryo extract. Bakar and Carrel (1926) obtained active fractions of the extract by precipitation with carbon dioxide and found that the activity was concentrated largely in the protein portion containing nucleoproteins and glycoproteins. It was further observed (Carrel and Bakar, 1926) that proteases and higher molecular weight protein degradation products also had very potent growth promoting properties. Growth promoting activity appeared to be associated particularly with fractions containing predominantly nucleoproteins of the ribonucleic acid type. Fractions relatively high in deoxyribonucleic acid appeared much less active. Active nucleoprotein fractions from adult chicken heart, brain, liver and spleen have been used but no indications of organ specificity were observed. The activity of the fraction also did not depend on their total nucleic acid content or on the age of the individuals from which they were prepared.

6.3.1.5 Preparation of Embryo Extract

Embryo extract is made from 10 to 11 day old embryos (before the calcifying mechanisms have become too active). The embryos are removed from the egg, then homogenized in a motor driven homogenizer. Six to eight embryos and a measured quantity of balanced salt solution (e.g. 2.0 ml per embryo) may be processed at one time. After homogenization, it is centrifuged and further diluted 10 to 20 times. Embryo extract may be stored indefinitely after it has been dried from the frozen state.

6.3.2 Complex Natural Media

Some of the complex natural media are as follows:

6.3.2.1 Supplemented Hanks-Simms Medium

Weller and co-workers (1952) in their earlier work with polioviruses made excellent use of a combination of three parts Hank's balanced salt and one part Simm's ox serum ultrafiltrate. For roller tube cultures of various human and animal tissues (embryonic, infant and adult), the complete medium consisted of Hanks-Simms solution (85%), beef embryo extract (10%), horse serum inactivated at 56 C for 30 minutes (5 to 20%), penicillin (50 mg/ml) and streptomycin (50 μg/ml).

6.3.2.2 Supplemented Bovine Amniotic Fluid Medium

Milovanic and co-workers (1957, 1958) used the following medium: Bovine amniotic fluid (37.5%), horse serum inactivated at 56°C for 30 minutes (20%), bovine embryo extract (5%), Hanks balanced salt solution (37.5%), streptomycin (100 μg/ml) , penicillin (100 μg/ml) and mycostatin (100 μg/ml).

6.3.2.3 Serum-supplemented Yeast Extract Medium

Various human cell lines and strains from other species have been successfully grown in this medium. The medium consists of: Yeast extract medium (76 parts) (composition: 10 parts of 1 per cent solution of Difco's yeastolate, 2.5 parts of 10 per cent glucose solution and 87.5 parts of Hanks balanced salt solution), human serum (20 parts) and 1.4 per cent sodium bicarbonate solution (4 parts).

6.3.2.4 Serum-supplemented Lactalbumin Hydrolysate and Yeast Extract Medium

This medium consists of Earle's saline containing lactalbumin hydrolysate (0.5.%), yeast extract (0.1.%) and human or ox serum (10-20%).

6.3.3 Chemically Defined Media

Earlier, nutritive media for the cultivation of animal cells *in vitro* were derived from the organisms and consisted of blood plasma, blood serum, tissue extracts, etc. The complexity and variability of these naturally occurring materials made it difficult to use them in experiments designed to determine the nutritive substances required by the cells and the effect of a particular substance upon them.

The first attempts to devise chemically defined media were made by Lewis and Lewis, Bakar and Carrel, Vogelaar and Erlichman. Carrel's discovery (1912) that extracts of embryonic tissues contained an abundance of growth promoting substances made it possible for the first time to propagate animal cells indefinitely and stimulated the search for the particular substances responsible.

Carrel and Baker (1926) reported that Witte's peptone, proteases and other degradation products when used with serum or plasma provided essential nutrients for fibroblasts, epitheial cells and blood monocytes. Vogelaar and

Erlichman (1933) prepared a feeding solution consisting of irradiated beef plasma, Witte's peptone, hemin, cystine, insulin, thyroxine, glucose and the salts of Tyrode's solution. They kept a strain of fibroblasts from the human thyroid in a state of active proliferation for three months. Bakar later on added vitamin A and D, ascorbic acid, glutathione and 10 per cent serum for the cultivation of epithelial cells. For blood monocytes certain B vitamins were also added.

Fischer's supplementary medium, V-614 consisted of dialyzed plasma, dialyzed embryo extract, Tyrode's solution, glucose, fructose diphosphate, glutamine, cystine, glutathione, tryptophan, phenylalanine, threonine, isoleucine, leucine, valine, arginine, histidine and lysine. Fischer further suggested that different cell types may have different amino acid requirements. Thus, osteoblasts were more sensitive than myoblasts to lysine deficiency. He also stated that animal tissues cultivated outside the body may require certain nutrients not required by the intact animal.

White (1946) for the first time made a serious attempt to cultivate animal tissues in a complete solution of 20 ingredients of known composition. He reported a feeding solution of 20 ingredients of known composition that supported relatively large masses of chick embryo heart tissues in a state of functional survival for several weeks.

6.3.3.1 Medium No. 199

Morgan *et al.* (1950) published the composition of a more adequate medium No. 199. The medium included almost a complete complement of aminoacids and vitamins as well as several nucleic acid constituents and certain intermediary metabolites and accessory growth factors. Glutamine was included because of the importance placed upon it by Fischer's group; and Tween - 80 was used as a water soluble source of fatty acid and as a means of dissolving the fat soluble vitamins and cholesterol in a minimal concentration of ethyl- alcohol. The medium also contained the salts of Earle's balanced salt solution, glucose, ferric nitrate and phenol red.

The other tissue culture media which are being used are as. follows:

6.3.3.2 Medium No. 612

It was observed that medium 199 had a very high oxidation-reduction potential; Healy and co-workers attempted to bring it near the physiological range by increasing the three reducing agents present in the medium namely cysteine, glutathione, and ascorbic acid considerably. Cysteine and glutathione increase the rate of cell multiplication and improve the appearance of the cells; ascorbic acid has no apparent effect. Healy increased the levels of cysteine and glutathione 2600 and 200 times respectively. The ascorbic acid level was increased 1000 times. He designated this medium as medium No. 612.

6.3.3.3 Medium No. 635

This medium was devised by omitting from medium No. 612 all the purines, prymidines as well as adenosinetriphosphate, adenylic acid, ribose and deoxyribose. This medium gives a better growth response than that of medium No. 612 but the cultures rarely survive more than 40 days.

6.3.3.4 Medium No. 858

This medium includes all the deoxyribonucleosides, coenzymes, and sodium glucuronate in addition to medium No. 635. This medium contains only L-form amino acids, and yields ten-fold increase in the population of culture cells in seven days. Addition of 10 to 20 per cent of horse serum yields 20 to 30 fold increase in seven days.

6.3.3.5 Medium No. 866

Medium No. 866 is similar to that of medium no. 858 supplemented with three fatty acids namely, linolenic acid and arachidonic acid. This medium does not improve the growth of culture cells.

6.3.3.6 Medium CMRL—1066

This medium is identical with medium No. 858 except that the fat soluble vitamins (A, D, E, and K), ferric nitrate and sodium bicarbonate included in medium No. 858 have been omitted. Five B vitamins (thiamine, riboflavin, niacin, niacinamide and sodium pantothenate) are added. It also contains 0.02 mg percent n-butyl parahydroxybenzoate, which offers protection from certain moulds. Antibiotics are added according to the need.

Eagle found that 12 amino acids are essential for the growth of both L-strain and HeLa-strain cultures even in the presence of small quantities of whole or dialyzed serum. These amino acids are arginine, cystine, histidine, isoleucine, leucine, lysine, methionine, phenylalanine, threonine, tryptophan, tyrosine, and valine. Recent attempts have been made to determine the vitamin requirements of cells cultivated in chemically defined media containing dialyzed. serum.

Glucose is generally added to tissue culture media as an energy source; other carbohydrates have also been tested. Harris and Kutsky have shown that chick heart fibroblasts can utilize D-fructose or D-mannose as well as D-glucose.

Interesting studies of the inorganic requirements of cells *in vitro* have also been conducted. Harris found that carbon dioxide is. beneficial for the outgrowth of cells from explanted chick embryo tissues. Eagle has shown that sodium, potassium, magnesium, calcium chloride and H_2PO_4 ions are essential for the survival of L-strain and HeLa cells.

6.3.4 Use of Sodium Bicarbonate and Antibiotics

Buffering of culture media for mammalian cells is usually provided by sodium bicarbonate. This dissociates in solution releasing carbondioxide into the atmosphere and hydroxyl ions into the medium. If dissociation occurs faster than the production of acid by the cells, then the medium will turn alkaline. Thus the buffering capacity of the culture medium is better maintained if the proportion of the CO_2 in the gas phase inside the culture vessel is high. This is reflected in the differences in the bicarbonate content of two balanced salt solutions shown in Table 6.2. Cells which release a lot of metabolic CO_2 are best cultured in supplemented Hanks' saline in a sealed container, where the CO_2 released helps to slow down the dissociation of sodium bicarbonate. Cells which do not produce much CO_2 do better in Earle's saline exposed to a gas mixture of 5 per cent CO_2 in air. Because of the difficulties associated with the use of bicarbonate buffers, a number of organic buffers have been introduced for animal cell culture. The most popular of these is HEPES (N 2 hydroxyethyl piperazine-N′-2 ethanesulphonic acid) which has a pKa of 7.3 at 37° C. Unfortunately this compound is too expensive for routine large scale use.

The media used to culture animal cells are rich in nutrients, so they are particularly susceptible to contamination with bacteria and fungi unless good aseptic techniques are practised. For this reason antibiotics are usually added: penicillin to prevent the growth of gram-negative cells and nystatin to inhibit fungi. Another problem with cell cultures is contamination with mycoplasmas, a group of bacteria which lack cell walls. Most of the contaminating mycoplasmas are non-pathogenic and probably originate from the oropharynx of laboratory staff but are derived from trypsin or serum. Tetracyclines, kanamycin and gentamycin can be used to inhibit most mycoplasmas.

6.4 Hybridomas And Monoclonal Antibodies (MABs)

Hybridoma refers to a hybrid cell line produced by the fusion of a normal lymphocyte antibody producing cell with a myeloma cell, (malignant tumours of bone marrow). This was first reported by Köhler and Milstein in 1974. Monoclonal antibody refers to an antibody preparation that contains only a single type of antibody molecules which are produced by hybridoma technology. These hybridomas have the ability to multiply rapidly and indefinitely *in vitro* and to produce an antibody of pre-determined specificity.

One animal cell product that is attracting ever-increasing attention is the monoclonal antibody. This is a specific antibody produced from a normally short-lived, antigen—activated B cell that has been immortalized by hybridizing it with a myeloma cell. Thus the hybrid retains the ability of the B cell to secrete an antibody and the ability of the myeloma cell to grow indefinitely. The advantage of the monoclonal antibody is that it is derived from a single cell and comprises of a uniform breed of antibody specific for a single antigen site (epitope). Traditional polyclonal antisera are derived from many cells and contain heterogeneous antibodies that are specific for all the epitopes in an antigen.

When a foreign macromolecule (antigen) is introduced into the circulatory system of a higher vertebrate it stimulates specific white blood cells, the lymphocytes, to produce antibodies that combine specifically with the macromolecule to facilitate its destruction within, or removal from, the body. The antibodies which are synthesized can be found in the globulin fraction of the proteins that circulate in the blood and hence are called immunoglobulins. All immunoglobulin molecules have a similar basic structure consisting of two heavy and two light chains held together by disulphide bonds. There are areas in heavy and light chains known as variable regions in which the amino acid sequence of the protein chain varies from one antibody to another. This variation occurs at the N-terminus of the peptide chains. Each different antibody will therefore have a different amino acid sequence and spatial arrangment and it is conceivable that every possible shape presented by an antigen can be accommodated by some antibody produced by the immune system.

When the immune system of an animal encounters a new antigen it does not respond to the entire surface of the antigen but to specific antigenic determinants (epitopes) located on it. Thus a protein antigen may possess several epitopes and would induce the formation of several different antibodies in the blood; this blood contains polyclonal antiserum with different antibodies. This is not very specific. Hence the use of a single antibody species which is very specific in its activity.

6.4.1 Antibody, Antigen and Lymphocytes

Antibodies are part of the body's defences against foreign invaders, including disease causing organisms. When the B lymphocytes (plasma cells) of the immune system are stimulated by the presence of an invading pathogen or other foreign material, they produce antibodies which are nothing but protein molecules that specifically recognize and bind to the substance that originally elicited their production. These protein molecules are immunoglobulins, accounting for about 20 per cent of the total plasma proteins and some beta-globulins. Immunoglobulins are glycoproteins composed of 82 to 96 per cent polypeptide and 4 to 8 per cent carbohydrate. The polypeptide part possesses the biological properties of antibodies. The antibody producing cells recognize the physico-chemical characteristics (electric charge, pattern or shape) of the particular antigen and produce an antibody that binds specifically to the antigen, thus effectively neutralising or destroying it.

Antigen is the substance that incites the immune system to form immune products specific for the substance. Chemically antigens are the proteins, polysaccharides or nucleic acids that are either soluble or particulate in nature. The antigens form the immune products and also interact with them. Antigens are also termed immunogens when the emphasis is on their ability to incite the formation of immune products (immunogenicity). An antigen is always a foreign substance for a host. It must be capable of inducing an antibody response in the host. The portion of the antigen that combines with the antibody is called its determinant group. Antigenic properties are common to toxins of plant origin such as ricin, robin, abrin, cortin etc., toxins of animal origin such as snake, spiders, scorpions etc., enzymes, native foreign proteins, various cellular components, bacteria and their toxins and virus, etc.

Lymphocytes are animal cells found in the bone marrow and foetus. They are found in yolk-sac, liver and thymus. They are found in two types, B and T lymphocytes. The T lymphocytes are mainly involved in cellular type of immunological response that is with cellular -immunity. B lymphocytes are mainly involved in the production of antibodies. It is a type of hormonal immunity. Both the lymphocytes are quite distinct and independent in their function, but they may help each other in antibody production. The production of antibody increases in the presence of T-lymphocytes- Thus T-lymphocytes act as helper cells. A small percentage (5%) of lymphocytes cannot be classified as 'T' or 'B' cells and are therefore, termed as null cells. Lymphocytes cannot be maintained in a culture medium independently. Myelomas produce large quantities of abnormal immunoglobulins (antibodies) in culture which have an identical structure.

6.4.2 The Discovery

Barski, Sorieul and Cornefort from France (1960) observed a new cell type during their culture experiments with two stocks of tumour mouse cells. This new cell type was produced by the fusion of the two parental stock cells and it was different from the cells of the parents both in morphological characteristics and growth patterns. Moreover, the chromosome numbers of these new cell types were equal to the total number of chromosomes of both the parents and they also contained chromosome markers that were peculiar to the parent cells. Ephrussi *et al.* (1964) confirmed the findings of Barski *et al;* they also succeeded in fusing other types of non-tumour mouse cells. The frequency of cell fusion was very low $10^{-4} - 10^{-6}$) but Okada (1958, 1962) was able to increase the frequency of fusion of animal tumour cells by using the Japanese haemagglutination virus (JHV). Okada and Tadokora (1962) showed that such a virus could be completely inactivated by ultraviolet radiation and yet retain the ability to induce cell fusion. Harris and Watkins (1965) used inactivated sendai virus to induce the fusion of human HeLa cells and tumour mouse cells. They were also able to induce somatic cell fusion between cells of different vertebrate classes.

Around this time Potter had induced a series of cancerous tumours in mice, which are derived from antibody producing cells. These cells produced the same type of antibody. Cotton and Milstein (1973) fused rat and mouse myeloma cells together and observed that the immunoglobulins produced by the hybrid cells consisted of various combinations of the polypetide chains produced by the parental lines.

Somatic cell fusion has been obtained between human and mouse cells, monkey and mouse cells, human HeLa cells and *Aedes aegypti* cells, mouse and chicken cells, plant and animal cells and so on. Fusion is usually induced by using fusing agents such as sendai virus and polyethylene glycol. In the case of fusion between cells belonging to different species or groups, the loss of chromosomes of one parental line was generally observed and the resulting hybrid cells were very useful for genetic analysis studies. Somatic cell fusion results in the production of a heterokaryon (a single cell with two kinds of nuclei). Properties of the cytoplasm influence the expression of genes in the nucleus because of the positive feedback between the nucleus and cytoplasm.

The monoclonal antibody story began in 1974 when Georges Köhler and Cesar Milstein were studying the role of gene mutations in generating antibody diversity. To start with, they wanted a line of cells that could be grown in culture and would produce a single kind of antibody molecule in response to a known antigen. Köhler and Milstein hit on the idea of fusing normal antibody-producing cells of known specificity with cells from the cancerous tumour cells, myeloma, so that they could obtain a permanent line of cells that made the antibody they wanted. To obtain the antibody producing cells of known specificity, Köhler injected mice with sheep red blood cells, which are very highly antigenic, harvested the B lymphocytes from the animal's spleens, and then fused the B cells with P3 myeloma cells (cell lines of Potter). When the resulting hybrid cells were cloned, some of the clones proved to produce antibodies that specifically recongize sheep red blood cells (Fig. 6.1). All hybrids of the same clone produced the same antibody molecules. Although the original hybridomas of Köhler and Milstein produced two antibodies, one from the myeloma cell and the other from the spleen cell, researchers now use myeloma cells that do not make any antibody of their own so that the only product of the hybridoma clone is the spleen-cell antibody.

Thus, Köhler and Milstein succeeded in isolating clones of cells capable of secreting a single molecular type of antibody and to maintain them in culture. These chimaeric cells (hybridomas) retained the property of immortality of the myeloma cells as well as that of secreting an antibody specific for a known antigen.

Not just any myeloma cell can be used. The myeloma cell used must have two particular properties. First, the myeloma cell should not secrete any antibody by itself; such cell lines are reported where a particular lymphocyte multiplies uncontrollably without any antibody production. Second, the myeloma cells used for fusion are specially selected by growing them in the presence of 8-azaguanine. Most of the cells are killed by this technique but a few survive and these resistant cells have a defect in-the enzyme hypoxanthin phosphoribosyl transferase (HPRT).

When HPRT—negative cells are grown in a mixture of hypoxanthine aminopterin and thyimdine (HAT medium) the cells will die because they can no longer synthesize DNA. The aminopterin blocks the main pathway for purine and pyrimidine biosynthesis. Normal cells can use the thymidine to make pyrimidines and, using HPRT, can convert the Hypoxanthine to purines. In a fusion mixture of lymphocytes and myeloma cells neith.er cell can grow in the HAT medium. The lymphocytes will survive for a few days before dying out; the myeloma cells will also die because they lack HPRT. However, the hybridoma cells will possess the ability of the myeloma cells to grow *in vitro* and the normal HPRT gene from the lymphocytes with which they have fused. Thus the hybridoma will grow successfully in HAT selection medium.

6.4.3 Making a Hybridoma

The starting point for making a hybridoma which secretes the desired MAB is to immunize an animal, e.g. a mouse, with the appropriate antigen. Normally the antigen is injected subcutaneously or into the peritoneal cavity along with an adjuvant to stimulate the immune system. The animal is injected on several occasions and with each successive immunization there is an increased stimulation of the B lymphocytes which are responding to the antigen. The final dose of antigen is given intravenously three days before the animal is killed. The intravenous injection ensures a high dose of antigen and three days after immunization the immune stimulated cells will grow maximally.

After the immunized animal is killed, the spleen is aseptically removed and gently disrupted to release the lymphocytes and red blood cells. The lymphocytes are separated from the red blood cells and spleenic fluid by density gradient centrifugations. After washing, the lymphocytes are mixed with an HPRT—negative myeloma cell line. The mixture of cells is exposed to the fusion-promoting agent polyethylene .glycol, but only for a few minutes since it is cytotoxic. The cells are then washed free of the polyethylene glycol by suspending the pellets in fresh media. The washed cells comprise a mixture of hybridomas, unfused myeloma cells and unfused lymphocytes. By using HAT growing medium the hybridomas can be selected.

If all the hybridomas that occurred after a fusion were grown together, then a polyclonal antibody mixture would be obtained. Consequently, single antibody producing hybridoma cells need to be isolated and grown individually. This is done by diluting a suspension of hybridoma cells to such an extent that individual aliquots contain, on an average, only one cell. The cells are then grown in fresh medium. Each clone is then examined to determine if it produces the desired antibody. The clones selected can be stored by freezing. At any time, a sample of one of these clones can be injected into animals or can be grown *in vitro* and the antibody can be produced. A scheme for the production of monoclonal antibody is presented herewith. It involves three

(i) Fusion and culture of hybridomas
(ii) Cloning and preservation of hybridomas
(iii) Production of antibodies.

6.4.3.1 Fusion and Culture of Hybridomas

(a) Inject an antigen into the body of a mouse through intravenous route 72 hours before use. On the day of fusion, collect the spleen and make a free cell suspension by injecting and flushing the spleen with sterile serum-free medium. Centrifuge the cells and resuspend in lysing solution. When sterile water is used, suspend the cells in 1 ml of water and immediately dilute 20 times by medium; any delay will result in the loss of plasmablasts and a consequent reduction in antibody producing hybrids.

(b) Maintain plasma cells in cell culture and seed into fresh flasks and medium 16-24 hours before the fusion process to ensure that they are in the early phase of growth at the time of fusion. At the time of use, collect the cells, centrifuge and resuspend in serum-free medium.

(c) Collect myeloma cells also and maintain in the culture medium.

(d) After the collection, max the myeloma and spleen cells in the appropriate ratio depending on the properties of the tumour cells. The ratio of spleen to tumour cells may vary from 5:1 to 2:1.

(e) Thereafter, centrifuge the cell suspension into a loose pellet at 1000 rpm for 10-15 minutes. Discard the supernatant and overlay the pellet with 1 ml of PEG. The two are Mix the two for three minutes so that pellet breaks up into uniform small clumps.

(f) Following fusion, dilute the cells in 30 ml of serum-free medium with the first 10 ml medium being added and mixed at one ml per minute. Slow dilution reduces the risk of osmotic disruption of the fused cells. Centrifuge the cells and resuspend in complete medium containing HAT and then dispense into 96-well tissue culture plates, 10 plates for each 10^8 splenocytes used in the fusion. Add 10^6 thymocytes to each well to serve as feeder-cells. The latter step has proven critical for optimizing the outgrowth of newly formed hybrids. Feeder-cells and 2-ME in the medium exert a synergistic effect.

(g) Incubate the cultures in a carbon dioxide incubator with high humidity for three or four days between changes of culture medium. Replace half the medium with fresh HAT medium every fourth day in case of rapidly growing cultures.

(h) Identify and mark the wells containing hybrid colonies (hybridomas) on day nine or ten and then allow the colonies to grow to 500 or more cells. In rapidly growing cultures, supernatants can be collected and assayed for antibody activities by day 12-14. Where appropriate, collect and test the supernatants from the largest colonies first; test the remainder two to four days later.

(i) When the antibody test is accomplished, the positive cell lines are transferred to 24 well plates. Feeder cells are added (3.5×10^6) to each well to promote cell growth. Maintain cells in static culture for a minimum of two weeks by removing 50-75 per cent of the hybrid cells every two to three days. This manoeuvre selects stable, rapidly growing antibody producing hybrids. Slow growing hybrids and hybrids that cease to synthesize antibody are eliminated.

(j) After two weeks, make duplicate cultures and allow the cells to overgrow and die. Collect the supernatant and assay for the presence of antibody. Take cultures producing antibodies of the desired specificity from the master plate and expand into six well plates (two to three wells for each cell lines). Harvest the cells twice for preservation in liquid nitrogen. Replenish the cultures with fresh medium and allow the cells to overgrow and die. Collect the final supernatant for further analysis. The six

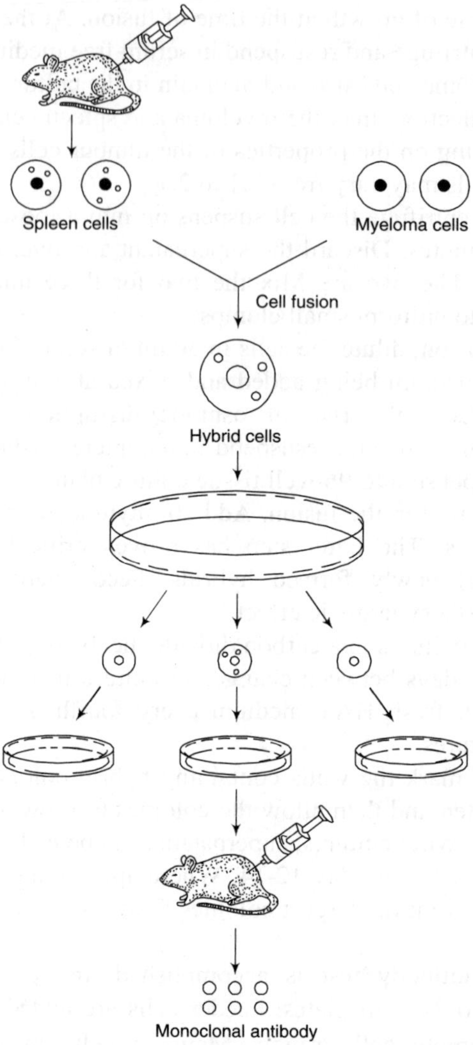

Figure 6.1

Production of monoclonal antibodies. A mouse is injected with any desired antigen to elicit antibody production. Antibody-producing cells are subsequently harvested from the animal's spleen and fused with mouse myeloma cells to form hybrid cells, which are grown in culture. Individual hybrids are then grown in culture to form clones, which are screened for the production of antibody that reacts with original antigen. Cells from clones that produce the monoclonal antibody may then be injected into the peritoneal cavity of another mouse where they form a tumour, the hybridoma. The tumor cells secrete the antibody into the fluid that accumulates in the mouse abdominal cavity. The monoclonal antibody is harvested from this fluid. Some cells of the monoclonal-anti body-producing clone can also be frozen for future use.

(***Source:*** *Marx, J.L. (Ed.). A Revolution in Biotechnology. © 1989 Cambridge: Cambridge University Press. Reprinted by permission.*)

well plates are essential for minimising labour and time during this phase of hybridoma production.

6.4.3.2 Cloning and Preservation of Hybridomas

(a) After the preliminary selection of hybrids is made, screen the final supernatants in detail to identify antibodies of interest. Take the parent cell lines from the freezer and clone by limiting dilution. When the viability is appropriate, clone the cell lines immediately. Take the remainder of the excess cells and culture them in a T 75 flask for one or two days. As soon as enough cells are present, harvest the cells and freeze one ampoule to replace the ampoule used for cloning. The culture should not be allowed to proliferate more than necessary to avoid change in composition of the cell line at this early stage of processing. As in the initial step, use feeder cells to promote growth.

(b) After six to eight days, mark wells containing a single colony and assay supernatants from the marked wells after 12-14 days. Transfer 24-48 positive cultures to 24 well plates and maintain in static culture as described earlier.

(c) After noting which cloned lines are stable, expand four to six clones of each cell line into six well plates for cell preservation and production of antibodies.

(d) Preserve four to six clones from each cell lines in liquid nitrogen.

6.4.3.3 Production of Antibodies

(a) Cloned cell lines are cultured *in vitro* in ascites from mice to produce antibodies.

(b) After the production, monoclonal antibodies are assayed in the supernatants of hybridomas by using a proper technique. The following techniques are in use for assaying monoclonal antibodies:

(i) Flow cytometry
(ii) Cytotoxicity
(iii) Enzyme-linked immunoabsorbant assay (ELISA)
(iv) Immunofluorescence
(v) Radioimmunoassay (RIA)

6.5 Applications

Monoclonal antibodies have proved to be extremely valuable for basic immunological and molecular research because of their specificity and high purity. They are used in such diverse applications like human therapy, commercial protein purification, suppressing immune responses, diagnosis of diseases, cancer therapy, diagnosis of allergy, hormone tests, purification of complex mixtures, structure of cell membrane, identification of specialized cells, preparation of vaccines and increasing the effectiveness of medicinal substances.

6.5.1 Gene cloning

One of the most difficult problems of gene cloning is identifying the cells that contain the desired gene. If a monoclonal antibody that recognizes the gene product is available, it can be used as a probe for detecting those cells that make the product and thereby help us to detect the gene.

6.5.2 Identifying Cell Types

Monoclonal antibodies contribute to the identification of many different types of cells that participate in immune responses and to unravel the interactions. For example, in the lymphocytes with B, helper T and suppressor T, the use of monoclonal antibodies has established that the various types of T cells carry antigens or markers on their surfaces that allow one type to be distinguished from another. The MABs have also helped to define the changes undergone by the T and B cells during development.

6.5.3 Suppressing Immune Responses

MABs are now being used to prevenl the rejection of transplanted kidneys. This antibody, which is marked under the name Orthoclone OKT-3 specifically reacts with OKT-3 'antigen that is found on all T cells. To prevent rejection of foreign tissues, kidney transplant patients are routinely given drugs to suppress the activities of their immune systems. Orthoclone OKT-3 attacks the, T cells that cause the rejection.

Several human diseases are caused by an apparent attack of the immune system on the tissues of the body. Investigators are attempting to determine whether MABs that are directed against immune cell components that may be involved in triggering the abnormal immune responses, could be used to treat such autoimmune conditions.

A human MAB against *E. coli* endotoxin has been produced which protects mice from bacteraemia. It is being tried out in humans also. An anti-T-cell MAB is available that has been used to remove T cells from the donor marrow prior to transplantation, leading to reduction in graft-versus-host disease.

6.5.4 Diagnosis of Diseases

The diagnostic applications of monoclonal antibodies are by far the most advanced, especially for tests that are performed on body fluids such as blood and urine samples. MAB is used to detect pregnancy as early as a week or two after conception by reacting with human chorionic gonadotrophin, a hormone secreted by the placenta and found in the urine of pregnant women. The diagnosis of venereal diseases is also being improved by the availability of MABs. Today MABs are available which can identify gonorrhoea (caused by *Neisseria gonorrhoeae)* and chlamydia infections (caused by *Chlamydia trachomatis)* in 15 to 20 minutes unlike three to seven days required by other methods earlier. MABs are also available that distinguish between the closely related herpes virus 1 and herpes virus 2.

6.5.5 Cancer Diagnosis and Therapy

The availability of MABs that recognize immune cell antigens has resulted in improved diagnosis of particular types of leukaemias and lymphomas. MABs are also being applied to the diagnosis of solid tumours, particularly the carcinomas of the lung, breast, colon, rectum etc. MABs are also used to examine blood, sputum or biopsy samples for cancer cells or for materials that have been released by cancer cells. Today special MABs are available for colorectal cancers, ovarian cancer, lung cancers.

Ultimately MABs may be used not just to detect cancer cells but to destroy them; clinical trials have shown that MABs have induced at least partial remissions. Recent studies have shown that conjugates, drugs and toxins with MABs can kill leukaemia cells.

6.5.6 Protein Purification

Monoclonal antibody affinity columns are readily prepared by coupling MABs to a cyanogen bromide-activated chromatography matrix, e.g Sepharose. MABs immobilized in this way are particularly valuable for the purification of proteins. Since the MAB has a unique specificity for the desired protein, the level of contamination by unwanted protein species usually is very low. Since the MAB antigen complex has a single binding affinity it is possible to elute the required protein in a single, sharp peak. The concentration of the required protein relative to total protein in a mixture can even be very low. This method is used commercially to purify recombinant-derived interferon-2. This method has its own limitation. 100% pure protein is difficult to achieve because there is always a tendency for small amounts of immunoglobulin to leak off the immunoaffinity column. Also MABs often do not distinguish between intact protein molecules and fragments containing the antigenic site.

6.6 Chimaeric Antibodies

In nature a complete gene for an antibody light chain is assembled by combining three separate DNA segments. Two of these make up the coding sequence for the variable region and the third encodes the constant region of the protein chain. Assembly of the heavy chain genes is similar except that three DNA sequences must be joined to form the gene segments coding for the variable region. By recombinant DNA technology, the genes for mouse and human heavy chain variable, heavy chain constant, light chain variable and light chain constant regions have been cloned and expressed in bacteria. Researchers have also produced chimaeric antibodies (hybrid antibodies which are partly human and partly mouse) in which the constant regions are of human origin and the variable regions are of mouse origin.

To construct a chimaeric antibody the genes for the light and heavy chains are made individually by recombinant DNA methods. Cloned gene sequences are already available for the constant regions of the two classes of human light chains and the five classes of human heavy chains. The gene sequences encoding the mouse variable regions are cloned from a hybridoma cell line that makes a monoclonal antibody of the desired specificity.

The cloned sequences for the light chain constant and variable regions are then joined, as are those for the heavy chain to form the complete genes. Once the genes from the chimaeric light and heavy chains are in hand, they are introduced together into mouse myeloma cells where the proteins are made and the complete antibody molecules are assembled.

6.7 Hazards Associated With MABs

The majority of mammalian cells contain in their chromosomes genetic information related to retroviruses (some of them cause cancer). Mice, and in particular the inbred strains used in laboratory studies, carry a number of different types of these viruses and murine cell lines frequently release virus. Retrovirus production has been noted in a number of myeloma cell lines and in hybridomas prepared from them. Due to dangers which those viruses can pose, regulatory authorities have stipulated that medicinal products containing MABs will not be approved unless the MABs and the hybridomas can be shown to be virus free. An alternative method of producing MABs, and one which eliminates the virological hazards, is to synthesize them in bacteria using recombinant DNA technology. This has already been achieved recently. Commercial application is awaited.

6.8 Transgenic Animals

The modification of germ cells by gene manipulation *in vitro* is referred to as transgenesis. Transgenic animals are created by introducing new DNA sequences into germ line via addition to the egg. In animal breeding, modification of germ cells and improvement of the animal are desired goals.

6.8.1 Gene Delivery Methods

Whether it is the somatic cells to be modified or germ cells to be modified, a method of introducing exogenous DNA into these cells is essential. As described already in Chapter Four, there are many methods currently available for this purpose. Out of these the most widely employed methods are (i) use of viral vectors, (ii) calcium phosphate-mediated DNA uptake, (iii) microinjection of eggs, (iv) fusion of DNA loaded membranous vesicles (e.g. liposomes) to target cells and (v) electroporation (DNA uptake mediated by electric current). None of these delivery methods fulfils the criteria of being able to transfect the majority of cells with the minimum cellular damage or mortality. Where somatic cells are to be modified the use of viral vectors or calcium phosphate-mediated uptake is recommended. For the modification of germ cells, microinjection is the method of choice. Whatever the DNA delivery method used one problem still remains; there is no control over where the donor DNA will integrate in the recipient genome and whether this will result in any pathological condition or not.

6.8.2 Production of Transgenic Mice

The aim of transgenesis is to produce animals with a heritable change in their genotype so that the benefits of gene manipulation can be passed on to their offspring. Most experiments dealing with the production of transgenic mice have made use of the mouse metallothionein (MMT) gene promoter. In an ideal transgenesis experiment, the promoter selected would be one which enables the normal cellular control patterns to be exerted on the gene of interest, i.e. the gene should be switched on and off at the correct time and in the correct tissues. Success of this kind has been achieved with transgenic mice carrying the human insulin gene. There has not been much success with regard to transgenic experiments with other animals.

An archetypal example of transgenesis in animals is the production of 'supermice' which are extra large as a result of the overproduction of human growth hormone. Although of great academic interest, such supermice have no commercial value. Other transgenic mice have been produced which systhesize human tissue plasminogen activator (tPA) and secrete it in their milk. Although this tPA is produced at a high concentration (50,000 mg/ml) and is biologically active, mice are unlikely to be acceptable as a pharmaceutical production system. Currently there are many human diseases for which animal models are lacking, thereby hindering the development of suitable therapeutic agents. By means of transgenesis a number of mice have been produced which carry genetic lesions identical to those existing in certain human inherited diseases (Table 6.4).

While transgenic mice are of interest as an experimental tool, the technique needs to be applied to farm animals if any commercial benefit is to ensue. Working with large domestic animals is much more difficult than with mice. First, they do not produce as many eggs. Second, reimplantation of manipulated embryos is more difficult because sheep and cattle will not give birth to more than two offsprings. Finally, the eggs of many domestic animals have such an opaque cytoplasm that it is impossible to see their pronuclei or nuclei without resorting to special techniques. So far, the enhanced growth of mice after the transfer of the human growth hormone gene is an effort that has not been as easy to mimic in other animals. Desirable features of transgenic farm animals include increased efficiency of feed utilization, leaner meat, more rapid growth to marketable size and increased disease resistance.

Table 6.4

Human disease equivalents derived from genetic alterations in the mouse (after Old, A. and Primrose, S. B. 1989)

	Genetic alternation	Method of genetic alternation	Human disease equivalent
1.	Introduction of mutant collagen gene into wild type mice	Nuclear microinjection of inducible minigene	Osteogenesis imperfecta
2.	Inactivation of mouse gene encoding hypoxanthineguanine phosphoribosyl transferase (HPRT)	Insertion of retrovirus into HPRT locus in embryonic stem cells	HPRT deficiency
3.	Mutation at locus for X-linked muscular dystrophy	Male mutagenesis followed by identification of female carriers	X-linked muscular dystrophy
4.	Introduction of activated human *ras* and *c-myc* oncogenes	Nuclear microinjection of inducible minigene	Induction of malignancy
5.	Introduction of mutant (z) allele of human a_1-anti-trypsin gene	Microinjection of DNA fragment bearing mutant allele	Neonatl hepatitis
6.	Introduction of HIV *tat* gene	Microinjection of DNA fragments	Kaposis sarcoma

6.9 Animal Cloning

Cloning is the production of a genetically identical duplicate of an organism. Etymologically the term cloning is derived from the Greek word *Klon*, which means a young shoot. Originally the word clone was used for new plants, which were obtained through cuttings of a parent plant. The new plants had identical characters like the parent plant.

Later scientists succeeded in establishing animal cell clones, where a single cell multiplied and produced identical cells in colonies. This was followed by the development of techniques where the two to eight celled embryo (blastomere) produced by the union of an egg and sperm was split and each cell was allowed to develop into individuals.

In 1950s Briggs and King transferred a nucleus from an embryo cell of a frog to an enucleated egg cell of a frog and placed in the womb of a frog. It gave birth to a tadpole, which died before developing into a frog. Similar attempts were also made in fruitfly *Drosophila* (1970s) and mice (1984) but normal adults could not be obtained. In October 1993 Hall and Stillman artificially split a human embryo into identical twins but it resulted in abnormal foetus. In March 1995, Ian Wilmut and his colleagues used the nuclear transfer technique to produce two lambs Megan and Morag. They took the nuclei from cultured cells that were derived from a nine-day-old embryo and fused one nucleus with one enucleated egg. The fused cell was implanted into the uterus, where it was allowed to develop into a complete organism. These two lambs were clones of the embryo from which the cultured cells were derived but not the clones of the animal. The cultured cells that were derived from embryo and used in their cloning experiments, could be reprogrammed to function like those in an early embryo, although they were supposed to be partially specialized or differentiated.

Dolly-The Sheep:The first cloned Mammal

Ian Wilmut, Keith Campbell and their colleagues at the Edinburgh Roslin Institute, used the technique of somatic cell nuclear transfer and produced the cloned animal Dolly in February 1997. The method involved transferring the nucleus from the udder cell of a normal 6 year old adult Finn Dorset Ewe (containing all the donor's genetic material) to an unfertilized egg of Scottish Black Face Ewe from which the maternal nucleus (all the genetic material) was removed. The fused cell (unfertilized egg with foreign nucleus) was activated with a short electric impulse to accept the nucleus, multiply and then it was implanted in the uterus of a surrogate mother Black Face Ewe, which gave birth to Dolly that was exactly similar to Finn Dorset Ewe (which donated the genetic material)

Till this time, it was believed that a mammal could not be reproduced asexually from an adult animal. Dolly was the first fully developed mammal to be born using the genetic material taken from a mature animal's somatic cell (nonreproductive) with the help of somatic cell nuclear transfer technique. Dolly contained the genetic material of only one parent in contrast to clones produced through artificial splitting of embryos

The scientists of Roslin Institute were engaged in 277 fusion attempts and they succeeded in producing 29 embryos. Only when the fusion is successful, an embryo develops. Out of the 29 embryos implanted into the uteri of surrogate sheep, only 13 became pregnant and only one gave birth to Dolly. The rest of the embryos died in the uteri. The researchers had spent 750,000 US dollars.

In March 1997 Don Wolf and his colleagues succeeded in producing two monkeys named Neti and Ditto by nuclear transfer technique from embryo to egg. In December 1997, Roslin Institute in collaboration with PPL Therapeutics produced two sheeps Molly and Polly using somatic fetus cells carrying a human gene for clotting factor IX. The clotting factor IX gene was linked to a sheep gene that increases milk production.

In 1998 University of Hawaii reported the production of 50 mice using nuclear transplant technique by transferring nucleus from adult cells to egg. Kato *et al*

(1998), Well *et al* (2000) and Kabota *et al* (2001) produced cows using nuclear transplant technique by transferring nucleus from adult cells to egg, from skin cell to egg and skin fibroblast culture, respectively. Cloning was also successfully achieved with fishes, mice, cows, sheep, goats, pigs, dogs, cats, etc. Genetically engineered animals produced through cloning are used to improve meat and milk production, to produce disease resistant animals, to produce biopharmaceuticals, to produce proteins, to produce tissues and organs, etc. For example transgenic cows having myelin basic protein human gene produce milk which contains myelin basic protein which helps to fight multiple sclerosis in humans. Aslo transgenic cows having human myostatin gene produce milk, which contains myostatin to treat patients with muscular dystrophy. Similarly sheep with a gene for alpha-1 antitrypsin, produce milk which contains alpha-1antitrypsin to treat patients with cystic fibrosis.

6.10 Human cloning

The success of cloning from different mammals opened up the possibility for human cloning. The same methodology could be used to produce human beings. Between 1998-2001, there were a few scientists (Severino Antinori, Brigitte Boisselier) who expressed their intentions to clone human beings. On October 13, 2001, scientists of Advanced Cell Technology, Massachusetts, USA, claimed that they had succeeded in cloning human embryos using somatic cell nuclear transfer technology with the intention of developing embryonic stem cells from such embryos. However these embryos did not survive long.

In February 2004, scientists from Seoul National University in South Korea, successfully cloned human embryos under the leadership of Woo Suk Hwang, using somatic cell nuclear transfer technology. 242 ova donated by 16 South Korean women were used for cloning. The nucleus of the cumulus cells taken from the ovaries of the same women was fused with the enucleated ovum with an electric pulse. Out of those 242 ova, 30 ova developed into human embryos, having the genotype of the donor somatic cell. Out of these only one proceeded to yield stem cells. Later his work was questioned for its ethical uprightness. In May 2005, the Newcastle University scientists successfully cloned human embryo from an adult human cell using the somatic cell nuclear transfer technique. In May 2005, the South Korean scientists from Seoul National University cloned human embryos using cells taken from certain patients. They obtained 31 embryos from 185 eggs of 18 women using adult cells taken from different patients - 6 adults and 3 children - with spinal cord injuries, juvenile diabetes and rare immune disorder. This study showed that embryonic stem cells can be derived from patients with various illnesses regardless of sex and age. Later the results were doubted by the scientific community.

If cloned embryos are transferred to the uterus of a woman as in the case of *in vitro* fertilization, then they may grow into full human beings.

6.10.1 Stem Cells

Stem Cells are unspecialized or undifferentiated cells that have the unique ability to give rise to many different cell types such as skin, liver, kidney, heart, neuron etc. They also possess the property of self-duplicating for indefinite period of time. Stem cells are of two types, namely, the embryonic stem cell and the adult stem cell. Embryonic stem cells are derived from the inner cell mass of the blastocyst stage of the embryo, i.e. before the blastocyst implants itself in the uterine wall. Embryonic stem cells are pluripotent. They are capable of self-renewal and they can differentiate into any cell type in the body. Adult stem cells are unspecialized and undifferentiated cells that are found to differentiate into cell types of the tissue of origin. Adult stem cells can be found in the bone marrow, blood stream, umbilical cord, conrnea and retina of the eye, dental pulp of the tooth, liver, skin, gastrointestinal tract and pancreas. It is rather difficult to make adult stem cells to produce the needed tissue for transplantation, etc. Hence the embryonic stem cells are considered as the most important source. Eventhough success had been achieved in the production of embryonic stem cells from mouse (Evans and Kaufman, 1981), non-human primates (Thomson *et al*, 1995) etc., it was only in 1998, embryonic stem cells from human embryos were obtained by Thomson and his colleagues from Wisconsin University, USA. These embryonic stem cells developed into desired tissues. Scientists believe that using such tissues developed from embryonic stem cells, of patients suffering from heart attack, diabetes, brain cell damage, spinal cord damage etc., it is possible to cure these diseases in adults.

Embryonic stem cell transfer is significantly employed for specific transgenic animal strains that are created for specific experimental or biomedical need. One such transgenic animal model is knock out mice. For creating a knockout mice the cultured pluripotent embryonic stem cells are trasfected with DNA frgments containing a mutant allele of the gene to be knocked out, as well as genes that can be used to select cells that have incorporated the altered DNA into their genome. Of those cells that take up the DNA, approximately one in 10,000 undergoes a process of homologous recombination in which the transfected DNA replaces the homologous DNA sequence that contains the normal alleles. Using this procedure, the embryonic stem cells with heterozygous nature are selected, injected into the blastocoel of a mouse blastocyst and then the embryo is implanted into the oviduct of a female mouse. The offsprings are heterozygous for the gene. Knockout mice provide a unique insight into the genetic basis of a human disease as well as a mechanism for studying various cellular activities in which the product of a particular gene might be engaged.

Study Outline

Animal Cell and Tissue Culture

In vitro cultivation of animal cells was shown in 1907. More recently the goal has been the production of human proteins of therapeutic value and monoclonal antibodies.

Culture

It is an art and an indispensable tool. In animals, isolation of free cells and cell aggregates from organs is considered to be a problem because it is difficult to release these cells from the supporting matrix without affecting the integrity of the cell membrane. The techniques used are mechanical (shaking the tissue with glass beads) and biochemical (incubation with enzymes). Culturing of these cells are done using primary cell line culture and monolayer culture. Maintaining and growing small parts or pieces or organs in vitro is called organ culture. It is used to maintain the architechture of tissue and to direct it towards normal development. One of its applications is the production of tissues for implantations in patients. Hybrid cells can be formed by the fusion of two different types of somatic cells.

Cell Growth

Primary cell lines and established cell lines have their own specific growth kinetics. The cultures exhibit lag phase, logarithmic phase and stationary phase.

Genetics of Culture Cells

Primary cell lines retain their diploid karyotype. Transformed cell lines show a great variation in the karyotype.

Metabolism

As there are variations in the cultural properties of the cell line they also show metabolic variation. For example, cells from liver derived hepatomas fail to synthesize normal liver enzymes but secrete liver product albumin. Tumour cells of the testis secrete androgen while pitUitary tumour cells secrete adrenocorticotrophic hormone and growth hormones.

Culture Media for Animals

A satisfactory medium should contain all the requirements with appropriate pH (7.0-7.3). It should be isotonic with cell cytoplasm and also sterile.

Hybridomas and Monoclonal Antibodies (MAB)

Hybridoma refers to a hybrid cell line produced by fusion of normal lymphocyte with a myeloma cell. Monoclonal antibody refers to an antibody preparation that contains only a single type of antibody molecule produced by hybridoma technology. The advantage of monoclonal antibody is that it is derived from a single cell and comprises of a uniform breed of antibody, specific for a single antigen site. The antibodies synthesized are associated with the globulin fraction of the protein in the blood. These are known as immunoglobulins. They have a different aminoacid sequence. When the immune system of the animal encounters a new antigen it does not respond to the entire surface of the antigen but to specific sites only. Thus it induces the formation of several antibodies in the blood.

Antibody, Antigen and Lymphocytes

Antibodies are a part of the body defences against foreign invaders including disease causing organisms. Antigen is the substance that incites the immune system to form immune product specific for the substance. An antigen is always a foreign substance for a host. It must be capable of inducing antibody response in the host. Lymphocytes are the animal cells found in the bone marrow and in foetus. They are found in yolk-sac, liver and thymus. They are of two types, B and T lymphocytes. Myelomas are the cells of certain malignant tumours (cancer) of bone marrow. They produce large quantities of immunoglobulins.

Applications

Monoclonal antibodies are extremely valuable for immunological and molecular research because of their high specificity and purity. They are used in diverse applications like human therapy, diagnosis of allergy, preparation of vaccines, purification of complex mixtures etc. In gene cloning, they are used as a probe detecting those cells that make the product and help to detect the gene. They help in the identification of many different cell types that participate in immune responses. MABs are used to prevent the rejection of transplanted kidneys. Detection of early pregnancy is done with the help of monoclonal antibodies and also the detection of particular type of leukaemias and lymphomas and solid tumour in lung, breast, colon, rectum etc. Monoclonal antibodies are used in the purification of recombinant derived interferon $\alpha 2$.

Hazards Associated with MABs

There is possibility of MABs containing viruses which may cause cancers. Hence regulatory authorities have stipulated that medicinal products containing MABs or products using MABs will not be approved unless the MABs and hybridomas can be shówn to be virus free.

Transgenic Animals

In vitro modification of germ cells by gene manipulation is referred to as transgenesis. Transgenic animals are created by introducing new DNA sequences into germ line via addition to the egg. There are several methods available for this purpose. The most widely employed methods use viral vectors, $CaPO_4$— mediated DNA uptake, microinjection, and electroporation.
Under culture

Animal cloning

Cloning is the production of a genetically identical duplicate of an organism. Using nuclear transfer and somatic cell nuclear techniques scientists have been able to clone sheep, cow, dog, cat, fish, mice, pig, etc. These transgenic animals are used to produce proteins in milk, tissues and organs, etc. which could be of benefit to human beings in treating diseases.

Human cloning

Success in animal cloning has opened the way for human cloning. Using similar methods as animal cloning, it is possible to clone humans. Embryonic stem cells are unspecialized and undifferentiated cells that have the unique ability to give rise to many different cell types. They can self-duplicate. Embryonic stem cells and adult stem cells can be obtained. Stem cells are useful in curing diseases.

Questions

(1) What are the various techniques used for the isolation of animal cells?
(2) Explain monolayer culture and primary cell line culture.
(3) What are the advantages of primary cell line culture?
(4) What are the growth kinetics of animal cells in culture?
(5) What is contact inhibition?
(6) Briefly state the metabolic changes of the cell line cultures.
(7) Describe the uses of monoclonal antibodies and hybridomas.
(8) What are antibodies, antigens and lymphocytes?
(9) Why are monoclonal antibodies hazardous at times?
(10) What is transgenesis? What are transgenic animals?
(11) How an animal is cloned?
(12) How was Dolly the sheep cloned?
(13) What are the success stories of human cloning?
(14) What are stem cells and their uses?
(15) What is knock out mice?

7
Agricultural Biotechnology

Introduction

Improvements in agricultural production, and the food and nutrition situation depend on land, water and energy resources. Research on the selection of new high yielding varieties started after the second world war and the selected new cultivars were disseminated all over the world during 1960-70. From the mid 1960s onwards, following the introduction of cultivars in several countries of Asia and Latin America, a green revolution was achieved. From 1970, a new type of research started with the aim of producing new varieties, not by cross-breeding or hybridization but using cell protoplast, tissue culture and genetic recombination techniques. The new plants produced by such techniques are supposed to be resistant to diseases, predators and drought and can be grown without fertilizers or pesticides.

Biotechnological research is increasingly contributing to the improved production and propagation of new cultivated varieties of plants that have a direct role in agricultural practices in relation to nutritional quality, food output and other useful substances. Some of the important aspects of agricultural biotechnology which fall under application and technique are:

(1) micropropagation for biomass energy production,
(2) production of disease-free and disease-resistant plants,
(3) induction and selection of mutants resistant to pests, pathogens, adverse soil conditions, drought, temperature, herbicides etc.
(4) production of haploids through anther culture,
(5) somatic hybrids and cybrids through the fusion of protoplasts,
(6) transformation through the uptake of foreign genomes,
(7) nitrogen fixation
(8) improving nutritional quality and
(9) increased yield of chemical compounds. Moreover, biotechnology enables faster multiplication of disease-free elite and rare stocks of forest and horticultural trees by micropropagation.

7.1 Micropropagation For Biomass Increase

Mass propagation of crop and forest plants is an important application of micropropagation techniques which involve the development of embryos from somatic cells in culture. Biotechnology of fruit and forest trees offers means not only for the rapid and mass multiplication of the existing stocks of germplasm for woody biomass energy production, but also for the conservation of important, superior and rare trees which are threatened with extinction. Due to rapid deforestation and depletion of genetic stocks, concerted efforts must be made to evolve methods for mass propagation, production of short duration trees with a rapid turnover of biomass, and the induction of genetic variability for the production of novel fruit and forest trees which are high-yielding, resistant to pests and diseases, and which display increased photosynthetic efficiency.

Because of the energy crisis, efforts are being made to look for alternatives to the conventional sources of energy. The conversion of solar energy for increased biomass production especially as firewood, is regarded as a promising source of bioenergy. Plant derived biomass provides as much as 15% of the world's energy needs. Wood is the largest biomass source of fuel energy. It is expected that the world's demand for wood will double by the end of the century. Also, with the ever increasing demand for paper, there is a pressure to develop fast-growing pulp wood plants for rapid turnover of the product. Attention is also being paid to fruit trees for an increased production of alcohol for use as a fuel. Harvesting solar energy through increased photosynthesis, and the bioformation of tree products for biomass energy production in the form of deposition of large quantities of cellulose, lignins and hemicellulose is being attempted.

Biomass production involves the use of fast growing plants to provide raw materials which can be converted by various processes to a range of energy-rich materials. A typical industrial use of biomass is the conversion of plant materials such as lignocellulose to alcohols, and on a smaller scale to biogas (Carbon dioxide and methane). The production of ethanol in combination with petroleum may help to satisfy the demand for fuel and thus arrest a total reliance on fossil fuels.

7.1.1 Fuel Resource

There are several ways in which plant material may be used as a substrate for the production of energy. Products of agricultural crops supply the major proportion of food for people and animals, in addition to certain raw materials. In this respect, it is worth noting that the total food materials produced on cultivated lands has been estimated to account for only 6 per cent of the total biomass derived from primary photosynthesis. The major proportion of the global primary photosynthetic production occurs in woodlands and forests (44%), and this is converted to usable energy by burning either to obtain heat, or to produce steam to drive machines and turbines which produce electricity. Other alternatives include the conversion or extraction of fuels and chemicals from primary products. Energy is also generated by feeding animals on grassland and the utilization of these to perform work. The move towards the use of biomass-derived fuels and chemicals has come about because unlike the fossil fuels such as petroleum and natural gas, biomass is, in the long run, completely renewable.

The useful components of biomass are sugars, starch and lignocellulose. Plants producing high levels of sugar include sugar-cane, sugar-beet and millet. These are perhaps the most suitable and readily available substrates for a wide variety of processes, especially those geared to produce alcohol. Plant products containing starch include the grain crops, particularly maize, rice and wheat, as well as potatoes and other root crops like sweet potato and cassava. Starch, however, must be first broken down by digestion or hydrolysis to mono and oligosaccharides, if it is to be used in fermentation processes.

These two sources of biomass represent a relatively small proportion of those available for use in chemical or energy fuel production programmes, competing with demand as food sources. (In Brazil, sugar-cane is specifically grown as a substrate for gasohol).

Undoubtedly, the major source of biomass for various biotechnological processes is lignocellulose derived from agriculture and forestry. Lignocellulose contains three major chemical components—lignin, cellulose and a collection of polysaccharides collectively known as hemicellulose. There are several energy conversion systems available for dealing with lignocellulose biomass substrates. Biomass can be burnt directly to yield energy or can be subjected to pyrolysis or gasification. These processes yield mainly methane, or with the necessary additional synthetic steps, methanol.

7.1.2 Micropropagation Technique

The world demand for wood in 2000 AD. is expected to be 300 million metric tonnes as compared to 130 million metric tonnes in 1970. This drastic increase is primarily due to its increasing use as fuel energy. In view of the urgent need for biofuel energy, micropropagation has far reaching implications in mass production, propagation and tree improvement programmes. By using *in vitro* techniques, a desired tree, selected on the basis of its past performance, may be vegetatively propagated and cloned at an enormously rapid rate, which by conventional methods of cutting, grafting and other silvicultural or horticultural practices may take years. This faster rate of multiplication enables rapid production of phytomass energy. Various aspects for which protoplast, cell, tissue and organ culture technology can be employed for the improvement of trees are given in Fig. 7.1.

Micropropagation involves three stages:

(a) establishment of cultures,

(b) regeneration of plants, and

(c) transfer of plants from test-tube to soil. The *in vitro* plant regeneration may be directly from the explants such as segments, buds, meristems etc. or indirectly via initiation and differentiation of callus. The first method ensures maintenance of the clones (clonal stability); the second method generally results

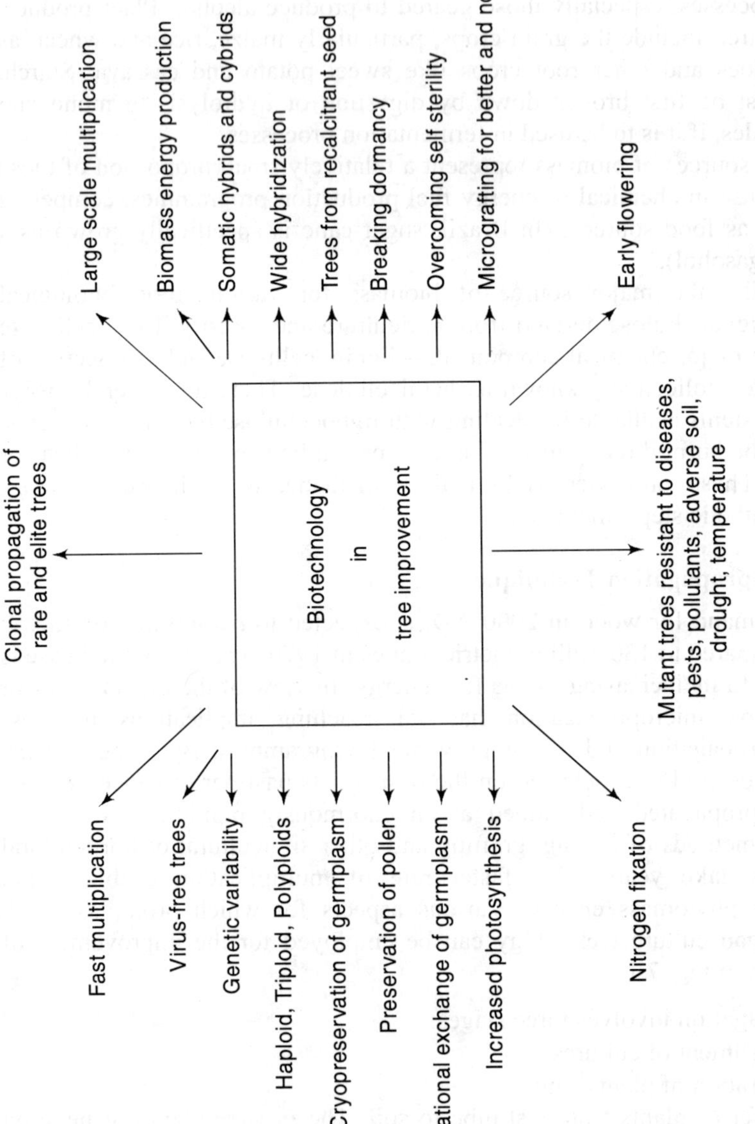

Figure 7.1

Various aspects for which protoplast, cell, tissue and organ culture technology can be employed for the improvement of trees.

in genetic variability. In the direct method, the explants from young and juvenile trees are easier to grow than those from mature and old trees. Moreover, there are considerable differences in the regeneration and morphogenetic potential of various parts of the plant. Embryo culture has been employed as a useful tool for direct regeneration in trees where seeds are dormant, recalcitrant, or where they abort at early stages of development. In the indirect method, the callus cultures on periodic subculturing, undergo genetic erosions, mutations, changes in ploidy etc. This is a novel and rich source of genetic variability. The advantage of callus culture is the enormous number of plants that can be produced from a single culture. A number of examples of the differentiation of tree species from callus cultures are known (Table 7.1).

Table 7.1

Some fruit and forest angiosperm tree species from which complete plants have been obtained

Species	Culture
Acacia koa	Shoot-tip
Acer rubrum	Shoot-tip callus
Aesculus hippocastanum	Anther
Albizzia lebbeck	Hypocotyl
Alnus glutinosa	Epicotyl
Alnus rubra	Shoot-tip
Ananas comosus	Axillary bud
Betula pendula	Stem
	Anther
Broussonetia kazinoki	Hypocotyl
Carica papaya	Shoot-tip
Castanea sativa	Embryonic axis
	Shoot apex
Citrus maxima	Stem callus
C. sinensis	Stem callus
Coffea arabica	Callus
Corylus avellana	Embryonic axis
Elaeis guincesis	Callus
Eucalyptus alba	Hypocotyl
E. citriodora	Lignotuber
E. grandis	Axillary bud
Hevea brasiliensis	Anther
Liquidambar styraciflua	Hypocotyl

Contd...

Species	Culture
Malus	Shoot apex
Morus alba	Shoot-tip
Musa	Shoot apex
Olea europaea	Stem
Paulownia taiwaniana	Stem
P. tomentosa	Embryo
Populus x canadensis	Shoot-tip
P. canescens	Shoot-tip
P. euroamericana	Shoot-tip
P. nigra	Anther
P. tremula	Stem
P. tremuloides	Stem
Populus hybrids	Anther
Prunus amygdalus	Callus
Prunus domestica	Root callus
Pyrus communis	Shoot-tip
Santalum album	Hypocotyl
Sapium sebiferum	Embryo, callus
Tectona grandis	Hypocotyl, stem, shoot-tip
Ulmus americana	Hypocotyl
Ulmus campestris	Callus

Induction of somatic embryogenesis is the most important mode of micropropagation. This enables us to produce millions of embryos which are regarded as 'seeds'. When these embryos are encapsulated, artificial seeds are produced. Micrografting is a relatively recent technique which involves the excision of the extreme tip of the shoot, preferably a dome (0.1-0.5 mm) and its eventual grafting on to the root stock. After this, the plants are transferred to the liquid medium, which ensures the harmonious development of the graft. This

Table 7.2

Some fruit tree species in which virus has been eliminated by micro-grafting.

Tree	Virus
Apple	Apple stem grooving
Apricot	Chlorotic leaf spot virus
Banana	Chlorotic leaf spot virus
Citrus	A number of viruses
Fig	Mosaic virus
Peach	Sharka virus
	Ringspot virus

technique helps us to eliminate viruses which infest trees and cause heavy losses both in the fruit yield and biomass production. Table 7.2 gives the names of some fruit tree species in which virus has been eliminated by micrografting.

7.1.3 Higher production of Phytomass by Increased Photosynthesis

Phytomass production depends on the plant type and its photosynthetic efficiency. In general, as compared to agricultural crops, trees are photosynthetically inactive and photosynthetic rates of single leaves in trees may be half of those in crops. Harvesting solar energy through increased photosynthesis, for biomass energy production in the form of deposition of cellulose, lignins and hemicellulose is being attempted. The photosynthetic efficiency could be increased in the less efficient trees by protoplast fusion and gene transfer.

7.2 Production Of Disease Free And Disease Resistant Plants

Substantial crop losses occur each year due to attacks by insect pests or microbial pathogens. Genetic engineering promises to have an enormous impact on the improvement of crop species. Plant breeding has played a major part in providing plants with better resistance to insect pest. Genetic transformation can rapidly accelerate plant breeding efforts for crop protection. Genetically engineering resistance to disease by recombinant DNA methods has been hampered by insufficient knowledge on the basis of pathogenicity and resistance mechanisms. Cloning of plant genes responsible for pest and disease resistance will help in elucidating some of the biological mechanisms of resistance.

7.2.1 Virus-Resistant Plants

A possible way to engineer disease resistant would be to isolate the resistant genes from plants that are resistant to a pathogen and to transfer them to susceptible plants. This approach is complicated by the fact that resistance could be a polygenic trait. Even if resistance is encoded by a single gene, identifying and isolating such a gene from the host could be very difficult, largely due to the complexity of the host-pathogen interactions. Still it is possible to produce plants that are resistant to disease, by transferring one or a few genes into them. Researchers have tried to use the *Agrobacterium* gene transfer system to produce tobacco and tomato plants with an increased resistance to tobacco mosaic virus.

In 1929 McKinney observed that tobacco plants infected with one strain of a virus resist infection by a second related strain. This phenomenon, termed cross protection, could be demonstrated with a number of viruses for which distinct strains could be found. This discovery led plant pathologists to embark on a search for viruses that cause mild symptoms or no symptoms at all, when they infect plants. Cross protection has been successfully applied in agriculture and has been effective with a number of viral diseases. Some of the examples include protection of citrus plants from Citrus tristeza virus, protection of glass house grown tomatoes from tobacco mosaic virus and protection of papaya plants from papaya ringspot virus. Application of cross protection to large scale agriculture has its drawbacks: (i) it requires the widespread distribution of a virus in the growing environment—a practice that many agriculturists find unsatisfactory. (ii) a virulent strain may evolve from the mild viral strain and produce greater crop loss than protection. (iii) infection by even a mild virus can cause small but significant decreases in crop yields. (iv) cross protection depends on isolating and characterizing an appropriate mild viral strain, which often requires a considerable effort.

There are different hypotheses to explain the molecular mechanisms of cross protection. One theory is that the first virus somehow interferes with the replication of R.NA of the second virus. Almost all plant viruses have RNA genomes and such an interference would effectively block their life-cycles. The interference might result because the RNAs of the two viruses are so closely related that RNA from the first can hybridize with a small amount of RNA from the second virus that would be present early in infection and prevent either its replication or translation into protein. Alternatively, the first virus might in some way 'use up' the machinery needed for RNA replication, thereby slowing or preventing the reproduction of the second virus. Another hypothesis suggests that cross protection blocks the establishment of an infection by the second virus. This may be done by preventing the virus from reorganizing or binding to its receptor on the cell surface, as a result the release of its RNA genome inside the cell might somehow be inhibited.

Although the mechanism of cross protection is not fully understood, several investigators have suggested that protection from viral disease could be achieved with the help of gene transfer. Scientists working with tobacco mosaic virus (TMV) were able to produce a DNA copy of the RNA genome of TMV and to identify and isolate the gene that encodes the viral coat protein. They joined the coat protein gene to other DNA sequences that supply the signals needed for the initiation and termination of transcription in plant cells. The resulting chimaeric gene was inserted into a Ti plasmid from which the tumour-inducing genes had been deleted. Then *Agrobacterium tumefaciens* was used to transfer the Ti plasmid with the chimaeric gene into tomato and tobacco cells. Plants were regenerated from the cells that had acquired the new DNA. The plants yielded seeds and the seeds were germinated. The young seedlings that had been transformed by the chimaeric gene did not develop any infection or the symptoms developed more slowly than the control plants.

Scientists also constructed an expression vector containing the 35S promoter from cauliflower mosaic virus (CaMV) , a cDNA encoding the coat protein gene of the U1 strain of TMV and a polyadenylation signal from nopaline synthase gene. This vector was introduced into tobacco and tomato cells and plants were regenerated. Progeny of self-fertilized transgenic plants expressing high levels of the coat protein gene did not develop any infection, or the disease symptoms developed more slowly than the controls. Also scientists have cloned RNA encoding the CP of alfalfa mosaic virus (A1MV) and engineered it into an expression vector downstream from the CaMV 35S promoter. The cDNA was flanked at the 3′ end by the nopaline synthase polyadenylation site. Leaf discs of tobacco and tomato were transformed with *A. tumefaciens* containing this construct, selected for kanamycin resistance and regenerated into plants. Progeny from a single transgenic tobacco plant did not develop any infection or the disease symptoms developed more slowly than the controls. The engincering of resistance against TMV in tobacco by expression of TMV coat protein gene has been achieved. Likewise resistance has been created against many other viruses in many plants. Resistance to specific viruses by expression of a negative-sense coat protein gene transcript has been shown for the potato leaf roll virus and potato virus X.

Genetically engineered cross protection generally provides an applicable way of producing virus resistant plants. Protection against fungal and bacterial pathogens might be obtained by transferring a fungal or bacterial gene for virulence into the target plants. Recently, a new class of bactericidal proteins (lysozyme, cecropins and attacins) have been identified in the pupae of the giant silk moth *Hylophora cecropia.* These lytic proteins have also shown a potent *in vitro* antifungal activity against pathogenic fungi, including *Phytophthora infestans*. Transgenic tobacco plants that express barley ribosome-inactivating protein (RIP), exhibited heightened protection against agronomically deleterious fungus *Rhizoctonia solani.* Similarly, tobacco pathogen related proteins (PR), namely PR-S and osmotin, have been shown to be serologieally related to zeamatin, an antifungal protein of maize.

7.2.2 Insect Resistant Plants

Another application of genetic engineering with important implications for crop improvement is the production of insect resistant plants. Progress in engineering insect resistance in transgenic plants has been achieved through the expression of the insect toxin gene of *Bacillus thuringiensis* in plants. (The parasporal protein crystals produced as spores by this bacterium have a natural insecticidal effect). Experiments have shown that the region essential for toxicity resides in the N-terminal portion of the protein, extending approximately from amino acid 29 to amino acid 610. A fragment of the toxin gene from *B. thuringiensis* subsp. *kurstaki* HD-1, encoding amino acids 1-725 was isolated and engineered by the addition of synthetic oligonucleotide linkers and inserted into the expression cassette vector pMON316 at the BglII site to create pMON9711. In pMON9711 the *B. thuringiensis* toxin gene is flanked by the CaMV 355 promoter and the 3′ end of the nopaline synthase gene. PMON 9711 also contains a chimaeric neomycin phosphotransferase gene which confers kanamycin resistance on transformed plant cells. Transgenic tomato plants regenerated from transformed tomato cells pMON9711 were resistant to insects.

Researchers have begun to explore new ways of using *B. thuringiensis* toxins for insect control. One approach that is now being tried involves introducing the cloned toxin genes into other bacteria that may survive longer in the environment than *B. thuringiensis.* Another approach is to construct plants with their own built-in insecticidal toxin. The purified protein produced by *B. thuringiensis* toxin gene is as toxic as the spore crystals. Recently scientists have used the Ti plasmid to introduce the cloned toxin gene into tobacco, tomato, potato and cotton plants. Soon, it may be possible to engineer genetically modified varieties of crop plants that have built-in insecticidal toxins specific for the insect pests that feed on the plants in question. Baculo virus and *B. thuringiensis* provide an alternative to chemicals for controlling insect pests of agronomically important plant species. Bt toxin is pathogenic to many lepidopteran, coleopteran and dipteran insects.

7.2.3 Herbicide Resistant Plants

Herbicide resistance can be achieved with several different means such as

(i) reduced herbicide uptake,
(ii) overproduction of the herbicide target site,
(iii) metabolism, modification, or conjugation of the herbicide,
(iv) mutual alterations in the herbicide target site, thus lowering the affinity to the herbicide,
(v) tissue culture,
(vi) gene amplification,
(vii) mutation, and
(viii) genetic engineering.

Herbicides are widely used in agriculture to control weeds. They inhibit plant growth by blocking the biosynthesis of essential amino acids. These include: glyphosate, N-(Phosphonomethyl)—glycine, which inhibits the synthesis of aromatic amino acids; the sulphonyl ureas and imidazolinones, which block branched-chain amino acid biosynthesis; and phosphinothricin which inhibits glutamine biosynthesis. If a cell is deprived of these amino acids, it will not be able to synthesize proteins and will die. Different experiments in plants have shown that EPSP (5-enolpyruvyl shikimate 3-phosphate) synthase is the primary target of the herbicide. Initial attempts to engineer glyphosate resistance in transgenic plants have employed two different strategies. In the first study, a mutant gene encoding glyphosate-resistant EPSP synthase was isolated from *Salmonella typhimurium.* The isolation of this gene allowed the construction of two chimaeric genes, one in which the EPSP synthase coding sequence was flanked by the regulatory regions from the octopine synthase gene, and the other in which the coding sequence was flanked by the mannopine synthase promoter and the *tml3′* region. The chimaeric genes were then introduced into tobacco cells using Ri plasmid vectors (Ri plasmids are root-inciting plasmids harboured by virulent *Agrobacterium rhizogenes* strains carrying genes essential for root production). Plants were regenerated from the transformed cells. The transformed plants carrying the chimaeric genes were two to three-fold more resistant to glyphosate than the control plants. In the second study, overproduction of the glyphosate-sensitive plant EPSP synthase in transgenic *Petunia* plants was shown to confer substantial resistance to glyphosate. The full-length cDNA clone encoding *Petunia* EPSP synthase was isolated from a glyphosate resistant *Petunia* cell line that overproduces (15-20 times more) the herbicide sensitive form of EPSP synthase. A chimaeric gene was constructed in which the coding sequence of the *Petunia* EPSP synthase precursor enzyme was placed under the control of the cauliflower mosaic virus 35S promoter. The chimaeric gene was introduced into *Petunia* cells. When *Petunia* cells were raised in culture and plants containing chimaeric gene were regenerated, they were found to survive glyphosate spraying.

The major difference between the two methods is that, in the first study, the bacterial enzyme was not targeted to chloroplasts whereas in the second study it was targeted to the chloroplast. Recent studies have shown that the plant EPSP synthase activity is localized in chloroplasts which represent a major site of aromatic amino acid biosynthesis. Genetically engineered herbicide resistance may have commercial utility in the near future. Transgenic plants have been obtained conferring herbicide resistance such as glyphosate, gluphosinate and biolaphos, 2,4-D, chlorsulphuron, sulphonylurea and bromoxynil. Scientists in the United States have bombarded wheat calluses using a minute particle gun, with bacterial plasmids containing bar genes which provide resistance to herbicide Basta and have produced transgenic herbicide resistant wheat plants. Before commercialization of herbicide resistant crop plants, factors such as potential loss in vigour and yield, herbicide performance, crop and chemical registration costs, potential for outcrossing to weed species and the potential for a crop becoming a weed should be considered.

7.3 Induction And Selection Of Mutants

The history of plant breeding has witnessed revolutionary changes since the time of natural selection. Today, biotechnology is used as a valuable tool for plant breeders.

7.3.1 Biochemical Mutants

The manipulations with cultured plant cells has resulted in the isolation of a number of variant cell lines. Variants resistant to antibiotics, amino acids, amino acid analogues, chlorate, nucleic acid base analogues, fungal toxin, environmental stresses (salinity, chilling, high temperature, aluminium toxicity etc.) and herbicides, have been successfully isolated through direct selection while indirect selection has been reported for auxotrophs. Table 7.3 enumerates the various biochemical mutants selected and where regeneration of complete plantlets has been achieved.

Table 7.3

List of some biochemical mutants/variants cell line of higher plants obtained by plant cell, tissue, and organ culture techniques. (after Mantell, S.H. et *al.,* 1985)

Phenotypes (resistant to chemical/environmental factor(s)/auxotrophy/autotrophy		Plant Species	Plant regeneration	Modes of inheritance
(1)	(2)	(3)	(4)	
1.	Resistant Mutants			
	Antibiotic resistance	*Petunia hybrida*	–	Not known
	Streptomycin	*Nicotiana tabacum*	+	Maternally inherited
		N. sylvestris	+	Not known
	Kanamycin	*N. sylvestris*	–	Not known
	Chloramphenicol	*N. sylvestris*	+	Semi-dominant
	Amino acid resistance			
	Threonine	*N. tabacum*	–	Not known
	Valine	*N. tabacum*	+	Sexual transmission (Dominant & Semidominant)
	Amino acid analogue resistance			

Contd...

Table 7.3 Contd...

Phenotypes (resistant to chemical/environmental factor(s)/auxotrophy/autotrophy		Plant Species	Plant regeneration	Modes of inheritance
(1)	(2)	(3)	(4)	
	5-methyltryptophan	*N. tabacum*	–	Not known
		Daucus carota	+	Not known
		D. carota	+	Not known
		Solanum tuberosum	–	Not known
	p-flurophenylalanine	*D. carota*	–	Not known
		N. tabacum	–	Not known
		Acer pseudoplata nus	–	Not known
	Ethionine	*D. carota*	–	Not known
		N. sylvestris	–	Not known
	S-2-aminoethylcystine and hydroxylysine	*N tabacutn*	–	Not known
	S-2-aminoethylcysteine	*Hordeum vulgare*	+	Sexually transmitted
		Oryza sativa	–	Not known
		D. carota	–	Not known
	Hydroxyproline	*D. carota*	–	Not known
	a-aminocaprylic acid and	*D. carota*	–	Not known
	Selenomethionine			
	p-fluorophenylalanine	*D. carota*	+	?
	+ ethionine			
	+ aminoethylcysteine +			
	5-methyltryptophan in combination			
	Methionine sulfoximine			
	Nucleic acid base analogue resistance			

Contd...

Table 7.3 Contd…

Phenotypes (resistant to chemical/environmental factor(s)/auxotrophy/autotrophy		Plant Species	Plant regeneration	Modes of inheritance
(1)	(2)	(3)	(4)	
	5-bromode oxyuridine	*N. tabacum*	+	Sexual transmission, semi Dominant (Mendelian trait)
		Glycine max	–	Not known
		A. pseudoplatanus	–	Not known
	8-azaguanine	*A. pseudoplatanus*	–	Not known
	N. tabacum	–	Not known	
	Aminopterine	*Datura innoxia*	+	Not known
	5-fluorouracil	*D. carota*	+	Not known
	Herbicide resistance			
	Picloram	*N. tabacum*	+	Dominant, semi-dominant allele of single nuclear gene
	Amitrole	*N. tabacum*	+	Not known
	N-phenylcarbamate	*N. tabacum*	+	Not known
	2,4-Dichlorophenoxy-acetic acid	*N. sylvestris*	–	Not known
		Citrus sinensis	+	Not known
		D. carota	–	Not known
	Fungal toxin resistance			
	Methionine sulfoximine	*N. tabacum*	+	Semi-dominant

Contd…

Table 7.3 Contd…

Phenotypes (resistant to chemical/environmental factor(s)/auxotrophy/autotrophy		Plant Species	Plant regeneration	Modes of inheritance
(1)	(2)	(3)	(4)	
	Helminthosporium maydis toxin	*Zea mays*	+	Maternally inherited
		Saccharum officinalis	+	Not known
	Chilling resistance	*N. sylvestris*	+	Not sexually transmitted
		Capsicum annum	–	Not known
	Sodium chloride resistance	*N. sylvestris*	–	Not known
		N. tabacum	+	Not known
		C. annuum	–	Not known
		Citrus sinensis	–	Not known
		D. innoxia	+	Not known
		Medicago sativa	–	Not known
		Kickxia ramosissima	+	Not known
	Aluminium resistance	*Lycopersicon esculentum*	–	Not known
	Mercury resistance	*P. hybrida*	–	Not known
	Chlorate resistance	*N. tabacum*	–	Not known
	Cycloheximide resistance	*D. carota*	+	Not known
		N. tabacum	+	Epigenetic
	Colchicine resistance	*D. carota*	–	Not known
	Abscisic acid resistance	*N. sylvestris*	–	Not known
2.	Auxotrophic Mutants Hypoxanthine Biotin p-aminobenzoic acid	*N. tabacum*	+	Leaky auxotrophs
	Arginine			
	Lysine			
	Proline			

Contd…

Table 7.3 Contd…

Phenotypes (resistant to chemical/environmental factor(s)/auxotrophy/autotrophy		Plant Species	Plant regeneration	Modes of inheritance
(1)	(2)	(3)	(4)	
	Auxin	*A. pseudoplatanus*	–	Not known
	Thiamine	*Arabidiopsis spp.*	+	Not known
	Prolien	*Z. mays*	+	Not known
3.	Autotrophic Mutants			
	Cytokinin	*N. tabacum*	+	Not known
	Auxin	*N. tabacum*	+	Not known
	D. *carota*	?	?	
4.	Visually Selected Mutants			
	Pigment mutants			
	Altered-carotene and lycopene concentrations	*D. carota*	–	Not known
	Altered anthocyanin levels	*D. carota*	–	Not known
	Altered pigmentation of plant body	*D. innoxia*	+	Not known
	Chlorophyll deficient	*N. sylvestris*	?	?
	Different carotenoid contents			
	contents	*D. carota*	+	Epigenetic

– Regeneration not achieved
+ Regeneration achieved
? Not clear

The criterion for antibiotic resistance was the ability of the cells to form either 'green type' or 'white type' callus on medium containing lethal doses of antibiotic. These lines varied in their degrees of resistance depending upon the extent of deformation in the ultrastructure of their chloroplasts and mitochondria. The probable mechanism attributed to streptomycin resistance is an alteration in the chloroplast or mitochondrial 70s ribosomes, as is known to occur in some microorganisms.

The synthesis of amino acids is controlled by feed-back inhibition in which the end-product amino acid inhibits the first step of its own synthesis.

Deregulation of the first step enzyme permits accumulation or overproduction of the end-product. So scientists have succeeded in selecting feed-back insensitive cells *in vitro*. Also cell lines that are resistant to analogues of specific amino acids have been selected. Cell lines that are resistant to fungal toxin, herbicide and environmental stresses, have been isolated.

Physical and chemical mutagens are used in the explants of different species to generate mutations. Table 7.4 lists the plant species and the explants used in mutation experiments.

Single cell and protoplast culture systems have proved to be valuable for mutagenesis since the presence of discrete cells in these avoids the development of excessive numbers of chimaeral mixtures of cells that are often obtained when multicellular tissues or organs are exposed to mutagens. Protoplasts are particularly suitable in this regard since they have less tendency to form aggregates (Fig. 7.2)

Table 7.4

Plant species and explants used in mutation experiments

Plant species	Explant
(a) Cereals:	
— wheat	anthers
— Rice	anthers
— Barley	anthers
(b) Legumes:	
— Pea	axillary buds
— Mungbean	axillary buds
— Soybean	axillary buds
— Chick pea	axillary buds
— Peanut	cotyledons
(c) Others:	
— Brassicas	anthers
— Tobacco	anthers
— Cucurbits	Cotyledons
— Potato	node cuttings, petioles and stem cuttings
— Garlic	shoot meristem
— Banana	corms with shoot tips, young leaves
— Tomato	hypocotyl, leaf segments pedicels etc.

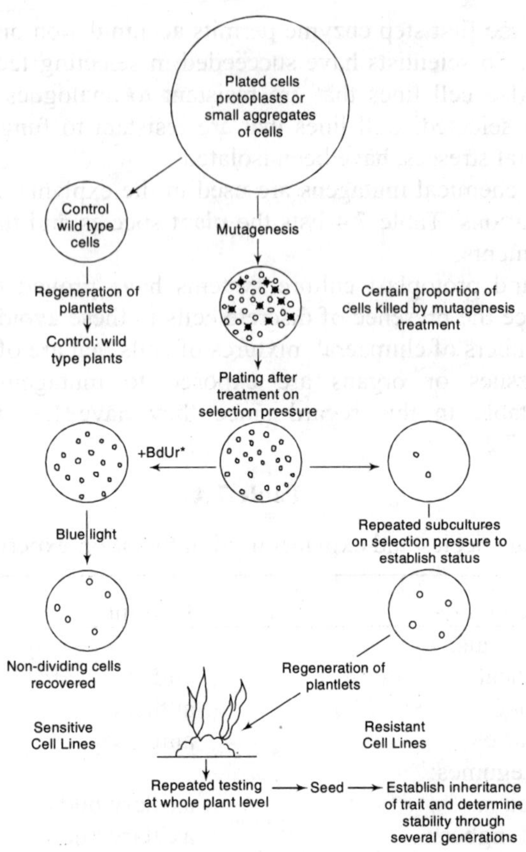

Figure 7.2

Stage employed in the selection of a mutant from a cell culture line. 5-Bromo-deoxyuridine is an analogue of thymine. Dividing cells incorporate the analogue in their DNA and these cells are killed on subsequent exposure to fluorescent light. Non-dividing (sensitive) cells survive and can be rescued.

(***Source:*** *Mantell, S.H.; Mathews, J.A.; McKee, R.A. Principles of Plant Biotechnology.* © *Oxford, Blackwell Scientific Publications. Reprinted by permission.*)

7.4 Production Through Haploid Technique

Haploids have played a significant role in the propagation and breeding of plants even though limited success has been achieved with regard to trees.

7.4.1 Major Economic Crops

Androgenesis has been observed in *Coffea arabica.* Anthers have been cultured in *Cocos nucifera* and scientists have obtained various stages of pollen embryos up to the torpedo stage. Anther culture of *Hevea brasiliensis* has been successful and plantlets have been produced.

Callus, embryoids, or plants have been obtained using anther culture in the following genera; *Anemone, Brassica, Camellia, Datura, Festuca, Hordeum, Hyoscyamus, Lotium, Lycopersicum, Nicotiana, Oryza, Paeonia, Petunia, Scopolia, Secale, Solanum, Triticale, Triticum* and *Zea.*

7.4.2 Fruit Crops

Rhizogenic callus has been obtained in *Prunus allium.* Callus was also observed in *P. armenica.* The anthers of the hybrid *Prunus* and *Pandora* also yielded callus. Callus from cherry cultivars, pollen embryos from apple cultivars, callus from grapevine and orange have been reported.

7.4.3 Forest Trees

By forest trees we generally mean those which can be exploited for their timber. Many species of *Populus* and their hybrids have produced callus from anther. Dihaploid callus has been obtained from *Ulmus americana.*

7.4.4 Ornamental Trees

Callus and plantlets have been obtained from a large number of species such as *Ginkgo biloba, Taxus baccata, Pinus resinosa, Cassia fistula, Sacaranda acutifolia.*

7.5 Somatic Hybrids

The liberation of protoplasts from their rigid cell walls renders them amenable to fusion. Together with the capacity to regenerate plants from these protoplasts, this provides a unique opportunity for the production of somatic hybrids. The attraction of the procedure is threefold: (i) it offers to extend the possibility of hybrid formation to widely unrelated forms unable to interact sexually; (ii) it offers an asexual means of effecting gene transfer either of whole genomes, or of partial genomes; (iii) traits can be transferred without the need for detailed knowledge of their precise genetic base. A number of plants have been regenerated through protoplast fusion technique.

With the successful production of hybrid plants at the tetraploid and hexaploid levels, both for inter and intraspecific fusions, the number of practical applications of fusion technology are increasing. Characters from wild species that are sexually incompatible have been introduced via fusion. Somatic hybridization provides the opportunity to combine dihaploid lines selected for different agronomic characters. This bypasses dihaploid sterility problems, and heterosis can be maximized without the reassortment of dominant characters at meiosis. Other approaches to genetic manipulation include the irradiation of donor protoplasts with useful characters, to fragment their genomes, followed by fusion to tetraploid acceptor protoplasts. Protoplast fusion also provides a means of transferring cytoplasmic traits into another genomic background. An interesting feature of somatic hybrids is that they normally exhibit a range of phenotypes because individual plants may possess chloroplasts from either parent and recombined mitochondria. A background of somaclonal variation may be added to this. Thus new combinations of genes may be obtained after fusion even from sexually compatible parents.

7.6 Transformation Through Uptake Of Foreign Genome

During the past few years, there has been a vast accumulation of knowledge regarding the structural and functional organization of genes in higher plants, and factors that control their expression. This increased interest in plant molecular biology has been greatly facilitated by the development of gene transfer systems which allow genes to be introduced into cells of a variety of plant species. As it is possible to regenerate fertile plants from single transformed cells, engineered genes integrated stably into plant chromosomes can serve as powerful tools to study important physiological and development processes. Of fundamental importance for stable transformation of plants has been the development of the *Agrobacterium* Ti plasmid system.

7.6.1 Transformation of Plants

The successful development of methods to transfer genes into plants was made possible by engineering genes to confer a selectable phenotype to transformed cells. The first such selectable marker gene for plant cells was a chimaeric construction using the bacterial cloning sequence for neomycin phosphotransferase with 5′ and 3′ sequences from the nopaline synthase gene from *Agrobacterium tumefaciens.* This gene construction permitted plant cells to grow on medium containing otherwise inhibitory concentrations of kanamycin. The other key requirements for producing transgenic plants are a DNA delivery method and procedures for regenerating whole plants from the transformed cells.

To make use of the natural gene transfer mechanism available in Ti plasmid, scientists have designed a shuttle vector that can replicate in *Escherichia coli* where recombinant DNA manipulations are easily handled, and is then transferred into *A. tumefaciens* in the preparation for transfer into plants. There are two basic modes of maintenance of the shuttle vectors in *Agrobacterium* either by integration into the Ti plasmid by recombination at a region of DNA homology or by autonomous replication in *trans* to the Ti plasmid. The former type of vector is referred to as a *cis* or integrating vector while the latter is called a *trans* or binary vector. In most cases, they accomplish the same goal of shuttling genes from *E. coli* to *A. tumefaciens* in a T DNA package that can then be transferred to plants.

The essential components of the vectors include plasmid functions for replication and/or integration in bacteria as well as spectinomycin and streptomycin resistant genes for genetic manipulations in bacteria. They also include a chimaeric selectable marker for plant antibiotic resistance such as neomycin phosphotransferase which makes transferred plant cells resistant to kanamycin, and a border sequence to identify the end of the new T DNA. There is also a scorable marker, the gene for nopaline synthase that provides a powerful genetic tool for monitoring the presence of T DNA in plants and their progeny. It also has a site to add the favourite gene.

Techniques to grow plant cells and tissues in culture and to regenerate intact plants from them provides the basis for the stable genetic modification of plants. The simplest and most widely practised approach is based on variations of the leaf disc technique where explants are infected with *Agrobacterium* strains and then selected and regenerated in a single step. In some instances, plant transformation is achieved through protoplasts which can take up exogenously added DNA. These protoplasts are cultured to give rise to callus and from callus mature plants are obtained. It is also possible to transfer genes into meristematic or reproductive tissues of intact plants.

7.6.2 Gene Expression

In general, it appears that regulated genes are expressed approximately in transgenic plants despite their integration at a different chromosomal location, and that *cis*-control elements programming their expression are in close proximity to the coding sequence. This implies that *trans*-acting proteins involved in regulating the expression of these genes are capable of finding their cognate sequences and activating transcription at different chromosomal locations. As the introduced genes are regulated appropriately in heterologous plants, species specificity does not appear to be a critical factor. This suggests a remarkable evolutionary conservation of regulatory factors governing tissue specific expression of genes.

Making use of the Ti plasmid system with the newly constructed vectors, scientists have been able to produce plants that are resistant to herbicide, viruses, insects and pests (Refer Section 7.2).

7.6.3 Transgenic Plants

Genetic engineering can be used to introduce into a plant, genes which do not exist in any member of the same plant family, or even in any plant. As discussed already in Chapter Four, different cloning vectors are used for introducing the foreign genes. If genetically engineered plants are to be used commercially, then the following requirements must be satisfied: (i) introduction of the gene(s) of interest to all plant cells; (ii) stable maintenance of the new genetic information, (iii) transmission of the new gene to subsequent generations and (iv) expression of the cloned genes in the correct cells at the correct time.

Ti plasmids of *Agrobacterium tumefaciens* have been used widely as effective vectors for obtaining transgenic plants, For a foreign gene to be expressed in plant cells it is essential that it be preceded by a promoter recognized by the host cell. Since opine synthesis is not essential, vectors have been constructed in which the foreign gene is placed under the control of the *nos* (nopaline synthase) promoter. The number of useful traits, mostly single gene, that have been engineered in crop plants is growing slowly. Until recently, many plant genes have been cloned, characterized and transferred into plant cells. These are: isopentyltransferase, fungal protection, nematode resistance, phaseolin gene, yeast ornithine decarboxylase, chalcone synthase, male sterility, cold resistance, virus resistance, glyphosate tolerance and production of antibodies. There is still an uphill task of identifying the sets of genes that regulate important agronomic traits in food crops such as yield, tillering, flowering characteristics, sterility, incompatibility and morphology. In 2004, transgenic plants were cultivated in 200 million acres of the world. Out of this, 144.5 million acres were used for herbicide tolerant plants, 38.5 million acres for insect resistant (Bt) plants, and 17.0 million acres for other transgenic plants.

Transgenic plants can be used as bioreactors for obtaining virtually unlimited quantities of commercially useful proteins, biologically active peptides and antibodies for large scale production. This is mainly due to the fact that techniques have been perfected to generate transgenic plants to the point where a foreign protein can be targeted to an organ of choice as well as to subcellular compartments.

7.7 Nitrogen Fixation

Nitrogen is extremely important in agriculture because it is a constituent of proteins, nucleic acids and other essential molecules in all organisms. Most of this nitrogen is derived from reduced or oxidized forms of nitrogen in the soil by growing plants, because plants and animals are unable to utilize nitrogen, which is abundant (nearly 80 per cent) in the atmosphere. Yields of many crops, particularly cereals, have been increased over the years by the application of large quantities of nitrogen fertilizers. This practice is expensive and leads to the eventual contamination of waterways with high levels of nitrates. The only other sources available to plants are from decomposing organic matter, soil reserves, biological nitrogen fixation, and from other sources such as automobile exhaust. Biological nitrogen fixation (enzymic conversion of N_2 gas to ammonia) is the most important source of fixed nitrogen entering the soils. A relatively small number of bacterial species have the special ability to reduce or fix atmospheric N_2 to form ammonia, a product that can be used by plants and other microbes as a building block for the synthesis of amino adds and other nitrogenous compounds. On a global scale the amounts of N_2 fixed by these bacteria are nearly 200 million tonnes each year.

The reduction of N_2 is catalyzed by the nitrogenase system, which is very similar in composition and function in all prokaryotes which produce it. Nitrogenase is found only in prokaryotic microorganisms and thus eukaryotes, such as plants, can benefit from N_2 fixation only if they interact with N_2-fixing species of microorganisms or obtain the fixed nitrogen after the death of the organisms. Nitrogenase functions only under anaerobic conditions because it is irreversibly inactivated by oxygen. The fixation of N_2 requires large amounts of energy, about 30 moles of ATP per mole of N_2 reduced, and thus acts as a major drain for energy produced by N_2 fixing microorganisms. The natural supply of nitrogen to certain plants is achieved by close associations between them and nitrogen-fixing microorganisms. Of the important crop species, only the legumes exhibit this phenomenon; nitrogen-fixing nodules are formed on their roots due to a symbiotic relationship with bacteria. Nodule formation depends on recognition between the appropriate bacterial strain and the legume host.

7.7.1 Nitrogen Fixing Organisms and Associations

The ability to fix N_2 is found in a wide range of prokaryotic microorganisms, some of which are listed in Table 7.5.

All these are simple non-nucleated prokaryotes. Nitrogen-fixers have not yet been found among nucleated eukaryotes. Genetic studies show that the structural genes are highly conserved in all known nitrogen-fixing species suggesting that the *nif* genes must have evolved and then spread throughout virtually all groups of prokaryotic microorganisms. Most important nitrogen-fixing associations that occur in nature, both in terms of the amounts of N_2 fixed and the benefits to particular crops, involve symbiotic associations in which plants provide specific structures in which the microoganisms are contained. The best known examples are root nodules which are induced by species of *Rhizobium* on leguminous plants, by the actinomycete *Frankia* on a range of woody and shrubby dicotyledonous plants, by the blue-green alga *Nostoc* on cycads, and the special pockets in the leaves of the water fern *Azolla* containing the blue-green alga *Anabaena.* In all these symbioses, the microoganisms live inside the plant as monocultures. They receive carbon compounds directly from the host and the fixed nitrogen is made available to the host.

7.7.2 Biochemistry of Nitrogenase

The special ability of nitrogen-fixing bacteria to reduce N_2 to ammonia depends on the possession of an enzyme system called the 'nitrogenase complex'. Current knowledge indicates that the nitrogenase complex is composed of six proteins and contains two different enzyme activities, one called simply nitrogenase and the other called nitrogenase reductase. The nitrogenase component of the

Table 7.5

Nitrogen-fixing prokaryotes of particular interest for genetic manipulation

Genus	Species	Group	Properties of interest
Azotobacter	*vinelandii*	Gram negative bacterium	Fixes N_2 in air; contains a protein that protects nitrogenase from oxygen damage
Azospirillum	—	Gram negative bacterium	Associated with roots of grasses and other plants
Rhizobium	—	Gram negative bacterium	Nodulates some leguminous plants; Fixes N_2 in legume root nodules.
Klebsiella	*pneumoni ae*	Gram negative bacterium	Model system for *nif* genetics. Genetics of *nif* well understood, particularly after transfer to *Escherichia coli*
Frankia	—	Gram negative actinomycete	Nodulates a range of unrelated shrubby and woody dicotyledonous plants; some species can be cultured.
Rhodospirill um *Rhodopseudo monas*	—	Gram negative bacteria	Purple green photosynthetic bacteria
Clostridium	—	Gram positive bacterium	Obligate anaerobe
Anabaena *Nostoc*	—	Filamentous blue green algae	Form symbiotic associations with a range of plants (*Cycads, Azolla*) fungi etc. Fixes N_2 in specialized cells called heterocysts
Methanococc us	—	Archae bacterium	—

complex contains four subunits, two copies each of two different proteins. Its structure also includes a cofactor, which contains the metals iron and molybdenum. The structure of the cofactor is unknown despite many years of study.

The precise details of how nitrogenase works are not completely clear. The N_2 almost certainly binds to the cofactor, after which it is reduced to ammonia by the addition of electrons and hydrogen ions. The hydrogen ions are obtained from water. The reduction of N_2 is energy-expensive; 20-30 molecules of adenosine triphosphate (ATP) are required to support the reduction of one molecule of nitrogen to ammonia. Nitrogenase reaction also reduces hydrogen ions to molecular hydrogen, H_2, which is given off as a gas. Nitrogenase reductase has a molecular weight of 60,000 and consists of two identical protein subunits. They have a characteristic brown colour because they contain clusters of iron and sulphur. This enzyme reduces nitrogenase, thereby replenishing the electrons used to reduce the N_2. The reductase acquires the electrons that it transfers from other proteins, the exact identities of which vary in the different nitrogen-fixing bacteria.

One very important point about nitrogenase is that it is poisoned by oxygen. When exposed to the atmosphere, the enzyme irreversibly loses half its activity in 3 seconds—a problem that seems to be common to the nitrogenases of all fixers. Bacteria of the *Clostridium* genus overcome this problem by an oxygen-free environment. *Klebsiella pneumoniae* lives with or without oxygen, but fixes nitrogen only when it grows anaerobically. In some blue-green algae, there is a temporal separation of nitrogen fixation which occurs at night, and photosynthesis, which takes place during the day. In *Anabaena,* the cells of the filaments are generally photosynthetic, but under conditions that favour nitrogen fixation some of them differentiate to produce morphologically distinct non-photosynthetic cells (heterocysts) that fix nitrogen.

7.7.3 Genetics of Free Living Nitrogen Fixation

The greatest advances in our understanding of biological nitrogen fixation have involved *Klebsiella pneumoniae,* which is closely related to the non-nitrogen-fixing bacterium *Escherichia coli.* Methods for genetic analysis in *E. coli* could be applied to *K. pneumoniae* and genes could be transferred between the two species and expressed in either of the two organisms. Experiments with mutants defective in nitrogen fixation (Nif-) showed that *nil* genes of *K. pneumoniae* are located on the chromosome, between genes for histidine biosynthesis (*his*) and shikimic acid uptake (*shi A*). This region was transferred to an *E. coli* strain which required histidine. *E. coli* recipients did not require histidine for growth and they had acquired the ability to fix nitrogen. This indicated that the *nif* genes of *K. pneumoniae* are clustered on the chromosomal DNA. *K. pneumoniae* devotes not less than 17 genes, which occupy about 33 kilobases of DNA in the *nif* gene cluster, for the reduction of N_2 to ammonia. RNA transcripts have been mapped and the promoter regions from the *nif* gene cluster have been cloned and sequenced so that the initiation point for each operon is now known.

The *nif H* gene specifies the nitrogenase reductase protein and the *nif* D and *nif K* genes encode the two protein components of nitrogenase. Five genes (*nif B, Q, V, N* and *E*) are involved in some as yet unspecified way in the synthesis of the iron-molybdenum cofactor and two genes (*nif F and J*) determine polypeptides needed for electron transfer to nitrogenase reductase. The genes (*nif M,* S *and V*) are required for the maturation of the complete, functional nitrogenase complex and, *nif A* and *nif C*, have been shown to regulate the expression of all the other *nif* genes. The functions of *nif X* and *nif Y* are as yet unknown. Several of *nif* genes of other nitrogen-fixing organisms have proved to be very similar in structure to those of *K. pneumoniae,* although in the other nitrogen-fixers the genes are usually scattered about the genome instead of being tightly clustered as they are in *K. pneumoniae.*

If nitrogen-fixing bacteria have a suitable source of fixed nitrogen, such as ammonia, glutamate or asparagine, the transcription of the *nif* genes is shut down so that the organisms do not waste the energy needed for synthesizing the proteins nor the A TP required for driving the reduction reaction. The genes are also not expressed when the cells are exposed to air. *Nif* gene regulation is very complex, involving both local control by genes within the *nif* complex and global control by regulatory genes located elsewhere in the genome. To start with, expression of the *nif* genes requires an RNA polymerase enzyme to transcribe the DNA into messenger RNA. RNA polymerase binds to the promoters during initiation of transcription. Sigma factors confer on RNA polymerase the ability to recognize the *nif* gene promoter and other gene promoters. The *ntr A, ntr B, ntr C* and *gln A* genes are part of a global system that regulates many aspects of nitrogen metabolism in bacteria. In the absence of nitrogen sources such as ammonia and glutamate, the *ntr C* product switches on genes that allow bacteria to use other nitrogen containing compounds that would normally be less favoured sources of the element. Among the genes switched on by the *ntr C* product is *nif A,* which then activates the *nif* gene complex. The product of the *ntr B* gene inhibits this *ntr* C mediated activation of the *nif* genes when ammonia concentrations are high. Finally, the *nif L* gene also contributes to the lack of expression of the *nif* genes in the presence of a nitrogen source such as ammonia or oxygen. When the *nif L* product is exposed to ammonia or oxygen it apparently prevents the *nif A* protein from inducing the transcription of the other *nif* genes.

7.7.4 Transfer of *nif* Genes from *K. pneumoniae* to Other Organisms

Nitrogenase activity in *E. coli* carrying the *nif* plasmid pRDI was found to be equivalent to that in the parent *K. pneumoniae* strain under suitable conditions. Transfer of pRDI to *Agrobacterium tumefaciens* did not result in nitrogen-fixing recombinants. Mutants of *Azotobacter vinelandii* lacking either nitrogenase component I or II regained these activties when pRDI was transferred to them. This is significant because *Azotobactersp.* are obligate aerobes which fix nitrogen in the presence of oxygen. A protein which binds to the enzyme complex protects the nitrogenase from oxygen inactivation. It would be of great interest to isolate the genes which encode this protein, since it might be possible to transfer the O_2 protection to other nitrogen-fixing systems, and to new hosts together with the *K. pneumoniae nif* genes. Another property of nitrogen fixation appears to be the evolution of hydrogen with concomitant ATP hydrolysis. Many

N_2 fixing bacteria have uptake hydrogenases which save energy by recycling H_2 to H_2O, releasing electrons. It would therefore be advantageous to introduce an uptake hydrogenase together with *nif* genes into new hosts which do not possess this function.

Any attempt to get *nif* genes expressed in eukaryotic cells will have to overcome considerable problems. There are basic differences in the organization, transcription and translation of genes in prokaryotes and eukaryotes. For instance, the promoter sequences recognized by the DNA-dependent RNA polymerases are different, as are the sites on the mRNA to which ribosomes bind and where translation is initiated. Furthermore, many bacteria have several genes transcribed from one promoter (as in the *nif* operon) resulting in polycistronic mRNA which has internal ribosome-binding sites for each gene, whereas eukaryotes almost invariably have monocistronic mRNAs with a binding site at the 5′ end. No internal ribosome-binding or re-initiation of protein synthesis occurs, unlike prokaryotes which can re-initiate translation within the mRNA.

Although the *nif* gene cluster from *K. pneumoniae* has been transferred to *Saccharomyces cerevisiae,* expression of the genes has not been reported. A vector system could be used to transfer nitrogen-fixing ability.

7.7.5 Symbiotic Nitrogen Fixation

The most important nitrogen-fixing bacteria, both agriculturally and ecologically, are those that interact with plants in symbiosis that may either be simple or complex. The bacterium *Azospirillum* lives around the root surfaces of grasses, although there are questions about whether the plants receive any significant contribution of nitrogen from this association. This is an example of simple association. The symbiosis of *Rhizobium* with legumes and *Frankia* with a variety of shrubs and trees are other examples. The *Rhizobium*-legume symbiosis often displays a host-range specificity. Particular legume species are nodulated only by certain species of bacteria (Table 7.6).

The rhizobia include two distinct subgroups which can be classified according to their behaviour in cultures as 'fast' or 'slow' growers. The slow-growing rhizobia are able to fix N_2 *in vitro* under micro-aerobic conditions, and for this reason, they have been recently classified as members of a new genus, the *Bradyrhizobium*.

Understanding symbiotic interactions requires analysis not just of the *nif* genes, but also of the special plant and bacterial genes that allow them to engage in such complex interactions. These bacteria have the unique capacity to recognize and invade particular legumes and induce in the host plant a coordinated response that include organized cell division and the synthesis of an array of proteins called nodulins. Bacteria in the form of 'bacteroids' turn on their *nif* genes and excrete the resulting ammonia to the host plant, which assimilates the

Table 7.6

Some *Rhizobium* species and their hosts

Bacterialspecies	Host plants	Comments
Rhizobium leguminosarum	Peas, *Vicia,* lentils	All these are very closely related to each other
R. trifolii	Clover, *Phaseolus* bean	–
R. loti	Lotus	Lotus is also nodulated by *Bradyrhizobium*
R. lupinii	Lupin	–
R. meliloti	Alfalfa	–
R. sesbania	*Sesbania*	Induces stem and root nodule on *Sesbania*. Also fixes nitrogen in free-living culture
R. fraedii	Soyabean	Induced non-fixing nodules on most soybean cultures.
Bradyrhizobium japonicum	Soyabean	Some strains fix nitrogen in free living culture.
B. 'Cowpea miscellany'	nodulates several tropical legumes including cowpea and also the non-legume *Parasponium*	Has the ability to nodulate a non-legume host

ammonia by condensing it with glutamic acid to form glutamine. The glutamine in turn is used to disseminate the fixed nitrogen to the rest of the plant.

The most abundant nodulin, leghaemoglobin, transports oxygen to the nitrogen fixing bacteroids. It causes the characteristic pink colouration of nitrogen-fixing nodules. The host genome specifies the protein portion of the leghaemoglobin molecule, whereas the bacteroid almost certainly makes the haem portion. The leghaemoglobin genes of the soybean are remarkably similar to the mammalian haemoglobin genes. Moreover, the root nodules formed on non-leguminous plants by *Frankia* also contain leghaemoglobin.

7.7.6 Genetic Analysis of Rhizobium

Isolation of the *nif* genes of *K. pneumoniae* has greatly aided in identifying the corresponding genes in *Rhizobium.* The nucleotide sequences of the *nif* genes of the different bacteria are so similar that the *K. pneumoniae* genes can be used as probes to 'fish out' the *nif* genes of other species. The *nif* genes of the fast-growing *Rhizobium* bacteria are located on large plasmids, called symbiotic plasmids. The same plasmids also contain the nod genes, which are needed for the bacteria to induce nodule formation by the host plant. In *Bradyrhizobium,* the *nif* and *nod* genes are on the bacterial chromosome.

The regulatory gene sequence that affects *nif* gene expression in *Rhizobium* species is clearly very similar to that in *K. pneumoniae.* The *Rhizobium* and *Klebsiella nif* promoters have similar sequences. In fact, transcription from the *Rhizobium nif* promoters can be activated by the *nif A* gene product of *K. pneumoniae.* Analysis of the rhizobial *nod* gene cluster has revealed some clues concerning the genes' functions and regulation. Eight genes, which are designated as *nod A* to *nod F, nod I* and *nod J* have been identified in the cluster. Mutations in *nod A, B, C and D* abolish nodulation, whereas mutations in the remaining four genes only delay the onset of nodule development and reduce the numbers formed. The *nod A, B,* C, *I* and *J* genes are transcribed as a single unit and appear to specify proteins that are associated with the bacterial membrane. The *nod E* and *F* genes are also transcribed together. The *nod D* gene has been shown to be regulatory, controlling the transcription both of itself and of the other *nod* genes in the cluster. When rhizobial bacteria are maintained in a minimal culture medium the *nod D* gene is expressed at high levels while the remaining *nod* genes are not transcribed. From the beginning of both the *nod A, B, C, I, J* and *nod F, E* regulatory units is a short, conserved DNA segment that may be involved in their regulation.

The host specificity of nodulation is plasmid-determined in *R. leguminosarum, R. phaseoli* and *R. trifolii.* A conjugative plasmid was identified. in R. *leguminosarum* and was shown to carry genes specifying both nodulation of *Pisum* and nitrogen fixation. This plasmid, pRL1JI is about 200 kb in size. A kanamycin resistant derivative, pJB5JI, has been made by introducing the transposon Tn5 into pRLlJI. It has facilitated transfer to many different *Rhizobium* species. A conjugative plasmid *carrying Trifolium* nodulation and N_2-fixation genes has been found in a *R. trifolii* strain which on transfer to *Agrobacterium tumefaciens* conferred the ability to nodulate clovers, although no nitrogen fixation was detected. An *A. tumefaciens* strain carrying pJB5JI has been shown to nodulate *Vicia hirsuta.* All these indicate that many of the genes involved in nodulation and nitrogen-fixation are plasmid encoded.

The construction of self-transmissible plasmids bearing *nif* genes made it possible to transfer the nitrogen-fixation ability to non-fixing species or to non-fixing mutants like *E. coli, Salmonella typhimurium, Serratia marcescens, Erwinia herbicola, Pseudomonas fluorescens* and *nif-mutants* of *Azotobacter vinelandii.* But this transfer does not always express in receptor cells.

7.7.7 Biofertilizers

The use of chemical fertilizers to increase grain production is the most common practice in farming. The consumption of these inorganic fertilizers which was only 0.05 million tonnes in 1951 has now crossed 10 million tonnes. The manufacture of these chemicals is very costly and depends on non-renewable fossil fuels. They also pollute the land and contribute to biological magnification. Hence, there is a great need to develop new methods by which other fertilizers could be used to enhance food grain production. Biofertilizers—living plants used as fertilizers—have become a means of supplementing the availability of the scarce resources of chemical fertilizers and also enriching the soil.

Nitrogen is the most essential macro-element for a proper and healthy crop. N_2 is the most limiting element in various types of Indian soils. The consumption of N_2 fertilizers in India is more than its production. This increasing need has necessitated the import of N_2-fertilizers from other countries. Cultivation of green manure producing crops especially leguminous species and addition of crop residues to the fields for enriching the soils are widely practised methods since long. Now-a-days due to plantation of most economically important crops like cereals, this practice has declined tremendously and thus the availability of crop residues for green leaf manuring has come to a limit. To overcome these problems, the use of biofertilizers is of great significance to the third world countries especially India.

The role of legumes in enriching the fertility of soil was known through the centuries. This is due to the association of most of the leguminous plants with symbiotic *Rhizobium* which form nodules and help in using atmospheric nitrogen. Taking a clue from this, scientists developed microbial inoculants which are carrier-based preparations containing beneficial microorganisms in a viable state intended for seed or soil application and designed to improve soil fertility and help plant growth by increasing the number and biological activity of desired microorganisms in the root environment. *Rhizobium* inoculant, *Azotobacter* inoculant, *Azospirillum* inoculant and blue-green algal inculant have been prepared. *Azolla* has been used as an organic manure. Phosphate solublizing microorganisms and mycorrhizal fungi have also found a place in biofertilizer technology.

Free living blue-green algae like *Nostoc, Anabaena* and *Aulosira* are grown in open water reservoirs to raise their biomass production. After sun-drying, the algal flakes are collected and spread over the rice fields generally one week after transplantation of rice seedlings. Rhizobial inoculants are prepared from the Rhizobia of the root nodules after isolating, culturing, mass-producing and inoculating them into peat powder which acts as the carrier and this is applied to the soil. Azotobacterinoculant is prepared from *Azotobacter* isolated from soil, cultured, mass-produced and inoculated into agar or peat powder which act as carriers and these are applied to the soil. *Azospirillum* inoculant is prepared from *Azospirillum* isolated from the soil as well as roots, cultured, mass-produced and inoculated into carriers such as farm yard manure alone or farm yard manure + soil or farm yard manure + charcoal and this is applied to the soil.

Rhizobium inoculants can add upto 60 kg N/ha in the legume pulses and legume oilseed crops. Blue green algae can add 25 kg N/ha to wet land rice soils. For the application of 500 kg of *Rhizobium* inoculant and 10 kg of blue green algae per ha, approximately 15,000 tonnes of *Rhizobium* culture and 0.17 million tonnes of blue-green algae are required.

Azolla fern is used as an organic input in rice fields. There are two methods by which *Azolla* can be utilized to grow a healthy crop of rice; (i) as a green manure prior to rice plantation, and (ii) by growing it along with the main crop for some time. The major problem for *Azolla* collection is that the material cannot be shipped by mail and has to be carried by hand. Nodulating legumes are used as green manure. Microorganisms which solublize phosphates are isolated from soil or rhizosphere, cultured, mass-produced and inoculated into peat powder carriers and applied in the soil. Mycorrhizal fungi belong to *Glomus, Gigaspora, Acaulospora, Sclerocystis* and *Endogone* genera. Ectomycorrhizal fungi are isolated from root, spores, rhizomorphs or sclerotia. These are cultured and used for inoculation. Using pure cultures as inoculum is time consuming and expensive. More often soil, root, mycorrhizal seedlings, spores and sporocarps are used as inoculants. Obligate endosymbionts have not been cultured.

After realizing the importance of biofertilizers for supplementing the use of chemical fertilizers and organic manures, the Government of India has initiated a National Chemical Project on the development and use of Biofertilizers. Under this project, one National, six Regional and 40 sub-centres are being set up. These centres are to produce 600 tonnes of BGA besides 375 tonnes of *Rhizobium*. However, *Azolla* is not included in this programme. It is essential to set up *Azolla* production units at state, district and block levels in China and Vietnam to provide fresh and healthy inocula to the farmers in time so that these can be multiplied further by the farmers for inoculation in their rice fields.

Till recently, improvement in yield and other capabilities of microalgae has been achieved by the selection of algal strains and improvements in culturing and processing procedures. Very little work has been done by adopting a genetic engineering approach to improve algae. Presently, cell fusion techniques are being tested to obtain algae with both autotrophic and heterotrophic properties. Biotechnical Resources (USA) has used mutated algal strains with a shorter doubling time, which can utilize varieties of carbohydrates like glucose, and reach a high productivity of even 100 g/l.

The particular genetic engineering technique to be used to transform specialized potentials of microalgae into realities depends, on the nature of the substance of interest and the nature of the genetic make-up of the organism. It is important to genetically transform cyanobacteria in a stable, facile, and predictable manner, in order to explore the full biotechnological potential of these organisms. Recombinant DNA and gene cloning techniques are the tools to improve the algal strains, but very little work has been done. The first step in this direction, i.e. the characterization of efficient gene transfer systems to introduce foreign DNA into cyanobacteria has been developed only recently.

7.8 Improving Nutritional Quality

Seed crops play important roles in human and animal nutrition worldwide. Eight species of cereals contribute over 50% of the total world food calorie requirements; seven species of grain legumes make a significant contribution in developing countries as important sources of protein. The nutritional problem with cereals and legumes is that they contain limited amounts of certain amino acids which are essential to human beings and monogastric animals. Most cereals are deficient in lysine and to a lesser extent threonine, while legumes are deficient in sulphur amino acids. Some seed crops, notably rice, have low overall protein levels, but a somewhat better amino acid balance.

Over hundreds of years these crops have been bred for increased yields, protein levels, improvement in specific characteristics (such as baking quality of wheat and malting quality of barley), and to a certain extent for nutritional quality. The four major categories of seed proteins are: albumins (soluble in water), globulins (soluble in salt solutions), prolamins (soluble in aqueous alcohol) and glutelins (soluble in dilute acid or alkali). The major storage proteins of cereals generally fall into the prolamin category. They are deficient in lysine, rich in proline, glutamine and asparagine and highly hydrophobic. Legumes, on the other hand, principally store globulins which are deficient in methionine and are much less hydrophobic. The main storage proteins of rice fall into the glutelin category, making the grain less deficient in lysine. Globulin forms the principal nitrogen store in oats.

There have been a variety of approaches to improve nutritional quality. Early attempts concentrated on screening existing cultivars for unusual amino acid compositions and using these in breeding programmes. Also mutagenesis has played a significant role. However, to date there have been no dramatic improvements in the nutritional quality of commercially grown cultivars of seed crops.

Can biotechnology be used to overcome some of these problems? The genes coding for a number of these storage proteins have been cloned. It has been suggested that nutritional improvement could be achieved by using site-directed mutagenesis with the objective of introducing more lysine or methionine codons into the gene' sequences. The engineered gene could then be replaced in the plant and allowed to express. There have been no reports of successful replacement of a storage protein gene into a crop plant as yet except one recent report indicating that a gene encoding the french bean protein, phaseolin, has been expressed in sunflower tissue culture. The gene had been inserted into the sunflower cells via an *Agrobacterium* plasmid.

7.9 Increased Yield Of Chemical Compounds

Plants are sources of an extremely wide range of chemical substances. Plant compounds such as pharmaceuticals (alkaloids, steroids, anthraquinones), enzymes (proteases), latex (isoprenoids), waxes (wax esters), pigments (stains and dyes), oils (fatty acids), agrochemicals (insecticides), cosmetics (essential oils), food additives (flavour compounds), and gums (polysaccharides) are of commerical importance. Some indication of the industries involved, their key products and the range of chemical structures utilized are given in Table 7.7.

Table 7.7

Natural products from plants and their associated industries

Industry	Product	Plant	Industrial uses
Pharmaceuticals	Coderine (alkaloid)	*Papaver somniferum*	Analgesic
	Diosgenin (steroid)	*Dioscorea deltoidea*	Antifertility agents
	Quinine (alkaloid)	*Cinchona ledgeriana*	Antimalarial
	Digoxin (cardiac glycoside)	*Digitalis lanata*	Cardiotonic
	Scopalamine (alkaloid)	*Datura stramonium*	Antihypersensitie
	Vincristine (alkaloid)	*Catharanthus roseus*	Antileukaemic
Agrochemicals	Pyrethrin	*Chrysanthemum cinerariifolium*	Insecticide
Food and drink	Quinine (alkaloid)	*Cinchona ledgeriana*	Bittering agent
Thaumatin (chalione)	Non-nutritive	*Thaumatococcus danielli*	sweetener
Cosmetics	Jasmine	*Jasminum* sp.	Perfume

(***Source:*** *Mantell, S.H.; Smith, H. Plant Biotechnology. © 1983 Cambridge, Cambridge University Press, Reprinted by permission.*)

Most of these compounds are secondary metabolites produced by plants as a consequence of different stages of cell, tissue and organ differentiation. The importance of plants as sources of chemicals for various industries makes, improvement of crop plants involved, the most important consideration. In such a situation *in vitro* techniques play an important role. Cell cultures may contribute in at least four major ways to the production of plant natural products; (i) as a new route of synthesis to established products, (ii) as a route of synthesis to a novel product from plants difficult to grow or establish (e.g. thebaine from *Papaver bracteatum*),(iii) as a source of novel chemicals (e.g. rutacultin from cultures of *Ruta*), (iv) as biotransformation systems, either on their own or as part of a larger chemical process. Various substances such as alkaloids, allergens, anthraquinones, antileukaemia agents, antitumour agents, antiviral agents, aromas, benzoquinones, carbohydrates, cardiac glycosides chalcones, dianthrones, enzymes, enzyme inhibitors, flavonoids, flavones, flavours, furanocoumarins, hormones, insecticides, latex, lipids, naphthoquinones, nucleic acids, nucleotides, oils, opiates, organic acids, peptides, perfumes, phenols, pigments, plant growth regulators, proteins, steroids and derivatives, tannins, terpenes and terpenoids and vitamins, have been produced from cell cultures. A major problem encountered is that the plant cells cannot be grown in large enough volumes in a sufficiently productive state to make them economically suitable sources except in some medicinal plants. Table 7.8 contains examples of the most successful levels of plant metabolite production in culture systems.

Table 7.8

Yields of some natural products in cell cultures and their equivalent amounts in whole plant tissue.

		Yield	
Natural product	Species	Cell culture yield	Whole plant
Anthraquinones	*Morinda citrifolia*	900 n mol g–1 dry wt	Root 110 n mol g^{-2} dry wt
Anthraquinones	*Cassia tora*	0.334% fresh wt.	0.209% seed, dry wt.
Ajmalicine and serpentine	*Catharanthus roseus*	1.3% dry wt.	0.26% dry wt.
Diosgenin	*Dioscorea deltoidea*	26 mg g^{-1}dry wt.	20 mg g^{-1} dry wt tuber
Nicotine	*Nicotiana tabacum*	3-4% dry wt.	2-5% dry wt
Ubiquinone	*Nicotiana tabacum*	0.5 mg g^{-1} dry wt	16 mg g^{-1} dry wt leaf

(***Source:*** (*Mantell, S.H.; Mathews, J.A.; McKee, R.A. Principles of Plant Biotechnology. © 1987 Oxford Blackwell Scientific Publications. Reprinted by permission.*)

The potential advantages of using plant tissue culture as sources of industrially important compounds are: (i) independence from various environmental factors (ii) the relative degree of control, (iii) consistency in the quality of the products, and (iv) land area can be saved for food and cash crops. By optimization of different cultural factors, it has been possible to increase accumulations of certain secondary metabolites in cell cultures without any need for high levels of tissue differentiation.

Plants have also been used as a source of enzymes: eg. sulphydryl proteases which include the papaya proteases from *Carica papaya,* bromelain from pineapple (*Ananas comosus*), ficin from fig (*Ficus glabrata*), the amylolytic enzymes from cereals, and α and β-amylases, the lipoxygenases of soya bean and the pectic enzymes of *Citrus* fruits. It may be possible, in future, to transfer the genes coding for a particular plant product into microbes using suitable vectors and thus produce these natural products on a large scale.

7.10 Genetically modified Food

Genetically modified food is a food product, which contains some genetic material, which is not belonging to itself originally and naturally. This food carries the genetic material, which has been introduced into it through genetic modification. So far many genetically modified foods have been produced using genetic engineering techniques. For example, tomato, corn, rice, wheat, bean varieties, fruits, etc. Genetically modified seeds help farmers to reduce chemical fertilizers, insecticides and herbicides. Vaccines can be produced in genetically modified food. There are some people who object to the use of genetically modified food, since they contain 'alien genes' which may affect others. However, it has been reported by some scientists that such genes do not affect others.

Study Outline

Micropropagation for Biomass Energy Production

Mass propagation of crop and forest plants is an important application of micropropagation techniques which involves the development of embryos from somatic cells in culture. Using *in vitro* techniques, a desired tree selected on the basis of its past performance may be vegetatively propagated and cloned at an enormously rapid pace for the production of phytomass energy. Micropropagation involves thrree stages (a) establishment of cultures, (b) regeneration of plants, (c) transfer of plants from test tube to soil. Embryo culture has been employed as a useful tool for direct regeneration in trees where seeds are dormant. Induction of somatic embryogenesis is the most important mode of micropropagation. This enables us to produce embryos which are regarded as seeds. Micrografting is relatively a recent technique which involves the removal of the extreme tip and grafting on to the root stock.

Production of Disease Free and Disease Resistant Plants

To make the plant disease resistant, the resistant genes from the plants are transferred to the susceptible plants. Researchers have tried to use *Agrobacterium* gene transfer system to produce tobacc;o and tomato plants with increased resistance to TMV. The phenomenon known as the "cross protection" has been successfully applied in agriculture to bring about disease resistance.

Insect Resistant Plants

Another important achievement of genetic engineering has been the production of insect resistant plants. Insect resistance in transgenic plants has been achieved through the expression of the insect toxin gene of *Bacillus thuringiensis* in plants. It is done by introducing the cloned toxin gene into plant cells.

Herbicide Resistant Plants

Herbicides are widely used to control weeds. They inhibit plant growth by blocking the biosynthesis of essential amino acids. These include glyphosate, N-(phosphonomethyl)- glycine, which inhibit the synthesis of aromatic amino acids. Glyphosphate resistance in tobacco plants has been obtained by isolating a resistant gene from *Salmonella typhimurium* and introducing this into tobacco cells through Ri plasmid vectors. Recently herbicide-resistant wheat has also been produced.

Induction and Selection of Mutants

Manipulations with cultured plant cells have resulted in the isolation of a number of variant cell lines. Physical and chemical mutagens are used in the explants of different species to generate mutations. Single cell and protoplast culture systems have proved to be valuable for mutagenesis.

Production of Haploids

Haploids have played a significant role in the propagation and breeding of plants. The advantages are: (i) haploids are homozygous; (ii) homozygotes have valuable recessive characters which are unexpressed in natural conditions (iii) the number of androgenic progeny can be large. Major economically important haploid crops observed are coffee plant, coconut, rubber, prunus, forest trees like *Populus, Ulnus* ornamental plants like *Ginko, Taxus* and *Cassia fistula*.

Somatic Hybrids

Somatic hybrids are produced from the fusion of protoplasts of two cells. It offers the possibility of hybrid formation of widely unrelated forms of plants. It is an asexual means of effecting gene transfer.

Transformation Through Uptake of Foreign Genome

Transfer of genes into plants was made possible by the use of *Agrobacterium tumefaciens* plasmids. To make use of the natural gene transfer mechanism available in Ti plasmid, scientists have designed a shuttle vector that can replicate in *E. coli* where recombinant DNA manipulations are easily handled. Techniques to grow plant cells and tissues in culture and to regenerate intact plants from them provide the basis for the stable genetic modification of plants. For a foreign gene to be expressed in plant cells, it is essential that it be preceeded by a promoter recognised by the host cell. Using these techniques, success has been achieved in overcoming male sterility, inducing pest resistance and virus resistance, inducing glyphosate tolerance and production of antibodies.

Nitrogen Fixation

Biological nitrogen fixation is the most important source of fixed nitrogen entering into the soil. The reduction of nitrogen is catalyzed by nitrogenase system present in all prokaryotes. The fixation of nitrogen requires a large amount of energy. The nitrogen-fixing nodules are formed in the roots of leguminous plants due to a symbiotic relationship with bacteria. The special ability of nitrogen-fixing bacteria is due to the presence of an enzyme system called nitrogenase complex. The construction of self transmissible plasmids bearing *nif* genes made it possible to transfer the nitrogen-fixing ability to non-nitrogen fixing plants.

Biofertilizers

Living plants used as biofertilizers have become a means of supplementing the availability of the scarce resources of chemical fertilizers and also enriching the soil. Leguminous plants enrich the fertility of the soil due to the association of the symbiotic nitrogen-fixing bacteria (*Rhizobium*) which form nodules. Other biofertilizers are *Azotobacter, Azospirillum,* blue green algae, and *Azolla;* phosphate solubilizing microorganisms and mycorrhizal fungi have also found a place in biofertilizer technology. Biotechnological endeavours have made significant contribution towards improving the nutritional quality of the seeds, and also to increase the yield of plants. Various techniques have also been employed to increase primary and secondary metabolites.

Questions

(1) What is biomass production?
(2) What is bioenergy?
(3) What is the importance of micropropagation? Explain its application.
(4) Explain cross protection?
(5) State the importance of *Bacillus thuringiensis*?
(6) What are the techniques involved in evolving insect resistant and herbicide resistant plants?
(7) Distinguish somatic hybrids.
(8) Describe the enzyme involvement in nitrogen fixation.
(9) What is the significance of haploids in the propagation and breeding of plants?
(10) What is the role *of nif* genes?
(11) What are the various attempts made so far to transfer nif genes to non-nitrogen fixing plants?
(12) What are biofertilizers? Explain with examples.
(13) What are the achievements made through biotechnology in increasing the crop yield, quality of seeds and plant metabolites?
(14) What is genetically modified food? Is it safe?

8
Industrial Biotechnology

Introduction

Industrial biotechnology means the commercial exploitation of a variety of processes and techniques related to micro-organisms, plants, animals and human beings. With the development of techniques such as genetic engineering, tissue culture, hybridoma, immobilisation of cells and enzymes, advanced fermentation systems and biocatalysts, industrial biotechnology has offered new horizons to revolutionize world economy. Industrial biotechnology has the potential to provide bulk chemicals and industrial products to meet the demands of the growing world population.

After the research work carried out by Pasteur on alcoholic, butyric and lactic fermentations, Weizmann's discovery of acetone-butanol fermentation during the First World War represented a major achievement in industrial biotechnology. The biosynthesis of penicillins using fermentation methods in the 1940 marked the beginning of the era of modem industrial biotechnology. Since then, an innumerable number of compounds have been produced. Today industrial biotechnology involves not only improved fermentation techniques and processes but also a host of other important fields such as food production, fine chemical production, therapeutic production etc. Biotechnology offers the possibility of producing, from widely available renewable resources, substances and compounds essential to life and the greater well-being of human beings.

8.1 Industrial Microbial Products

Since the beginning of recorded history, microorganisms have been used for the benefit of human beings in many different ways. The important characteristics that have made microbes useful in industry are: CO their ability to grow rapidly on easily available cheap raw materials; on their ability to maintain a physiological constancy; (iii) their ability to bring about biochemical transformations under simple culture conditions; and (iv) high ratio of surface area to volume which facilitates the rapid uptake of nutrients required to support high rates of metabolism and biosynthesis.

8.1.1 Fermentation Products

Microbiologists tend to interpret fermentation as any process for the production of a product by the mass culture of microorganisms, whereas biochemists interpret it as an energy-generating process in which organic compounds act as both electron donors and terminal electron acceptors. The central part of a fermentation process is the growth of the industrial organism in an environment which stimulates the synthesis of the desired commercial products. This is carried out in a fermenter which is essentially a large vessel (ranging in size from 1000 to 1.5 million dm3) in which the organism may be maintained at the required temperature, pH, dissolved oxygen concentration and substrate concentration. However the actual culturing of the organism in the fermenter is only one of the number of stages in a fermentation process, as indicatcrd in Fig. 8.1.

The medium on which the organism is to be grown has to be formulated from its raw materials and sterilized; the fermenter has to be sterilized and inoculated with a viable, metabolically active culture which is capable of producing the required product. After growth, the culture fluid has to be harvested, the cells separated from the supernatant and the product has to be extracted from the relevant fraction (either the cells or the cell-free supernatant) and purified. For any fermentation to be successful and possible, first of all we must obtain a productive organism, and its productivity must be raised to economic levels by medium improvement, mutation, recombination and process design. Products of microbial fermentation and metabolism include primary metabolites, secondary metabolites, enzymes and proteins, capsular polysaccharides and the cellular biomass itself (known as single-cell protein).

8.1.2 Microbial Biomass and Single-Cell Proteins

The most obvious microbial product of commercial significance is probably microbial biomass (the microbial cells themselves). Yeast cells, used in the baking industry, have been produced commercially since the early 1900s, and yeast was also produced as human food in Germany during the First World War. Although the production of baker's yeast by fermentation has continued, the First World War production of microbial biomass as human food or animal feed was not investigated in any great depth until the 1960s. During this time, the biochemical diversity of microorganisms was exploited by the utilization of a wide variety of organisms capable of growing on a range of carbon sources including hydrocarbons for the production of single cell proteins (SCP). British Petroleum developed its technology to the extent of constructing a commercial plant for the production of yeast biomass from n-alkanes. Imperial Chemical Industries produced bacterial biomass *(Methylophilus methylotrophus)* from methanol and eventually established the Pruteen process for the production of high grade protein as an animal feed. Table 8.1 gives some of the applications of microbial cells.

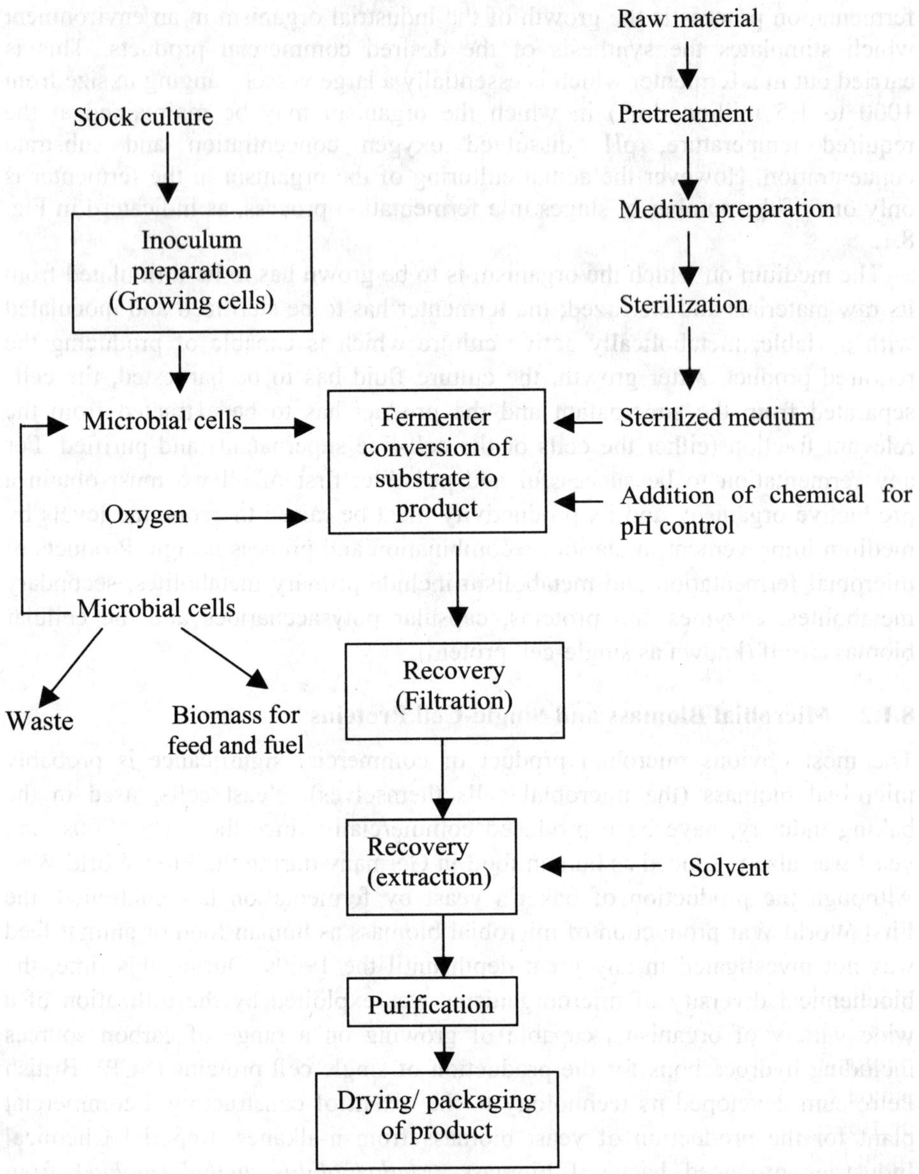

Figure 8.1.
Steps involved in the process of fermentation

Table 8.1

Some applications of microbial cells

Organism	Application
Bacillus thuringiensis and related organisms	Microbial insecticide
Lactobacillus sp., *Streptococcus cremoris* and related species	Starter cultures for the manufacture of dairy products e.g. yoghurt, cheese.
Penicillium roquefortii and related species	Inocula for the production of blue veined cheese
Rhizobium sp.	Inoculants for adding to legume seeds to promote nodulation and nitrogen fixation
Pseudomonas syringae (Many different organisms)	Creation of artificial snow. Ice-nucleation defective mutants for the prevention of frost damage to crops. Single-cell protein production

Microbial cells themselves are the desired end-product. Most of them have rather specialized applications, e.g. the production of *Penicillium roquefortii* spores. The characteristic flavour of blue cheese is due to the metabolic products of *P. roquefortii* growing in milk fats. Strain selection has resulted in the identification of several isolates with particularly desirable properties for cheese manufacture.

Single-cell proteins (SCP) are the dried cells of microorganisms such as algae, certain bacteria, yeast; moulds and higher fungi that are grown in large-scale culture systems as protein for human or animal consumption. The products also contain other nutrients, including carbohydrates, fats, vitamins and minerals. The development in single-cell protein production from ancient times to 1985 is given in Table 8.2.

Advances in scientific knowledge regarding the physiology, nutrition and genetics of microorganisms have led to significant improvements in single-cell protein production from a wide range of microorganisms and raw materials. Both photosynthetic and non-photosynthetic microorganisms have been used for single-cell protein production. At a minimum, these organisms require a carbon and energy source, a nitrogen source, and supplies of other nutrient elements, including Phosphorous, Sulphur, Iron, Calcium, Magnesium, Manganese, Sodium, Potassium and trace elements, for growth in a water environment. Some organisms cannot synthesize amino acids, vitamins and other cellular constituents from simple carbon and nitrogen sources, and in that event these substances must also be supplied for the organism to grow.

Table 8.2
Development in single-cell protein production

Period	Organism	Technical Development
2500 BC	*Saccharomyces cerevisiae*	Top fermenting yeast recovered for baking
1781-82	*Saccharomyces cerevisiae*	Compressed yeast prepared from brewer's yeast
1860	*Saccharomyces cerevisiae*	Vienna process aerated, malted grain mash substrate
1868	*Saccharomyces cerevisiae*	Introduction of compressed yeast manufacturing into US
1874	*Saccharomyces cerevisiae*	Continuous aerations
1900	*Saccharomyces cerevisiae*	Centrifuge used for yeast separation
1914-18	*Saccharomyces cerevisiae*	Incremental feeding, molasses, ammonium salts
1918-19	*Endomyces vernalis*	Fat production from sulphite liquor
1920	*Aspergillus fumigatus*	Growth on straw and inorganic N for animal feed
1936	*Saccharomyces cerevisiae*	Heiskenskjold process using sulphite liquor
1936		Seholler-Tornesch process for fodder yeast from wood sugar.
1941-45	*Candida utilis*	Production of food yeast from sulphite liquor and wood sugar.
	Geotrichum candidum (Oidium lactis)	Production of fat
1946-54	*Candida utilis*	Continuous process yeast from sulphite liquor-Waldof fermenters
1948-53	*Chlarella* sp.	Production of algae in open circulation systems
1959	*Saccharomyces cerevisiae*	Continuous production of bakers yeast on commercial scale.
1954-63	*Morchella* sp.	Submerged culture of mushroom mycelium
1958-64	*Kluyveromyces fragilis*	Fragilis food yeast from cheese whey
1959-72	*Candida lipolytica*	Feed yeast from hydrocarbons, n-paraffins, gas oil, air lift.
	Candida tropicalis	
1963-74	Fungi	Fungi from spent sulphite liquor, Pekils process

Contd…

Period	Organism	Technical Development
1970-74	*Candida utilis*	Food yeast from ethanol
1971-75	*K.fragilis*	Continuous production of fragilis yeast and/ or ethanol from cheese whey
1979-80	*Methylophilus methylotrophus*	Continuous production of bacterial single-cell protein from methanol on a commercial scale
1983-85	*Candida utilis, K.fragilis S.cerevisiae*	High cell density direct dry process for single-cell protein production from ethanol and carbohydrates.

Among algae, *Chlarella* sp., *Scenedesmus acutus* and *Spirulina maxima* are cultivated for single-cell proteins. Large pond areas are needed because the algal growth occurs mainly in the top 20 to 30 centimetres where the light intensity is the greatest. Usually the pond waters are agitated either continuously or intermittently by pumps, paddle wheels or windmills to prevent the algae from settling. This ensures that the cells are uniformly exposed to light and nutrients.

Candida utilis, Candida guillienmandis, Kluyveromyces fragilis and *Rhodopseudomonas* sp. have been used for single-cell protein production. Bacteria have also been used, because they multiply very fast and are capable of growing on a variety of raw materials ranging from carbohydrates such as starch and sugars, to gaseous and liquid hydrocarbons such as methane and petroleum fractions, to petrochemicals such as methanol and ethanol. Acid to neutral (5.0 to 7.0) pH is preferred. Bacterial single-cell protein may be produced in conventional batch systems in which all the nutrients are supplied to the fermenter initially; the cells are harvested when they have consumed the nutrients and stopped growing. In the more advanced production methods, the nutrients are supplied continuously in the concentrations needed to support bacterial growth and the cells are harvested continuously once the population reaches the desired concentration.

Yeast is also used for the production of single-cell protein. Yeast fermentations may be operated either in the batch or continuous mode, or by fed-batch mode. In fed-batch process the substrate and other nutrients are added in an incremental manner to meet the growth requirements of the yeast while maintaining very low nutrient concentrations in the growth medium at any time. This method yields 3.5 to 4.5 per cent dry weight of product compared with the 1.0 to 1.5 dry weight of products yielded by batch cultivation. Yeasts have certain advantages over bacteria for the production of single-cell protein. The yeasts tolerate a more acid environment, in the range of 3.5 to 4.5 instead of the near-neutral pHs preferred by bacteria. Also yeast cell diameters are about 0.0005 centimetres as compared with 0.0001 centimetres for bacteria.

Among higher fungi, *Fusarium graminearum, Penicillium cyclopium, Trichoderma harzianum, Paeeilomyees varioti, Chaetomium cellulolyticum* are used in the production of single-cell proteins. The present-day production of mould single-cell protein is achieved by methods similar to those used for the production of the yeast products. The simple sugars or the raw materials that contain them are suitable substrates for a variety of moulds. The growth rates of moulds and higher fungi are usually slower than those of bacteria and yeasts. Most of them are cultivated at a pH below 5.0. Batch, fed-batch or continuous process can be used for the production of mould single-cell protein.

The protein percentages for the various single-cell protein pruducts are crude values based on measurements of the total nitrogen contents of the materials. A significant fraction is contributed by nucleic acids. In addition, single-cell protein may be deficient in certain essential amino acids that animals cannot synthesize for themselves. Single-cell proteins will most probably be used in human foods primarily as protein supplements or as ingredients that perform specific functions— acting as flavours or leavening agents etc.

8.1.3 Insecticides

The widespread use of agrochemicals has allowed human beings to achieve an unprecedented control over pests and has contributed towards the present-day's high agricultural productivity. However the potential toxic effects on human beings and the environment and the rapid development of resistance in the target pests has led to a reconsideration of the real value of chemical insecticides.

Consequently interest has turned to certain microoganisms which are natural pesticides. Although over 100 bacteria, fungi and viruses that infect insects have been described, only very few are in commercial production. The most widely used is *Bacillus thuringiensis* which produces intracellularly a proteinaceous crystal toxic to insects. After ingestion by susceptible insects the crystalline toxin dissolves in the alkaline environment of the midgut where it inhibits ion transport leading to cessation of feeding and death. The nature and potency of the toxin crystals varies amongst bacterial serotypes and different strains are required to control different pests. Greater knowledge about the biological basis of toxicity may result in the use of protein engineering to develop a single strain which is pathogenic to a wide variety of insects.

8.1.4 Starter Cultures

A major application of microbial cells is the addition of starter cultures to milk for the production of fermented products such as cheese, yoghurt, sour cream etc. The basic reason for converting milk into products such as cheese is to preserve the valuable nutrients in milk. For thousands of years, human beings depended upon the natural contaminating flora in milk for the synthesis of lactic acid and flavours and the formation of the desired product. However, the widespread thermal processing of milk, e.g. pasteurization, to destroy pathogens such as causative agents of tuberculosis and brucellosis alters the microbial flora of milk and it no longer naturally undergoes a lactic fermentation.

Consequently, starter cultures have to be added and these are generally frozen or lyophilized cell concentrates of either pure cultures of lactic acid bacteria or selected mixtures. When these bacteria are added to milk they cleave the lactose to glucose and galactose and these are metabolized to lactic acid. The acid coagulates the milk proteins, principally casein, to form a continuous solid curd in which fat globules, water and water-soluble materials are entrapped. The curd is then pressed to expel the fluid whey, shaped and left to mature. Gene manipulation can help in the production of better microbes by increasing plasmid stability, since the ability to grow on lactose and to degrade casein are plasmid-mediated traits. Starter cultures are also used in the preparation of fermented meat products such as salami.

8.1.5 Bacterial Vaccines

Clinically, bacterial cells are used for the production of vaccines. Some vaccines, e.g. those for diphtheria and tetanus, are purified exotoxins which have been rendered non-toxic by treatment with heat or formalin. However, most bacterial vaccines, such as those for cholera, whooping cough, plague, typhoid, paratyphoid fever and typhus fever are simply suspensions of killed bacteria. After growth, the bacteria are killed with heat or chemical agents such as phenol, acetone or formalin. Only the vaccine for immunization against tuberculosis uses live cells; in this vaccine, an attenuated strain of *Mycobacterium bovis* is used.

The vaccines prepared from live, attenuated organisms often give life-long protection; vaccines prepared from killed cells have to be injected repeatedly according to carefully balanced immunization schedule. Recently a novel way of attenuating *Vibrio cholera* has been developed. Using recombinant DNA technology a portion of the gene for cholera enterotoxin was deleted. The modified protein produced is immunogenetic but non-toxic. The other development in the production of bacterial vaccines is to use subcellular components of the cell as immunogens; e.g. pili on the surface of Gram-negative bacteria are involved in the adsorption of the bacteria to animal cells. Purified pili are being tested as vaccines for *Neisseria gonorrhoeae. V. cholera* and enteropathogenic strains of *E. coli.*

8.1.6 Primary Metabolites

Primary metabolites are low molecular weight compounds (1500 daltons) necessary for microbial growth; some of them are the building blocks of macromolecules, while others participate in the synthesis of coenzymes. Among the most important in industry are aminoacids, organic acids, purine and pyrimidine nucleotides, solvents and vitamins. Microbial cells, like the cells of other living beings, do not overproduce primary metabolites, as this would be a wasteful process that decreases survival ability. There are, however, microbial strains that show aberrations in their regulation of production of these metabolites and they are the starting strains for industrial processes. To obtain overproducing strains it is necessary to subvert the cellular regulatory mechanisms. Metabolic regulation is achieved in two ways: by feedback inhibition of the activity of key enzymes by the end-product of a biosynthetic pathway and repression of the synthesis of the enzymes in a pathway by the end-product. Overproduction can also be facilitated by eliminating competing biochemical reactions. Table 8.3 summarises economically important essential primary metabolites produced by fermentation.

Table 8.3
Economically important, essential primary metabolites produced by fermentation

Metabolite	Use
Amino acids	
L-Glutamate	Flavour enhancer
L-Threonine	Food supplement
L-Lysine	Food supplement
L-Phenylalanine	Manufacture of Aspartame (artificial sweetener)
L-Tryptophan	Food supplement
L-Sorbose	Food supplement
Vitamins	
Riboflavin (vitamin B2)	Food supplement
Vitamin B12	Food supplement and feed additive
Nucleotides	
Inosine-5'-monophosphate	Flavour enhancer
Guanosine-5'-monophosphate	Flavour enhancer
Pigments	
B-carotene	Precursor of Vitamin A

(***Source:*** *Primrose, SB. Modern Biotechnology.* © 1987 *Oxford, Blackwell Scientific Publications. Reprinted by permission.)*

Bacteria such as *Ashbya gossypii, Gluconobacter suboxydans, Propionibacterium shermanii, Brevibacterium flavum, Corynebacterium glutamicum* and *Pseudomonas denitrificans* are involved in the industrial production of primary metabolites.

8.1.7 Secondary Metabolites

Secondary metabolites, also called idiolites, are low molecular weight compounds synthesized by microorganisms late in the growth cycle. They are not required for growth. These secondary metabolites include antibiotics, alkaloids, plant growth hormones, pigments and toxins. Since many of them, e.g. antibiotics, are inhibitory to other organisms they may impart an ecological advantage on the producing organism. The best known secondary metabolites are antibiotics. Over 4500 antibiotics have been described of which the majority are produced by actinomycetes. Six genera of filamentous fungi produce about 1000 distinct antibiotics. Two genera of bacteria synthesize 500 antibiotics; three genera of actinomycetes produce about 3000 antibiotics; Actinomycetes are actually gram positive bacteria which show fungus-like growth. Figure 8.2 gives the structures of some representative antibiotics.

Two approaches have been used to obtain enhance yield of products. One of these is the random mutation and selection procedure. The other involves screening of hundreds of culture medium additives as possible precursors of the desired product. Both approaches have been very successful but both are labour intensive. This is where the recombinant DNA technology is extremely helpful. Genes controlling the entire biosynthetic pathway can be cloned. Different methods are used for the selection of genes to be cloned.

8.1 .8 Polysaccharides

The industrial value of polysaccharides lies in their capacity for altering the rheoloical properties of aqueous solutions, either through gelling or by the alteration of their flow characteristics. Many polysaccharides are thixotropic, i.e. the solutions are characterized by high viscosity at low stress and decreased viscosity when stress is applied. Such characteristics make them useful in a variety of industries (Table 8.4).

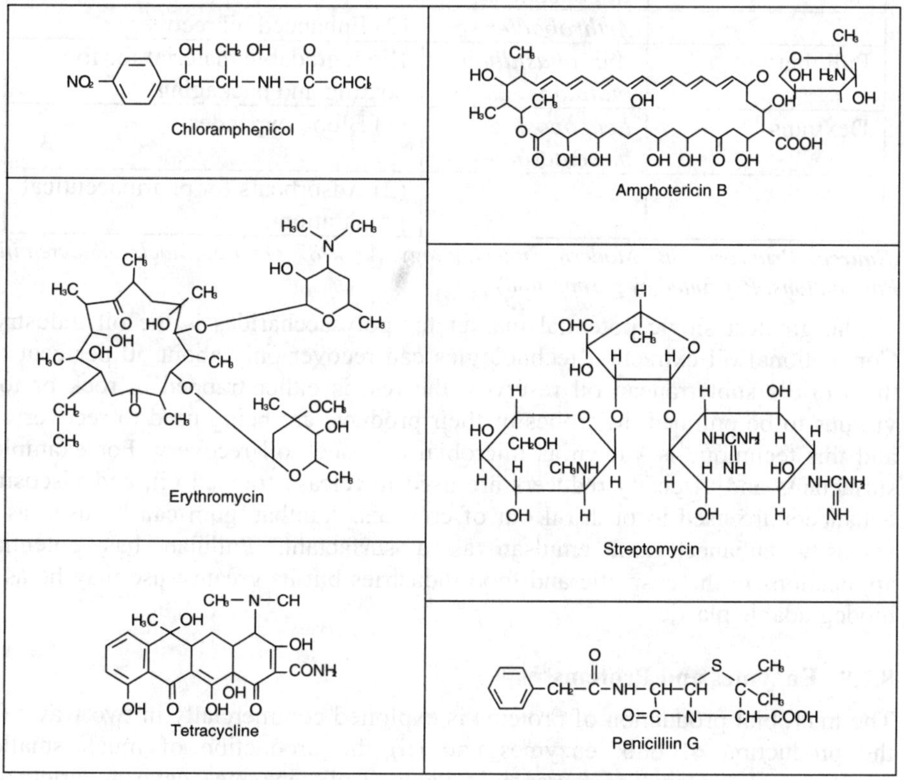

Figure 8.2
Structures of some representative antibiotics.

Table 8.4

Commercially available microbial polysaccharides and their uses

Polysaccharides	Producing Organism	Uses
Xanthan gum	*Xanthomonas campestris*	(1) Food dditive for stabilizing liquid suspensions and gelling soft foods e.g. ice cream, cheese, spreads
		(2) Lubrication e.g. toothpaste preparation
		(3) Enhanced oil recovery
Gellan	*Pseudomonas* sp.	Solidification of food products
Emulsan	*Acinetobacter calcoaceticus*	(1) Cleaning oil spills
	Arthrobacter sp.	(2) Enhanced oil recovery
Pullulan	*Aureobasidium pullulans*	Biodegradable material for food coating and packaging
Dextrans	*Leuconostoc mesenteroides*	(1) Blood expander
		(2) Adsorbents for pharmaceutical preparations

(***Source***: *Primrose, SB. Modern Biotechnology. © 1987 Oxford, Blackwell Scientific Publications. Reprinted by permission.*)

The greatest single potential market for polysaccharides is the oil industry. Conventional oil extraction technologies can recover only about 50 per cent of the world's subterranean oil reserves; the rest is either trapped in rock or too viscous to be pumped. Microbes or their products are being used to recover oil and this technique is known as microbial enhanced oil recovery. For example, surfactants and viscosity reducers are used to release trapped oil, and viscosity enhancers are used to push oil out of crevices. Xanthan gum can be used as a viscosity enhancer and emulsan as a surfactant. Pullulan has potential applications in the cosmetic and food industries but its greatest use may be as a biodegradable plastic.

8.1.9 Enzymes and Proteins

The microbial production of proteins is exploited commercially in two ways: (i) the production of bulk enzymes and (ii) the production of much smaller quantities of proteins of therapeutic value. Bulk enzymes have a variety of applications (Table 8.5).

Table 8.5

Sources and applications of some microbial enzymes

Enzyme	Source	Application
Amylase	*Aspergillus niger*	Baking: Flour supplement
	Aspergillus oryzae	Brewing: Mashing
	Bacillus subtilus	Food: Precooked foods, syrup
		Pharamaceuticals: Digestive aids
		Starch: Cold-water laundry
		Textiles: Desizing agent
Cellulase	*Aspergillus niger*	Food: Liquid coffee concentrate
Dextransucrase	*Leuconostoc mesenteroids*	Pharameceuticals: Dextran
Glucoamylase	*Aspergillus niger* *Rhizopus* sp.	Starch hydrolysis
Glucose isomerase	*Arthobacter* sp. *Bacillus* sp.	High-fructose corn syrup
Glucose oxidase	*A. niger*	Food: Glucose removal from egg solids
		Pharmaceuticals: Test papers
Invertase	*Saccharomyces cerevisiae*	Candy: Prevents granulation in soft center
		Food: Artificial honey
Lactase	*Saccharomyces fragilis*	Dairy: Prevents crystallization of lactose in ice cream and concentrated milk
Lipase	A. *niger*	Dairy: Flavour production in cheese
Pectinase	*Aspergillus* sp.	Clarification of wines, fruit juices
Penicillin acylase	*Escherichia coli*	Preparation of 6-aminopenicillanic acid
Protease, acid	*Aspergillus* sp.	Calf rennet substitute
Protease; alkaline	*Aspergillus oryzae*	Detergent additive, beer stabilizer, breadmaking meat tenderizer
	Bacillus sp.	Dehairing of hides

Contd...

Table 8.5 Contd...

Enzyme	Source	Application
Protease, neutral	*Bacillus amyloliquefaciens*	Liquefication of brewing adjuncts
Pullulanase	*Klebsiella aerogens*	Starch hydrolysis
Streptodornase	*Streptococcus pyogenes*	Pharmaceuticals: Reagent, wound debridement

*(**Source:** Primrose, S.B. Modem Biotechnology.* @ 1987 *Oxford, Blackwell Scientific Publications. Reprinted by permission.)*

Recombinant DNA technology can be used for the improved production of enzymes and proteins. Cloning can also be used to provide alternative sources of enzymes which are in short supply. One protein which is not an enzyme but which can be produced in, bulk is bovine growth hormone. Administration of this hormone to cows significantly increases their milk yield. This hormone also has an effect on fish. Recombinant DNA technology is being used to construct microorganisms which synthesize human proteins with therapeutic potential. Recombinant DNA technique has been used to manipulate the cellulase genes of a thermophilic actinomycete, *Thernomonospora,* which grows rapidly at 65°C and has one of the most active cellulase complexes yet found. This helps in the quick production of cellulose from lignocellulose substrate. Some human proteins with therapeutic potential are given in Table 8.6.

Table 8.6

Some human proteins with therapeutic potential

Interferons	Treatment of virus infections and cancer
Human growth hormone	Pituitary dwarfism
Insulin	Diabetes
Tissue plasminogen activator	Thrombosis
Urokinase	Thrombosis
Epidermal growth factor (urogastrone)	Wound healing
Interleukin-2	Cancer therapy
Relaxin	Facilitation of childbirth
al-antitrypsin	Emphsema
Tumour necrosis factor	Cancer therapy
Erythropoietin	Treatment of anaemia
Lung surfactant protein	Treatment of respiratory distress syndrome

(***Source***: *Prim rose, S.B. Modern Biotechnology.* © 1987 *Oxford, Blackwell Scientific Publications. Reprinted by permission.*)

Enzyme have a variety of commercial applications in analytical, wine, textile, photographic, pharmaceutical, food, leather, dairy, and paper industries.

8.1.10 Fuels

Microbial production of synthetic fuels has the potential for helping to meet world energy demands. Important fuels produced by microorganisms include ethanol, methane, hydrogen and hydrocarbons. The bacterium *Zymomonas mobilis* ferments carbohydrates forming alcohol twice as rapidly as yeasts. *Thermoanaerobacter ethanolicus* is more efficient than the organism currently used for the fermentative production of ethanol. Methane can be used for the generation of mechanical, electrical and heat energy. It can be produced by the anaerobic decomposition of waste materials. Bacteria such as *Clostridia* sp., *Bacteroides* sp., *Selenomonas* sp., and *Butyrovibrio* sp., are involved in this.

8.1.11 Microbial Mining

Microbial mining by the process of bioleaching recovers metals from ores that are not suitable for direct smelting because of their low metal content. Physical and chemical properties of a metallic ore are altered by microorganisms in bioleaching so that the metal can be extracted. Currently leaching is restricted to copper and uranium ores but the commonest organism involved, *Thiobacillus ferrooxidans,* can also effect the solubilization of Cobalt, Nickel, Zinc and Lead.

The application of leaching process to uranium mining is of particular interest because of the possibility of *in situ* mining. Instead of using conventional techniques to haul uranium ore to the surface, microbial suspensions can extract the metal from its source. Water is percolated through underground shafts where the bacteria dissolve the metals. The solution is then pumped to the surface where the metal is recovered. The bacteria do not directly attack the uranium minerals; instead they generate ferric ion from pyrite and soluble ferrous ions. Ferric ions readily attack minerals incorporating quadrivalent uranium, converting this ion to hexavalent uranium, which is soluble in dilute sulphuric acid. This procedure is already being used in Canadian uranium mines. It has been suggested that extending this practice to most mines has significant environmental benefits because of minimal disruption of the land surface. The deeper and lower grade deposits could be mined more readily by this method.

8.1.12 Bioconversion

Bioconversion consists of the conversion of a metabolite to a structurally related compound by microbial cells. One of the oldest bioconversions is that of ethyl alcohol to acetic acid, which takes place during the manufacture of vinegar. Bioconversions are very specific because they concern a single type of reaction and a compound of a defined structure (stereospecificity). They convert isopropanol to acetone, glycerol to dihydroxyacetone, L-tyrosine to L-dihydroxyphenylalanine, glucose to gluconic acid and then to 2-ketogluconic or to 5-ketogluconic acid, and sorbitol to L-sorbose. The synthesis of steroid hormones is based on the method of bioconversion. Microorganisms could also be used to manufacture raw materials of steroids.

Bioconversion sometimes needs mixed cultures or sequential addition of microbial strains or species, each of which carry out a specific step. The use of immobilized cells, which are more stable than either enzymes or cell cultures, has made it possible to increase the yield of bioconversion at a lower cost.

8.1.13 Food Products

Microorganisms are involved in the production of different kinds of food. Cheese and other dairy products, nondairy fermentations, alcoholic beverages and vinegar etc., make use of fermentation processes. Table 8.7 and 8.8 give the names of food products and the organisms involved.

8.1.14 Cell and Enzyme Immobilization

Microorganisms act as a catalyst in any fermentation where a product other than biomass is obtained. When the culture medium is removed from the fermenter the catalyst is either destroyed by subsequent downstream processing or discarded. One solution is to immobilize the microorganisms or even the appropriate enzyme. In this process the cells are firmly bonded to the support matrix and the enzymes are made to function. Three methods are available for immobilization: (a) *physical binding,* (b) *cross-linking* (c) *entrapment* (Fig. 8.3). In practice, combinations of methods can be used.

Table 8.7

Production of Alcoholic Beverages by Yeasts

Beverage	Yeast	Method of Preparation	Function of Yeast
Root beer (pre 1905 and home made)	*Saccharomyces cerevisiae*	Molasses, sassafras bark, wintergreen bark and sarasaparilla root added for flavour; add yeast incubate aerobically.	Converts sugar into carbon dioxide; by aerobic metabolism; 0.03% alcohol
Beer	S. *carlsbergensis* (*bottom yeast*)	Germinated barley releases starches and amylase enzymes (malting). Enzymes in malt hydrolyze starch to fermentable sugars (mashing). liquid (wort) sterilized. Hops (flowers) added for flavour. Yeast added incubated at 37-49°C.	Converts sugar into alcohol and carbon dioxide; 4.0% alcohol. Yeast grow on bottom of fermenting vessel.

Contd...

Table 8.7 Contd…

Beverage	Yeast	Method of Preparation	Function of Yeast
Ale	S. *cerevisiae* (*top yeast*)	As in beer; included at 50-70°C	Converts sugar into alcohol; 6% alcohol. Yeast grow at top of fermentation vessel.
Sake	S. *cerevisiae*	Aspergillus oryzae converts starch in steamed rice into sugar; yeast added; incubated at 20°c.	Converts sugar into alcohol; 14%-16% alcohol.
Wine natural	S. *cerevisiae*	Strain of grape provides various flavours and sugar concentrations. Grapes crushed into must; sulfur dioxide added to inhibit wild yeast; yeast added. Red wines; incubated at 25°c. Aged in oak for 3-5 years and in bottle for 5-15 years. White wines; incubated at 10-15°c. Aged 2-3 years in bottle.	Converts grape-sugar into alcohol; 14% or less alcohol.
Wine sherry	S. *cerevisiae* S. *beticus or* S. *bayanus*	As natural wine with additional surface growth (flor) at 27°c. Alcohol added to 18%-21 %.	S. beticus grows as surface film producing aldehydes from alcohol.
Wine, sparkling (champagne)	S. *cerevisiae*	As natural wine with secondary fermentation in bottle. 2.5% sugar and yeast added to bottled wine; incubated at 15°C; bottle inverted to collect yeast in neck.	In secondary fermentation produce carbon dioxide; yeast settle quickly.

Contd…

Table 8.7 Contd...

Beverage	Yeast	Method of Preparation	Function of Yeast
Distilled beverages			
Rum Jamaica	*Wild yeast*	Cane molasses inoculated from previous fermentation. Oak-ageing adds colour.	Converts sugar to alcohal; 50%-95% alcohal
		Distilled to concentrate.	
Brandy	s. *cerevisiae*	Fruits pressed; yeast added. Distilled to concentrate alcohol, blended with other brandies.	Converts sugar into alcohol 40-43% alcohol.
Whisky	s. *cerevisiae*	Wort (see beer) .is fermented by yeast. Distilled to concentrate alcohol; aged in charred oak barrels.	Converts sugar to alcohol; 50-95% alcohol.

Table 8.8

Some Fermented Foods and Related Products'

Foods and Products	Raw Ingredients	fermenting Organisms
Dairy products		
Cheeses (ripened)	Milk curd	*Streptococcus spp. Leuconestoc spp.*
Kefir	Milk streptococcus lactis	*Lactobacillus bulgaricus, Candida spp. Streptococcus lactis*
Kumisa	Raw mare's milk	*L. bulgaricus, Lactobacillus leichmannii, Candida spp.*
Taette	Milk	*S. lactis var. taette*
Yogurt	Milk, Milk solids	*Streptotoccus thermophilus, L. bulgaricus*
Meat and Fish Products		
Country-cured hams.	Pork hams	*Aspergillus, Penicillium spp.*

Contd...

Foods and Products	Raw Ingredients	fermenting Organisms
Dry sausages	Pork, beef	Pediococcus *cervisiae*
Fish sauces	Small fish	*Halophilic Bacillus spp.*
Izushi	Fresh fish, rice, vegetables	*Lactobacillus spp.*
Nonbeverage		
Plant Products		
Cocoa beans	Cocoa fruits (pods)	*Candida krusei, Geotrichum* spp.
Coffee beans	Coffee cherries	*Edwinia dissolvens* *Saccharomyces spp.*
Foods and Products	Raw ingredients	*Fermenting Organisms*
Kimchi	Cabbage and other vegetables	*Lactic-acid bacteria*
Miso	Soyabeans	*Aspergillus oryzae, Saccharomyces rouxii*
Olives	Green olives	*Leuconostoc mesenteroides, Lactobacilll.!s plantarum*
Poi	Taro roots	*Lactic-acid bacteria*
Sauerkraut	Cabbage	*L. mesenteroides, L. plantarum*
Soy sauce (shoyu)	Soyabeans	A. *orzyae or Aspergillus soyae; S. rouxii*
Tempeh	Soyabeans	*Lactobacillus delbrueckiia Rhizopus oligosporus; Rhizopus* oryzae
Breads	Idli	Rice and bean flour
Leuconostoc mesenteroides	Rolls, cakes, etc.	Wheat flours
Saccharomyces cerevisiae	San Francisco	
Sourdough bread	*Wheat flour*	*Saccharomyces exiguus,*
Sour pumpernickel	*Wheat flour*	*Lactobacillus sanfranciscos L mesenteroides*

Physical binding is the oldest immobilization technique but the least satisfactory. Cells or enzymes are mixed with an adsorbent and then packed in a column. Cells immobilized in this way have a tendency to autolyse. Enzymes and microbial cells can be immobilized by cross-linking them with bi-or multi-functional reagents such as gluctaralaehyde or toluene di-isocyanate. They can also be bonded to insoluble matrices using the same reagents. Although good retention of cells and enzymes is obtained with this method, it can be accompanied by an extensive loss of enzyme activity.

The most extensively used method of cell immobilization involves entrapment in a polymer matrix. Matrices which have been employed include collagen, gelatin, agar, alginate, carrageenan, polytacrylamide, cellulose triacetate and pblysyrene. Immobilized catalysts are used for the commercial production of D, L, aminoacids, high-fructose corn syrup, 6-amino penicillanic acid, urocanic acid, malic acid and aspartic acid. Cells of *Escherichia coli, Achromobacter liqueidum* and *Brevibacterium flavium* are used in immobilization.

8.2 Industrial Plant Products

For centuries, plants have been a valuable source of chemicals and they are currently seen as a source of low volume, chemicals of great value to the pharmaceutical, perfume and fine chemical industries. Even today 25 per cent of all drugs prescribed are derived from plants; quinine, codeine, diosgenin and digoxin are notable examples. A typical industrial use of biomass is the conversion of plant materials such as lignocellulose to alcohols, and on a smaller scale to biogas.

8.2.1 Alcohol Production

The useful components of plant biomass are sugars, starch and lignocellulose. Plants producing high levels of sugars include sugar-cane, sugar-beet and millet. They are used as substrates in the production of alcohol. Plant products containing starch include grain crops, particularly maize, rice and wheat, as well as the potatoes and other root crops like sweet potato and cassava. Starch is broken down to mono and oligosaccharides and is used in the fermentation process. Agriculture and forestry produce great amounts of lignocellulose which contains lignin, cellulose and hemicellulose. These raw materials are used in the fermentation process. Chapter 10 gives further details 10.2.3.1).

8.2.2 Chemical Resource

Plants are sources of an extremely wide range of chemical substances. The main groups of plant compounds of use to industry are listed in Table 8.9.

Table 8.9

Major groups of compounds with commercial importance which are derived from plants.

Compound group	Type and examples
Pharmaceuticals	Alkaloids, steroids, anthraquinones
Enzymes	Proteases (e.g. papain)
latex	Isoprenoids (e.g. rubber)
Waxes	Wax esters (e.g. jojoba)
Pigments	Stains and dyes
Oils	Fatty acids (e.g. seed oils)

Contd...

Compound group	Type and examples
Agrochemicals	Insecticides (e.g. pyrethrins)
Cosmetic substances	Essential oils (e.g. monoterpenes)
Food additives	Flavour compounds, non-nutritive sweeteners (e.g. thaumatin)
Gums	Polysaccharides (e.g. gum arabic)

(***Source:*** *Mantell, SH.; Mathews, J.A.; McKee, RA. Principles of Plant Biotechnology.* © 1987 *Oxford, Blackwell Scientific Publications. Reprinted by pennission.*)

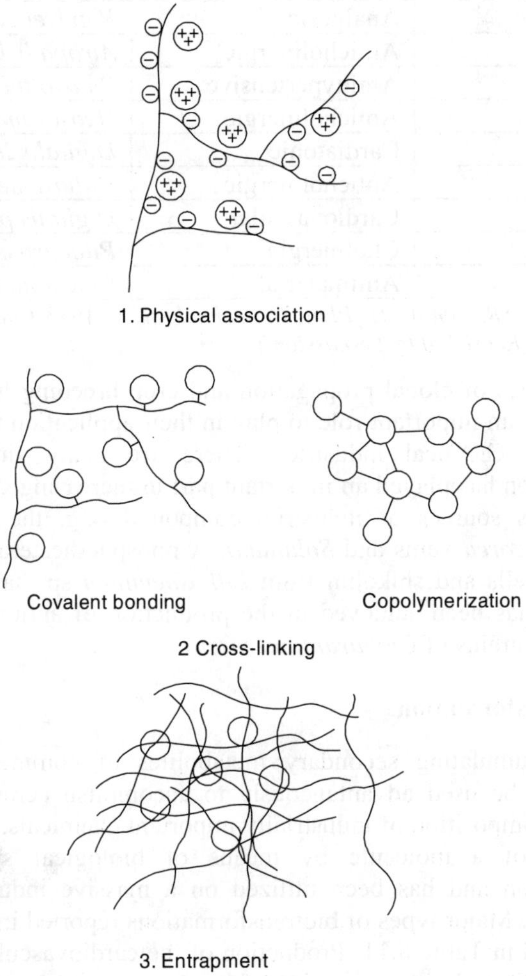

Figure 8.3

The three basic methods of cell and enzyme immobilization. The tinted circles represent enzyme molecules or microbial cells.

(***Source:*** *Primrose, S.B. Modern Biotechnology.* © 1987 *Oxford, Blackwell Scientific Publications Reprinted by permission.*)

The majority of commercially important compounds. (Table 8.10) are secondary metabolites produced by plants as a consequence of different stages of cell, tissue and organ differentiation.

Table 8.10

The ten most prescribed me dicinals from plant sources

Medicinal agent	Activity	Plan
Steroids from diosgenin	Anti-fertility agents	*Dioscorea deltoidea*
Codeine	Analgesic	*Papaver somniferum*
Atropine	Anticholinergic	*Atropa belladonna*
Reserpine	Antihypertensive	*Rauwolfia serpentina*
Hyoscyamine	Anticholinergic	*Hyoscyamus niger*
Digoxin	Cardiatonic	*Digitalis lanata*
Scopolamine	Anticholinergic	*Datura metel*
Digitoxin	Cardiovascular	*Digitalis purpurea*
Pilocarpine	Cholinergic	*Pilocarpus jaborandi*
Quinidine	Antimalarial	*Cinchona ledgeriana*

(***Source:*** *Mantel, SR.; Smith, H. Plant Biotechnology.* © 1983 *Cambridge: Cambridge University Press. Reprinted by permission.*)

The techniques of clonal propagation and crop breeding using tissue culture techniques have an important role to play in their application to plants of special significance to chemical industries. There are many situations in which micropropagation has played an important part in increasing stocks of wild plant species used as sources of industrial compound (e.g. the steroid producing species of *Dioscorea* yams and *Solanum),* A phosphodiesterase and ubiquinone from tobacco cells and shikonin from *Lithospennium* sp. have been produced. Some success has been achieved in the production of antitumour alkaloids by productive cell strains of *Catharanthus roseus.*

8.2.3 Biotransformation

Besides accumulating secondary metabolites of commercial significance, plant cells can be used advantageously to accomplish certain changes in the structure and composition of industrially important chemicals. The conversion of a small part of a molecule by means of biological systems is termed biotransformation and has been utilized on a massive industrial scale in the steroid industry. Major types of biotransformations reported in plant cell cultures are summarized in Table 8.11. Production of the cardiovascular steroid, digoxin from digitoxin from digitoxin obtained from *Digitalis* sp. has been achieved in a large scale by biotransformation.

The extraction of useful compounds from plant biomass presupposes the destruction of cells, as in the case of microorganisms. But it is desirable to avoid this destruction because a given mass of plant cells is much more costly to obtain

Table 8.11

Biotransformations which can be achieved by plant cultures

Reactions	Substrate	Product
Reduction	C = C	CH_2—CH_2
	C = C CO	CH_2—CH_2 or CH_2—CH_2—CHOH
	CO	CH_2OH
	CHO	CH_2OH
Oxidation	CH	CH_2OH
	CH_2OH	or COOH
		CHO
	CHOH	CO
	= S	S = O
Hydroxylation	CH	C—OH
	CH_2	CH—OH
Epoxidation	CH = CH	—HC—CH— O
Glycosylation	OH	O-glucose
	COOH	COO-glucose
	NH	N-acetate
Methylation and demethylation	OH	O—OH
	N	N—CH
	N—CH_3	= NH
Isomerization	transdextra—OH	cis Laevo-rotation—OH

(*Source: Mantell, SH.*; *Mathews, J.A.*; *McKee, RA. Principles of Plant Biotechnology.* © 1987 *Oxford, Blackwell Scientific Publications.Reprinted by permission.*)

than an equivalent mass of bacteria or yeasts. Immobilizing plant cells within polymers seems to be the most practical solution for the complete biosynthesis of useful compounds as well as for the bioconversion of a given substance. The cells must remain alive in these polymers for a sufficient duration so that the exploitation is cost effective. Also, it should be possible to recover the synthesized metabolites easily, because these generally accumulate in the cell vacuoles instead of being exsorbed into the culture medium. According to many specialists, this is the major problem posed by the utilization of plant cells in the production of useful compounds.

Another difficulty is the availability of sufficient quantities of homogenous plant material and stable strains, and this takes months or even years, depending on the species involved. Moreover the biochemical diversity found in cell cultures cannot be induced with certainty and a highly varied collection of strains must be maintained in order to stand a chance of discovering a new substance.

Another requirement is the use of highly specific screening methods, which can serve to identify accurately all the substances produced so as to isolate original compounds present in minute quantities.

Plant tissue culture has particularly important applications to certain industries like the pharmaceutical and food industries which require specific, highly purified substances. These may be produced by (i) biosynthesis of specific groups of compounds as conventional sources, or (ii) biotransformation of specific compounds to ones of a more desirable (valuable) type taking advantage of specific enzymes in living cells.

8.2.4 Enzymes

Only a limited number of plants yield commercially important enzymes. The bulk of enzymes used commercially are obtained from microbial sources, and are produced by fermentation processes. However, there are still several plant enzymes which have not yet been replaced by substitutes from microorganisms. Among these are the plant sulphydryl proteases which include the papaya proteases from *Carica papaya,* the main member being papain; bromelain from pineapple *(Ananas cosmosus)* and ficin from fig *(Ficus glabrata).* Other enzymes derived from plants-including the amylolytic enzymes from cerals, and β-amylase, the lipoxygenases of soybean, and the pectic enzymes of citrus fruits are all used in industrial processes, although they are now replaced by similar bacterial and fungal enzymes. Papain is used in meat tenderizing, protein hydrolysates in beer chill-proofing, baking etc. Bromelain is used in meat tenderizing, digestic aid, clinical applications etc. Ficin is used in meat tenderizing, protein hydrolysates etc. Plants such as tomato, soybean, wheat, maize, barley, beans, apple, alfalfa, egg plant, peas, peanut, potatoes, rape, squash and cauliflower contain lipoxygenases. Genetic engineering technology is being used to improve the yield of these enzymes.

8.3 Industrial Animal Products

Cultured animal cells produce a wide range of biological products of commercial interest including immunoregulators, antibodies, polypeptide growth factors, enzymes and hormones. These are already being used in the manufacture of virus vaccines, tissue plasminogen activator (an enzyme which facilitates the destruction of blood clots), interferon-α (for the treatment of cancer), monoclonal antibodies and tumour specific antigens (for inclusion in diagnostic kits). The possibility of growing fibroblasts in culture from burns patients is being considered. These cultured cells could be used as a reconstituent skin to facilitate wound healing. Another potential application of cultured cells is their use in evaluating new drugs and toxic chemicals.

8.3.1 Production of Viral Vaccines

The oldest commercial application of animal cell cultures is for the production of viral vaccines and it could be argued that globally, with the possible exception of antibiotics, they have provided greater benefit than any other pharmaceutical product. Table 8.12 lists the major human and veterinary virus vaccines and the cell cultures used in their production.

Table 8.12

Major human and veterinary virus vaccines and the cell cultures used

Human Vaccines		Veterinary Vaccines	
Virus	Cells used for culture	Virus	Cells used for culture
Measles	Chick embryo fibroblasts	Canine distemper	Chick embryo fibroblasts or Dog kidney cells
Polio (inactivated)	Monkey kidney cells	Canine hepatitis	Dog kidney cells
Polio (live)	Monkey kidney or human diploid cells	Foot and Mouth disease	Bovine kidney cells
Rabies	Human diploid cells	Rabies	Duck embryo or chick embryo
Rubella	Rabbit kidney, duck embryo or human diploid cells	Feline palneucopenia	Cat kidney cells
		Marek's disease	Chick embryo cel

(***Source:*** *Primrose, S.B. Modern Biotechnology.* © 1987 *Oxford, Blackwell Scientific Publications. Reprinted by permission.*)

Table 8.13

Proteins overproduced by some mammalian cell line

Product	Cell line	Source
Acetylcholine-sterase	BP4 1 AS	Murine neuroblastoma
Interferon-α	Namalwa	Human blood
Interferon- β	Flow 7000	Human embryonic foreskin
Interleukin	EL4 CL 14	Murine blood
Plasminogen	GPK	Guinea pig heratocyte
activator	BEB	Human breast
Urokinase	HT 1080	Human fibrosarcoma

(***Source:*** *Primrose, S.B. Modern Biotechnology.* © 1987 *Oxford, Blackwell Scientific Publications. Reprinted by permission.*)

8.3.2 Production of High-value Therapeutics

There are many human proteins which have long been believed or known to have therapeutic potential but which are in short supply. A more satisfactory alternative would be to grow in large-scale culture, cells derived from the tissue which normally synthesizes the desired protein.

Table 8.13 listed some examples. The disadvantage with this method is that such cultured cells produce only low levels of the therapeutic protein. This problem is overcome by using recombinant DNA technology.

8.3.3 Production of Therapeutics and Vaccines in Recombinant Mammalian Cells

A whole range of proteins of potential value to the pharmaceutical industry has now been produced in cultured, recombinant mammalian cells (Table 8.14). None of these substances have been marketed so far.

Table 8.14

Some mammalian proteins overproduced in cells in culture as a result of *in vitro* manipulation

Protein	Size	Use
Tissue plasminogen activator	527 amino acids	Thrombosis
Interleukin 2	133 amino acids	Cancer therapy
Tumour necrosis factor	157 amino acids	Cancer therapy
Factor VIII	2332 amino acids	Haemophilia
Factor IX	415 amino acids	Christmas disease
Erythropoietin	166 amino acids	Anaemia

(***Source:*** *Primrose, S.B. Modern Biotechnology* 1987. *Oxford Blackwell Scientific Publications. Reprinted by permission*)

8.3.4 Production of Human Insulin

In 1916, Sir Edward Sharpy-Schafer, while studying the Islets of Langherans of the pancreas, discovered and named the substance secreted, insulin. The antidiabetic role of insulin was reported in 1921 by Banting and Best in Canada. Insulin was for the first time successfully applied to a diabetic nine year old boy in 1922. It was immediately produced by Eli Lilly in 1923 and animal insulin (from Pancreas) was marketed. About 800-1000 kilo grams of pancreas produce 100 grams of insulin. Since then it has been produced commercially by several pharmaceutical concerns.

In 1979, of the 60 million diabetics in the world, 4 million were treated with insulin. In the United States, the number of diabetics who needed insulin shots were around 1.8 million in 1979, among whom 1,00,000 were children; this number increases by 6 per cent every year. In France, at the same time one million diabetics were recorded, of whom 1,50,000 needed insulin.

Genentech company took the initiative to synthesize human insulin from bacteria. 18 and 11 oligonucleotides coding for A arid B chains of insulin were assembled to make each gene. Each synthetic gene was linked to a plasmid near the end of a beta-galactosidase gene of *E.coli* (strain K 12). The two polypeptides were cleaved from the enzyme, purified and linked *in vitro* to form the complete insulin molecule. The amount of insulin initially made was 1,00,000 molecules per bacterial cell.

In the history of protein chemistry the year 1954 is a landmark, since Frederick Sanger and his co-workers at Cambridge University finally succeeded in achieving the first complete description of the structure of a protein molecule insulin.

Insulin is one of the smallest proteins. However, its formula is sufficiently formidable. The molecule of the animal (cattle) insulin is made up of 777 atoms, in the proportions 254 carbon, 377 hydrogen, 65 nitrogen, 75 oxygen and 6 sulphur ($C_{254}H_{377}O_{75}S_6$). The total number of amino acid units in the molecule is 51 in two polypeptide chains, 21 and 30 amino acids. units long (containing 17 different types). It is made up of two polypeptide chains A and B. It has already been synthesized.

The two polypeptide chains of insulin were originally. derived from pre pro insulin (with 109 amino acids). As preproinsulin is synthesized in the beta cells of pancreas, the first 23 amino acids serve as a signal to allow the passage of the molecule through the cell membrane. These amino acids are cleared off leaving the chain of pro insulin (86 amino acids). The proinsulin molecule folds up to bring the first and last segments of the chain together and the central portion of the molecule is cut out by enzymes to leave insulin: the role of this central portion is to align the two chains of insulin correctly.

In 1980, Novo Industry (Denmark) was able to transform swine insulin into 99 per cent pure human insulin by replacing the alanine residue which is the thirtieth amino acid of the B chain.

The economics of the market for insulin may be fundamentally altered by the application of microbiological techniques. The insulin currently used in diabetes therapy is extracted from the pancreas of cattle and swine. The insulin of these species differ slightly from human insulin in their amino acid sequence. Although animal insulins are effective in controlling the major symptoms of diabetes, they do not prevent some of the ancillary effects including deterioration of the kidneys and the retina. More than 20 per cernt of the diabetics all over the world are dependent on bovine and porcine insulin injection. Porcine insulin is similar to human insulin in that the C-terminal threonine on the alpha chain is replaced by alanine, while bovine is different at three positions. Besides bovine shows a greater immunogeneticity as compared to porcine. All patients treated with injections of bovine insulin develop circulating anti-insulin antibodies which are responsible for subcutaneous fat atrophy and also neutralize insulin in the circulation. Consequently the patient needs a higher dose in due course. Moreover, some diabetics are allergic to animal hormones.

Roberto Crea, Adam Kraszewski, Taddaki Hirose and Keiichi Itakura of the Hope National Medical Centre in California also synthesized genes coding for insulin polypeptide. Eighteen fragments of a few nucleotides each were assembled to make the gene for the longer chain and 11 fragments were joined into a gene for the shorter chain. Each synthetic gene was linked to a plasmid near the end of the beta galactosidase gene of *E.coli.* After gene expression and the translation of mRNA into protein,the two polypeptides were cleaved from the enzyme and linked to form the complete insulin molecule. Approximately 1 × 105 insulin molecules were synthesized per *E.coli* cell.

Other workers (Gilbert and Vitta-Komaroft) also separated mRNA from the beta cells of the pancreas of rat; complementary DNA was prepared with the help of reverse transcriptase, and a copy of this DNA was inserted into pBR322 plasmid in the middle of gene for penicillinase. The plasmid also contained the. structural genes for proinsulin. The hybrid protein synthesized in the bacterial cell was penicillinase + proinsulin from which insulin could be separated by trypsin.

If human insulin manufactured by. bacteria proves effective in controlling these pathologies, it will almost certainly gain a substantial share of the world market for insulin. Eli Lilly of the United States is already in the forefront for human insulin production by gene transfer mechanisms. A conservative estimate is that if the yields can be increased to the level of those of other industrial processes that employ *E.coli,* more than 1000 litres of fermentation broth could yield 200 grams of purified insulin. This is the amount extracted from some 1,600 kilograms of animal pancreatic glands. Eli Lilly has started selling Humulin, the commercially produced human insulin since 1982, and it has been approved by United States Food and Drug Administration Department.

8.3.5 Production of Interferon

Isaacs and Lindermann first isolated interferon at the National Institute of Medical Research near London, in 1957. It is a protein released in minute quantities by animal and human cells when a virus penetrates an organism. Interferon appears to the body's first line of defense against viral attacks. The first investigations had shown that interferon could help to cure viral diseases such as the common cold, hepatitis and herpes zoster (shingles). In addition to its role to boosting immunity, interferon also acts to inhibit the multiplication of abnormal cells, which would explain its antitumour effect. In 1978, Cantell and his co-workers at the Central Laboratory of Public Health in Helsinki processed 50,000 litres of human blood to produce about a tenth of a gram of pure interferon. It has been calculated that processing of 2 litres of human blood, can produce about 4 million units of interferon. (A unit is the amount of interferon that will protect 50 per cent of the cells in culture against virus infection).

When interferon was discovered, it was possible to interfere with viral replication without necessarily endangering cellular metabolism and many thought that interferon might prove to be a useful *antiviral agent.* However, a major problem was in the material supply and it remained so until the cloning of interferon genes in *E.coli* in the late 1970s.

The term interferon originated in connection with viral interference and it generated a lot of interest because of the enormous potential of its action against viral invasion. It consists of a group of small proteins secreted by cells in response to viral infection. It can also be produced when sensitized lymphocytes are exposed to a particular antigen under laboratory conditions. Interferon can be produced by treating the cells with double stranded RNA. It is produced by most body cells on exposure to viruses and triggers a reaction that neutralizes not only the viruses that induced its formation but also many other viruses.

Interferon are a group of small proteins with molecular weights between 20,000-30,000 daltons, and are broadly classified on the basis of physicochemical and antigenic properties into three types:

Interferon - (IFN - α)

Interferon - (IFN - β)

Interferon - (IFN - γ)

Subtypes of any interferon are classified as IFN 1 or IFN 2. α Interferon (originally referred to as leucocyte interferon) is best understood and was the first interferon to be purified. It is produced by separating WBCs from human blood and exposing them to Sendai Virus. The viral capsid stimulates a human cell chromosome (presumably number 5) to produce interferon. However, these interferons are unable to affect viral replication in the cell in which they are produced. These interferons are absorbed by adjacent cells where they induce chromosome number 21 to produce an unknown protein that binds to mRNA molecules specified by the virus. Interferon is finally released in the culture medium and is purified using monoclonal antibodies. It seems that IFN - α consists of a family of at least five proteins with different but homologous amino acid sequences (IFN α1- IFN α5). The complete amino acid sequence of IFN α1 (166 amino acids) and IFN α2 (165 amino acids) was determined in 1980. Partial sequence analysis of IFN-β has also been made. Interferon-γ is produced by sensitized lymphocytes in response to the sensitizing antigen or to non-specific mitogens. It is a mediator of cellular immunity and is one of the major lymphokines. Interferon is a very powerful antiviral agent (effective at concentrations at 10^{-12} to 10^{-14} moles per litre). Apparently interferon does not prevent a virus from infecting the cell, but inhibits its intracellular replication. It acts as a hormone and triggers the synthesis of several enzymes such as protein kinase and phosphodiesterase. These enzymes in turn inhibit viral replication by degradation of mRNA and protein synthesis.

One of the major problems that had to be overcome in obtaining interferon from cultured cells was the extremely low concentration of interferon made by the cells. The production process starts with the growing of a particular cell line for about a week in a nutrient medium. At that stage little or no interferon is being synthesized. The nutrient is then replaced with an inducer medium that typically contains a mixture of polyinosine-cytosine RNA (a synthetic double-stranded RNA) and diethylaminoethyl dextran). The two compounds induce the cells to start manufacturing interferon. Before the cells begin to excrete interferon, the medium is replaced once again with a medium containing additional substances (such as insulin and guano-sinephosphate or low concentrations of serum albumin) that have been found to increase the yield of interferon or to increase its stability. Finally, the medium is' collected, concentrated, dialyzed and freeze dried. The resulting material contains only about 0.1 per cent of pure interferon; hence other purification methods are needed. One of the most effective and specific is immuno affinity chromatography. Monoclonal antibodies with an affinity for a particular type of interferon can be attached to polysaccharide beads, which are placed in a glass column. When the crude interferon solution is passed through the coloumn, the interferon molecules are adsorbed on the beads while the impurities pass through the column. The interferon is released from the column by altering the pH of the column with a suitable washing solution. By this method it can be purified by 5,000 fold.

Human interferon was successfully produced in 1980 by two American scientists Gilbert and Weissmann by cloning the genes in colon bacilli. Similar results were also obtained by Japanese workers a few months later, with a comparatively higher yield. Their work triggered a wave of experimentation in Israel (Weizmann Institute) and France (Pasteur Institute). At the same time the nucleotide sequence of the genes of IFN-α and IFN-β was determined by Taniguchi from Japan, Houghton from England and Derynck ffom Belgium. Both IFN-α (Leucocyte interferon) and IFN-β (Fibroplastic interferon) had quite a similar structure and 14 different genes coding for human IFN-α are known as reported by Weissmann from Biogen.

The molecular biology of the synthesis of interferon took a vital position when human leucocyte interferon was engineered by yeast cells for the first time. A DNA sequence coding for human leucocyte interferon (LeIF-D) was attached to the yeast alcohol dehydrogeqase gene in a plasmid and introduced into cells of *Saccharomyces cerevisiae* (The plasmid could also replicate independently in *E.coli*). These yeast cells could synthesize about a million molecules of interferon (on a per cell basis) and the yield was several fold higher than that produced earlier by Japanese workers (About 10,000 per cell). The production was relatively slow in *E.coli* (1×10^5 per cell) because in yeast it is easy to grow and replicate glycoproteins derived from mammalian cells. In yeast the mechanism of glycosylation (addition of carbohydrate group) is similar to that in animal cells. The DNA sequence for γ interferon has also been determined and is different from α interferon. However, in contrast to β interferon, t interferon gene is split with three introns and four exons located on human chromosome(12), γ interferon gene has also been cloned in *E.coli*.

In 1982, a host of scientists from Imperial Chemical Industries (lCI) and University of Leicester in England reported the complete synthesis of a gene coding for human leucocyte interferon (IFN-α1) comprising 514 nucleotides, being the largest gene synthesized. The synthetic gene has been demonstrated to function normally when integrated into a plasmid and introduced into *E.coli* and *Methylophilus methylotrophus*. Genetic recombination techniques were used by several research institutions and industrial companies to produce various types of interferon.

Table 8.15 summarizes the list of various companies and the types of interferon.

Interferon is important for the following reasons:

(1) Interferon has a direct role to play in regulating the immune system and suppresses the multiplication of both β and γ lymphocytes *in vitro.* It is also known to inhibit antibodies (formation) *in vitro.*

(2) Interferon has been known to inhibit multiplication of cancerous cells. It is assumed that interferon kills the cancerous cells by increasing host immunity. There are special type of cells known as natural killer cells (NK) which are specialized lymphocytes and offer major resistance against the formation and multiplication of cancerous cells. Basically, NK cells differ from lymphocytes and macrophages. Interferon is now considered to stimulate the activity of NK cells both by increasing the potential ability of pre-existing cells and by the induction of new cells.

(3) Interferon is very effective against viral diseases. As a matter of fact, it acts directly by stopping the virus. It has been used for quite a while in Russia, for the treatment of common colds and influenza. It has also been tried against hepatitis and herpes zoster. Interferon can be inoculated by intravenous, intramuscular injections or even as a nasal spray (as done in former U.S.S.R.).

Table 8.15

Various biotech companies producing interferon

Company	Country	Types
Cetus and Shell	USA	α_2
Biogen	USA	β
Collaborative genetics	USA	β
Genetech	USA	α, β, γ
Dauchi Seiyaku	USA	γ
Kyowa Hakro koygo	Japan	γ
Toray Industries	Japan	β, γ
Pasteur Institute	France	β
Transgene	France	γ
Searle	UK	β
Kaligen AB	Sweden	γ, β
Weizmann Institute	Israel	β

8.3.6 Production of Somatostatin

Hormones are chemical substances produced in particular cells that function metabolically by interaction with a target cell or organ elsewhere in the system. Many hormones are proteins. Recent studies have provided important new insights regarding protein hormone biosynthesis and function. Some important hormones and their triggering functions are listed-in Table 8.16.

Initially it was thought that hormones bind directly to specific rate limiting enzymes, thereby either activating or inactivating them. However, this idea has now been abandoned and the concept of a receptor introduced.

Receptors are proteins that bind a hormone with high specificity and affinity. All hormones act by binding to macromolecular receptors that are located either on the cell membrane or inside of responsive cells. The receptors for all polypeptide hormones and most amino acid derivatives are located on the cell membrane. The first human peptide hormone to be synthesized in a bacterial cell was somatostatin, which has been studied in detail by workers from the Hope National Medical Centre, at the University of California in San Francisco.

Table 8.16

Several Hormones with Regulatory Functions

Metatonin	Regulates circadian rythms
Somatoliberin	Stimulates somatotropin secretion
Somatostatin	Stimulates gastrin ,secretion and stimulates stomatotropin secretion
Lipotropin	Fatty acid release from adipocytes
Somatotropin	General anabolic fffects, stimulates the release of growth factors \
Thyroxine and Triodothyromine	General stimulation of many cellular reactions
Pastrin	Stimulates secretion from stomach and pancreatic secretion
Secretin	Regulates pancreas secretion
Insulin	Glucose uptake, lipogenesis, General anabolic effects
Glucagen	Glycogenolysis, release of lipia
Estrogen	Maintenance of pregnancy
Androgen	Maturation and function of secondary sex organs
Relaxin	Muscle tone
Ephinephrine	Smooth muscle contraction, heart function, glycogenolysis and lipid release.

Somatostatin is one of a group of hormones made in the hypothalamus at the base of the brain. The somatostatin gene is inserted into the bacteria by means of an expression vector constructed partly from a plasmid. Somatostatin is a hypothalamic hormone, 14 amino acid units long, that controls the release of several hormones from the pituitary. The gene is synthesized from eight blocks of single-stranded DNA fragments made up of a few nucleotides each. The fragments has overlapping complementary sequences to allow for correct assembly of the gene. Of the 52 base pairs in the gene, 42 make up the code for somatostatin; the remainder provide the two "sticky ends" that allow the gene to be inserted into the plasmid and include the information needed for proper expression of the gene and recovery of the hormones.

The expression vector was constructed from the plasmid pBR322, to which was added the control region and most of the betagalactosidase gene from the bacterial lac operon. Betagalactosidase is an enzyme involved in lactose metabolism; the control region contains the regulatory elements needed for expression of thc bcta galactosidase gene. The somatostatin gene was inserted into the plasmid next to the betagalactosidase gene. After the plasmid was introduced into cells of the bacterium *Escherichia coli,* the human hormone was synthesized as a short peptide tail at the end of the enzyme. Cleavage with cyanogen bromide freed the hormone, which has been shown to be identical with the molecule in human beings. The synthesis of many hormones is ultimately regulated by the brain through neurohormones. Somatostatin is then transported in the blood to the pituitary gland, where it acts to inhibit the release of insulin and human growth hormone.

In November 1977, Boyer, co-founder of the Genetech company (established in 1976 in San Francisco), first announced the synthesis of a complex molecule, somatostatin, by bacteria, the genome of which had been modified (10,000 somatostatin molecules per bacterial cell). One hundred grams of colon bacillus cells in an eight litre fermenter produced five milligrams of somatostatin; the same quantity was previously extracted by Guillemin and Schally from 100 tonnes of sheep brains.

8.3.7 Production of Human Growth Hormone (Somatotropin)

A deficiency of the pituitary growth hormone(Somatotropin) results in a form of dwarfism that can be cured by administering the hormone. The hormone is species specific and its main source has been human cadavers. It has been demonstrated that an intramuscular dose of 6-10 mg per week can increase the stature by more than 6 cms during the first year of treatment. Recently somatotropin gene was synthetically produced by a combination of chemical synthesis and isolation of natural molecules. This is a polypeptide of 191 amino acids (worked out in detail by Goeddel and workers at Genetech). The segment of gene that codes for the first 24 amino acids of the peptide was constructed chemically from blocks of nucleotide. Recombinant hGH plasmid was constructed by usual genetic engineering techniques. Reverse transcriptase was employed to copy the gene for the hormone from mRNA obtained from human pituitary tissues. Restriction endonucleases cutout the needed fragment and DNA ligase was then used to join the natural and synthetic fragments. The complete gene was inserted into a modified version of plasmid pBR322 incorporating the *lac* operon. The synthetic part of the growth-hormone gene had been constructed with its own initiation codon(ATG). The hormone could, therefore, be produced independently in bacterial cells, without the need for attachment to a bacterial protein. This growth hormone may have many clinical uses, but the extremely limited availability of the substance is a serious constraint. Microbiological production may not only increase the commercial availability of the drug but may also make it possible to investigate in detail its potential applications.

Human growth hormone (hGH) or somatotropin is secreted by the anterior lobe of the pituitary gland. It was isolated and purified in 1963 by Roos and his co-workers from the pituitary glands of cadavers. A deficiency of this hormone results in pituitary dwarfism, the incidence of which is reckoned to be about seven to ten per million of population. In 1981, it was possible to extract from a pituitary gland of a cadaver 4 to 6 milligrams of somatotropin in the form of the final pharmaceutical product. The supplies were inadequate for the treatment of pituitary dwarfisms in the industrialized countries. In 1978, Genetech company isolated a strain of *E.coli* K 12 which was able to produce this hormone by genetic engineering. Through this, a litre of bacterial culture broth yielded in 7 hours a quantity of hormone equivalent to that extracted from 60 pituitaries.

8.3.8 Production of Other Hormones

With the advent of techniques of recombinant DNA and gene cloning, several other human hormones are being produced on a commercial scale by isolating specific DNA sequencies coding for those proteins/hormones (Table 8.17). This is likely to enable clinical applications and improve economic provision for their utility in several deficiencies. Therefore, production of Beta-endorphin (a 31 amino acids brain opiod) by genetically engineered colon bacilli has been widely acclaimed. Workers from Australian National University, Canberra, University of California, San Francisco, and University of Columbia, New York were able to clone the DNA of beta-endorphin in *E.coli* and transcribed it along with β-galactosidase. The beta-endorphin which was released from the hybrid protein and purified had the biological activities of endorphins and reacted specifically to antiserum against beta-endorphin.

Table 8.17

Some Other Hormones produced by Inserting and Gene Cloning in Bacteria. (after Trehan, K., 1990).

Hormone	Functions
Somatomedia A	Stimulates the fixation of sulphur in cartilage
Somatomedia B	Stimulating the synthesis of DNA in cyclical cells
Somatomedia C	Stimulates the incorporation of proline into collagen and of uridine into DNA
(Hypothetic Growth hormonereleasing Factor)	Could make up the deficiency of Somatotropin
Throotropin (THRF)	Regulates thyroid gland
Pancreas growth Hormone-releasing factor (hpGRF)	Possible treatment of pituitary dwarfism to accelerate the factor reconstitution of tissues of patients with severe burns
Thymopoietin	Thymic hormone

8.4 FERMENTATION OR BIOPROCESS TECHNOLOGY

Microorganisms have been used for the production of foods such as cheese, yoghurt, fermented pickles, and beverages such as beer, wine and derived spirits. This has been possible due to the role of fermentation technology. Today fermentation technology is recognized as bioprocess technology.

Bioprocessing involves a multitude of complex enzyme catalyzed reactions within specific microorganisms and these reactions are critically dependent on the physical and chemical conditions that exist in their immediate environment. Successul biprocessing will take place only when all the essential factors work together optimally.

Bioprocess technology is used in the following ways

(i) To produce various products related to food and beverages

(ii) To overproduce essential primary metabolites such as acetic and lactic acids, glycerol, acetone, butyl alcohol, organic acids, amino acids, vitamins and polysaccharides;

(iii) To produce secondary metabolites (metabolites that do not appear to have an obvious role in the metabolism of the producer organism) such as penicillin, streptomycin, cephalosporin, gibberellins, etc.

(iv) To produce many forms of industrially useful enzymes, e.g. exocellular enzymes such as invertase, asparaginase, restriction endonuclease, etc.

(v) To use cells derived from higher plants and animals to produce many important products, e.g. plant cell cultures are used to produce flavours, perfumes and drugs; animal cell culture is used to produce vaccines, antibodies, protein molecules such as interferon, interleukins etc.

Bioprocess technology uses essentially very similar product formation stages, no matter what organism is selected, what medium is employed and what product is formed. Usually, large numbers of cells are grown under defined controlled conditions. The organisms must be cultivated and motivated to form the desired products by means of a physical and technical containment system (bioreactor), and the correct medium composition and environmental growth regulating parameters, such as temperature and aeration.

In its simplest form the bioprocess can be seen as just mixing of microorganisms with a nutrient broth and allowing the components to react, e.g. yeast cells with a sugar solution to give alcohol. More advanced and sophisticated processes operating at large scale need to control the entire system so that the bioprocess can proceed efficiently and be readily and exactly repeated with the same amounts of raw materials and inoculum to produce precisely the same amount of product. The proper exploitation of an organism's potential to form distinct products of defined quality and in large amounts will need a detailed knowledge of the biochemical mechanisms of product formation.

8.4.1 Microbial culture

The growth of any organism is seen as the increase of cell material expressed in terms of mass or cell number. Growth results from a highly complicated and coordinated series of enzyme-catalyzed biological steps. Growth of a cell normally depends on the availability and transport of necessary nutrients and subsequent uptake. It also depends on environmental parameters such temperature, pH and aeration which have to be optimally maintained.

The amount of biomass or specific cellular component in a bioreactor can be determined gravimetrically (by dry weight, wet weight, DNA or protein) or numerically for unicellular systems (by number of cells). Doubling time refers to the duration of time required for the doubling in the weight of biomass. Generation time refers to the period necessary for the doubling of cell numbers. Depending on the size of the cell and complexity, the average doubling times vary. For exmple, for bacteria 0.25-1hr; for yeast 1-2hr; for mould fungi 2-6.5 hr; for plant cells 20-70 hr; for animal cells 15-48 hr.

There are three main ways of growing microorganisms in a bioreactor, namely batch, semi-continuous and continuous. Inside a bioreactor reactions can occur with static or agitated cultures, in the presence or absence of oxygen, and in liquid or low moisture conditions. Microorganisms can be free or attached to surfaces by immobilization or by natural adherence.

8.4.1.1 Batch culture

In a batch culture the microorganisms are inoculated into a fixed volume of medium and as growth takes place nutrients are consumed and products of growth (biomass, metabolites) accumulate. Ultimately, cell multiplication stops because of exhaustion or limitation of nutrients and accumulation of toxic excreted waste products from the cells.

There are six growth characteristics in a batch culture of a microorganism: 1, lag phase, 2, transient acceleration, 3, exponential phase, 4, deceleration phase, 5, stationary phase and 6, death phase.

The initial lag phase is a time of no apparent growth but cells are in the process of adapting to the environmental conditions and are biochemically and metabolically very active.

In the transient phase the cells begin to grow. In the exponential phase cells multiply at maximum possible rate because there is an ideal environment for growth, the nutrients are available in plenty and there are no growth inhibiting substances or wastes.

In the deceleration phase, growth rate decreases as nutrient conditions change due to accumulation of growth inhibiting substances which are produced by the cells. In the stationary phase no growth takes place because of lack of nutrients and the change in the environmental conditions. In the death phase the growth completely stops due to above reasons and cell lysis occurs. Hence most biotechnological batch processes are stopped before this stage.

Usually in industrial usage, batch cultivation has been operated to optimize the organism and then to allow it to perform specific biochemical transformations such as end-product formation (e.g. amino acids, enzymes) or decomposition of substances (sewage treatment, bioremediation). Many important products such as antibiotics are optimally formed during the stationery phase of the growth cycle in batch cultivation. The life of a batch culture can be prolonged by various substrate feed methods such as i) gradual addition of concentrated components of the nutrient, and ii) addition of medium to the culture and withdrawal of an equal volume of used cell-free medium.

8.4.1.2 Continuous culture

Continuous culture gives a balanced growth with little fluctuation of nutrients, metabolites, cell numbers or biomass. This is done by the addition of fresh medium into the batch system at the exponential phase of growth and the removal of used medium with cells or organisms. Continuous culture permits organisms to grow under unchanging (steady state) conditions in which growth occurs at a constant rate and in a constant environment. Factors such as pH and the concentrations of nutrients and metabolic products that change during batch culture are almost constant in continuous culture.

8.4.2 Fermenter/Bioreactor

A container is required to provide the correct environment for optimization of organism growth and metabolic activity for every biotechnological process. Such container is referred to as fermenter or bioreactor. There are different kinds of containers from simple, stirred or non-stirred, open to complex, aseptic, integrated types involving varying levels of computer inputs.

There are two distinct types of bioreactor system, namely non-aseptic and aseptic. In non-aseptic system it is not absolutely essential to operate with entirely pure cultlures, e.g. brewing, effluent disposal etc.

In aseptic system, it is absolutely essential to operate with entirely pure cultures for successful product formation, e.g. antibiotics, vitamins etc.

Within the bioreactor microorganisms are suspended in the aquous nutrient medium containing the necessary substrates for growth of the organism and required product formation. All nutrients, including oxygen, must be provided to diffuse into each cell, and waste products such as heat, CO_2 and spent metabolites be removed. Fermentation reactions involve a gas phase (containing N_2, O_2, and CO_2), one or more liquid phases (aquous medium and liquid substrate) and solid microphase (the microorganisms and solid substances).

Some important operating guidelines should be followed to achieve optimization of the bioreactor system.

(i) The bioreactor shoud be designed to exclude entrance of contaminating organisms as well as to contain the desired organisms

(ii) The volume of culture should remain constant, i.e., there should be no leakage or evaporation

(iii) The dissolved oxygen level must be maintained above critical levels of aeration and culture agitation for aerobic organisms

(iv) Environmental parameters such as temperature, pH etc. must be controlled; and the culture volume must be mixed well

(v) The material used to construct bioreactor should be resistant to corrosion, nontoxic and withstand high pressure.

8.4.2.1 Scale-up

Normally, fermentation processes are developed in three stages or scales. In the initial stage, basic screening procedures are carried out using relatively simple microbiological techniques, such as Petri dishes, flasks, etc. This is followed by a pilot scale investigation to determine the optimal operating conditions in a volume capacity of 5 to 200 litres. The final stage is the transfer of the study to plant or production scale and final economic realization.

In all fermentation processes, quality of water should be of prime importance since it affects microbial growth and the production of specific bioproducts. Availability and type of nutrient can exert strong physiological control over fermentation reactors and product fermentation. The basic nutritional requirements are an energy source or carbon source, a nitrogen source, inorganic elements and some specific growth factors. Sterilization practices for media must achieve maximum kill of contaminating microorganisms with minimum temperature damage to medium components.

In some biotechnological processes solid substrates such as cereal grains, legume seeds, wheat bran, lignocellulose materials such as straws, sawdust or wood shavings, and a wide range of plant and animal materials are used for the growth of microorganisms.

Large-scale production of suspension cell cultures of many plant species has been achieved, e.g. nicotine, alkaloids and ginseng. It is now possible that large-scale fermentation programmes may be able to produce commercially acceptable levels of certain high value plant products such as digitalis, jasmine, spearmint, codeine, etc.

There is an increasing use of animal cell cultivation for industrial-level production of high value products such as vaccines, interferons, hormones, insulin, plasminogen and various antibodies. The main problems that occur in mass cultivation of mammalian cells include the extreme sensitivity of cells to impurities in water, the cost and quality control of media and the need to avoid contamination by microorganisms.

Attachment culture and suspension culture are combined together by the use of microcarrier beads. In principle, the anchorage-dependent cells attach to special DEAE-Sephadex beads (having a surface area of $7cm^2\ mg^{-1}$) that are able to float in suspension. Many cell types have been grown in this manner, with successful production of viruses and human interferon.

8.4.2.2 Downstream processing

Downstream processing refers to extraction and purification of the desired end-product from the cell grown in a bioreactor. It is primarily concerned with initial separation of the bioreactor broth into a liquid phase and a solid phase and subsequent concentration and purification of the product. The steps involved are separation (filtration, centrifuagation, flotation, disruption), concentration (solubilization, extraction, thermal processing, membrane filtration, precipitation), purification (crystallization, chromatography), modification and drying.

Final products of the downstream purification stages should have some degree of stability for commercial distribution. Stability is best achieved for most products by using some form of drying. In practice this is achieved for most products by spray-drying, fluidized-bed drying or freeze-drying. The method of choice is product and cost dependent. Products sold in the dry form include organic acids, amino acids, antibiotics, polysaccharides, enzymes, single cell proteins, etc.

Many products cannot easily be supplied in dry form and hence only liquid preparations have to be done. At such times, care must be taken to avoid microbial contamination and deterioration. If the product is proteinaceous, care also should be taken to avoid denaturation.

8.5 Enzyme Technology

Enzyme technology refers to the use of enzymes in industrial processes in which their unique ability to perform their specific chemical transformations in isolation is utilized. Enzyme technology embraces the production, isolation, purification, use in soluble form, immobilization and use in bioreactors.

8.5.1 Enzymes

Enzymes are complex protein molecules present in living cells, where they act as catalysts in bringing about chemical changes in substances. Although enzymes are formed only in living cells, many can be separated from the cells and can continue to function *in vitro*. W. Kuhre coined the word 'enzyme' in 1878.

An enzyme is active because of its catalytic nature. An enzyme carries out its activity without being consumed in the reaction, while the reaction occurs at a very much higher rate when the enzyme is present. Enzymes are highly specific; they function only on substrates. A minute amount of enzyme can react with a large amount of substrate. The catalytic function of the enzyme is due not only to its primary molecular structure but also to the intricate folding configuration of the whole enzyme molecule. If the configuration is disturbed by change in pH or variation in temperature, the activity can be lost. Enzymes are non-toxic and biodegradable.

8.5.2 Applications

For many years, processes such as brewing, bread-making and the production of cheese have involved the unrecognized use of enzymes. Yeast fermentations and processes for conversion of starch to sugar had been going on for many years. The year 1896 saw the true beginnings of modern microbial enzyme technology, with the first marketing of takadiastase in the west. Takadiastase is a crude mixture of hydrolytic enzymes prepared by growing the fungus *Aspergillus oryzae* on wheat bran.

Earlier, in leather industry hides were softened (baking) by using dog faeces and pigeon droppings. Around 1900, Otto Rohm, a German chemist determined that the active components in dog faeces were proteases - enzymes that degrade proteins. He demonstraded that extracts from animal organs that produced similar enzymes could be used instead of the faeces. Soon pig and cow pancreases provided these enzymes.

From 1955 rapid development in enzyme technology occurred. The use of microorganisms in the production of enzymes gained ground. Today highly purified enzymes are used in industrial processing, clinical medicine and laboratory practice. Highly purified enzymes are very costly.

Most of the enzymes used on an industrial scale are extracellular enzymes, i.e. enzymes that are normally excreted by the microorganisms to act upon their substrate in an external environment, and are analogous to the digestive enzymes of human beings and animals. Thus, when microorganisms produce enzymes to split large external molecules into an assimilable form the enzymes are usually excreted into the fermentation media.

In this way the fermentation broth from the cultivation of certain microorganisms, e.g. bacteria, yeasts or filamentous fungi, then becomes a major source of enzymes such as proteases, amylases, etc. Some intracellular enzymes such as glucose oxidase for food preservation, asparaginase for cancer therapy and penicillin acylase for antibiotic conversion are now produced industrially.

The use of enzymes in detergents has been in practice for many years. Enzymes used in detergents improve washing results. While proteases have dominated the detergent market, there is increasing use of amylases and lipases for the removal of starches and fats. Cellulase and lipolase also have entered the detergent market.

8.5.3 Engineering of Enzymes

Genetic engineering is helpful to transfer useful genes of enzymes from one organism to another. If a good candidate enzyme for industrial use is identified, it can be cloned into a microorganism. This can be used in industrial fermentation. For example lipolase enzyme to remove fat stains in fabrics was first identified in fungus *Humicola languinosa* but the levels of enzyme production was inappropriate for commercial production. The gene for lipolase was cloned into *Aspergillus oryzae* and commercial level of enzyme production was achieved by NOVO Nordisk A/S.

8.5.4 Protein Engineering

Protein engineering is helpful to alter the performance of enzyme molecules. Protein engineering of enzymes involves the creation of a three-dimensional graphical model of the purified enzyme obtained from X-ray chrystallographic data. Depending on the requirement, charges to the enzyme structure can be done and then the corresponding changes in the gene can be made. Mutagenesis plays a very important role in this. A successful example of protein engineering is that of the enzyme phospholipase A2, which was modified structurally to resist higher concentrations of acid.

8.5.5 Immobilized enzymes

Enzymes are attached to insoluble polymers such as membranes and particles, acting as supports or carriers for the enzyme activity. The enzymes are physically confined during a continuous catalytic process and may be recovered from the reaction mixture and used over and over again, thus improving the economy of the process. Some enzymes that are rapidly inactivated by heat when in cell-free form become heat stable by attachment to inert polymeric supports. Whole microbial cells can be immobilized inside polyacrylamide beads and used for a wide range of catalytic functions.

Immobilized enzymes are more stable than the soluble forms of enzymes; they are able to be reused in the purified, semi-purified or whole-cell form. Physical and chemical methods are used for enzyme immobilization. Physically, enzymes may be adsorbed onto an insoluble matrix, entrapped within a gel, or encapsulated within a microcapsule or behind a semi-permeable membrane. Chemically, enzymes can be covalently attached to solid supports or cross-linked. Immobilized whole microbial cells are being utilized greatly.

Immobilized penicillin acylase is used to prepare 6-amino penicillanic acid from naturally produced penicillin G or V. Immobilized glucose isomerase is used for the industrial production of high fructose syrups by partial isomerization of glucose derived from starch. Another important use of immobilized enzymes is aminoacylase production of amino acids.

8.5.6 Artificial Enzymes

Artificial enzymes or synzymes are synthetic polymers that may be protein or non-protein molecules having catalytic activities. Synzyme has also two functional sites, one substrate binding site and a catalytically effective site. Derivatized myoglobin and cyclodextrin are examples.

8.5.7 Ribozyme

Ribozymes are the modified RNA molecules that have the capability of catalysing certain chemical reactions. Ribozymes function as true catalysts enhancing the rate of chemical reactions without any net change to themselves. The catalytic activity of ribozymes arises due to their three-dimensional structure, which enables them to generate the substrate-specific binding site, similar to enzymes.

Ribozymes contain stretches of nucleotides that allow them to base-pair with a complementary RNA and they have a catalytic site that is able to cleave the backbone of the complementary RNA. Ribozymes are useful to fight against chronic diseases.

8.5.8 Biosensors

Biosensor is an analytical device that involves the combination of biologically active material displaying characteristic specificity with chemical or electronic sensor to convert a biological compound into an electrical signal. These electrical signals are amplified, interpreted and displayed to measure the concentration of compound present in the solution.

In design, the biosensor (enzyme electrode) is composed of a given electrochemical sensor in close contact with a thin permeable enzyme membrane capable of reacting specifically with the given substrates. The embedded enzymes in the membrane produce O_2, hydrogen ions, ammonium ions, CO_2, heat, light or even electrons depending upon the enzymic reaction occurring, which are readily detected by the specific sensor. The magnitude of the response determines the concentration of the substrate.

The biological component in a biosensor can also be antibody, nucleic acid, a microbial cell, etc. Biosensors are of various types depending on the physical changes that occur in the vicinity of the sensor such as heat, electric potential, movement of electrons, light, change in mass, etc. Biosensors have been constructed to measure almost anything from blood glucose level to the freshness of fish. Biosensors have a great role to play in the world economy.

Study Outline

Industrial Biotechnology

The commercial exploitation of a variety of processes and techniques related to microorganisms, plants, animals and hQman beings is known as industrial biotechnology.

Fermentation Production

Products of microbial fermentation and metabolism include primary metabolites, secondary metabolites, enzymes, proteins, polysaccharides and cellular biomass (single cell proteins).

Microbial Biomass and Single Cell Protein

Microbial product of commercial significance is the microbial biomass (the microbial cells themselves) e.g. commercially produced yeast cells, bacteria (*Methylophilus methylotroph us*), flavouring cheese from fungal biomass (*Penicillium roquefortii*). Single cell proteins are the dried cells of microorganisms such as algae, certain bacteria, yeasts, moulds and some higher fungi. The protein percentages for various single cell proteins are high.

Insecticides

Due to the hazardous effect of agrochemicals on plants and human beings, attention has been diverted towards the use of natural insecticides. For example *Bacillus thuringiensis* which intracellularly produces a proteinaceous crystal, toxic to insects, is being used as a natural insecticide.

Bacterial Vaccines

Bacterial cells are used for the production of vaccines. They give life-long protection against diseases like cholera, diptheria, whooping cough, plague, tetanus etc.

Primary Metabolites

They are low molecular weight compounds necessary for microbial growth e.g. amino acids, organic acids, purine, pyrimidines, vitamins and nucleotides.

Secondary Metabolites

They are low molecular weight compounds synthesized by microorganisms late in the growth cycle. e.g. antibiotics, alkaloids, plant growth hormones, pigments and toxins.

Polysaccharides

Many polysaccharides are characterized by high viscosity at low stress and low viscosity when stress is applied. Such characteristics make them useful in industries. e.g. Xanthan Gum, Gellan, Emulsan, Pullulan and Dextrans.

Enzymes and Proteins

Recombimnt DNA technology can be used for the improved production of enzymes and proteins. It is used to construct microorganisms which synthesize. human proteins with therapeutic potentials. Enzymes have a variety of commercial applications such as textile, photographic, pharmaceutical, food, leather, dairy and paper industries.

Fuels

Important fuels produced by microorganisms include ethanol, methane, hydrogen and hydrocarbons, e.g. *Zymomonas mobilis* ferments carbohydrates to alcohol. *Tbermoanaerobacter ethanolicus* is more efficient in the production of alcohol.

Microbial Mining

Microbial mining by the process of bioleaching recovers metals from ores that are not suitable for direct smelting because of their low metal content. The commonest organism involved is *Thiobacillus ferooxidans,* which can effect the solubilization of cobalt, nickel, lime and lead.

Bioconversion

It consists of the conversion of a metabolite to a structurally related compound by microlial cells. One of the oldest bioconversions is that of ethyl alcohol to acetic acid. Bio conversions are specific because they concern a single type of reaction and compound of defined structure. Steroid hormone synthesis is based on the method of bioconversion.

Food products

Microorganisms are involved in the production of food products like cheese, and other dairy products, non dairy fermentations, alcoholic beverages, vinegar etc.

Cells and Enzyme Immobilization

By the process of immobilization, the cells are firmly bonded to the support matrix and enzymes are made to function. Three methods are available: (a) physical binding, (b) cross-linking and (c) entrapment. The most widely used method involves entrapment in a polymer matrix. Matrices that have been used include collagen, gelatin, agar alginate, polyacrylamide and polystyrene. Cells of *E. coli, Achromobactet: liquidum* and *Brevibacterium flavium* are used in immobilization.

Industrial Plant Products

Plants producing high levels of sugar include, sugar-cane, sugar-beet and millet. They are lused as substrates in the production of alcohol. Plants are, sources of an extremely wide range of chemical substances specially secondary metabolites.

Biotransformation

Plant cells can be used to accomplish certain changes in the structure and composition of industrially important chemicals. This conversion by means of a biological system is termed biotransformation, e.g., digoxin and digitoxin from *Digitalis.*

Enzymes

Only a limited number of plants yield commercially important enzymes. Important among these are the plant sulphydryl proteases that include protease from *Papaya,* the main member being papain, bromelain from pineapple and ficin from fig.

Industrial Animal Products

Cultured animal cells produce a wide range of biological products of commercial interest including immunoregulators, antibodies, polypeptides, growth factors, enzymes and hormones. These products are used to manufacture viral vaccines, tissue plasminogen, interferon, monoclonal antibodies and tumour specific antigens. There are many human proteins which have long been believed to have therapeutic potential but which are in short supply. A whole range of proteins of potential value to the pharmaceutical industry has now been produced in cultured, recombinant mammalian cells. Human insulin, interferon, somatostatin, somatotropin and other hormones are produced by recombinant DNA technology.

Production of Viral Vaccines, High-value Therapeutics

With the possible exception of antibiotics, viral vaccines have provided greater benefit than any other pharmaceutical product. Many high-value therapeutics are produced industrially.

Production of Human Insulin

Insulin was discovered in 1916; in 1954 Sanger and his co-workers described the structure of insulin. It is made up of 777 atoms in two polypeptide chains. Originally insulin was obtained from Hog pancreas cells. Now human insulin is produced from bacteria using recombinant methods.

Production of Interferon

Interferon is the body's first line of defense against viral attack. It is produced by most body cells on exposure to viruses. There are three types of interferons. Human interferon was successfully produced in 1980. Interferon has a direct role to play in regulating the immune system.

Production of Somatostatin, Somatotropin and other Hormones.

These hormones have been sucessfully produced using recombinant DNA technology. Several other human hormones are produced commercially.

Fermentation or Bioprocess Technology

Bioprocess involves a multitude of complex enzyme catalysed reactions within specific microorganisms in relation to the environmental conditions. It is useful to produce various products. The organisms are cultivated to form the desired products by means of a physical and technical containment system (bioreactor) and the correct medium composition and environmental growth regulating parameters such as temperature and aeration.

There are three ways of growing microorganisms in a bioreactor, namely batch, semi-continuous and continuous culture. There are six growth phases for a microorganism, namely, lag phase, transient acceleration phase, exponential phase, deceleration phase, stationery phase and death phase.

A fermenter or bioreactor is a container that provides the correct environment for optimisation of organism growth and metabolic activity for every biotechnological process. Scale-up operation helps in multiplying the product in large-scale. Downstream processing refers to extraction and purification of the desired end-product from the cell growth in a bioreactor.

Enzyme technology

Enzyme technology refers to the use of enzymes in industrial processes in which their unique ability to perform their specific chemical transformations in isolation is utilized. An enzyme carries out its activity without being consumed in the reaction, while the reaction occurs at a very much higher rate when the enzyme is present. Enzymes have many applications.

Enzymes can be engineered by transferring useful genes of enzymes from one organism to another. Protein engineering is helpful to alter the performance of enzyme molecules. Immobilized enzymes are used for a wide range of catalytic functions. Artificial enzymes are synthetic polymer molecules having catalytic activities. Ribozymes are the modified RNA molecules that have the capability of catalyzing certain chemical reactions. Biosensor is an analytical device that involves the combination of biologically active material displaying characteristic specificity with chemical or electronic sensor to convert a biological compound into an electrical signal.

Questions

(1) What are the various industrial microbial products?
(2) What is microbial biomass? What is its significance?
(3) Give examples of single cell proteins and their uses.
(4) What is the role of *Bacillus thuringiensis* in insect control?
(5) Give examples of bacterial and viral vaccines and their preparation.
(6) List the names of primary and secondary metabolites and their industrial uses.
(7) What is bioconversion?
(8) Explain the techniques of cell and enzyme immobilization and its uses.
(9) What is the significance of biotransformation?
(10) Give a few examples of industrially important animal products.
(11) How is humulin produced?
(12) What is the importance of Interferon?
(13) What are the roles of human hormones?
(14) What is bioprocess technology?
(15) What are the uses of bioprocess technology?
(16) What are the different phases of microbial growth?
(17) What is batch culture?
(18) What is a bioreactor?
(19) What are the guidelines for bioreactor operation?
(20) What is scale-up operation?
(21) What is downstream processing?
(22) What are the applications of enzyme technology?
(23) What is enzyme engineering?
(24) What is protein engineering?
(25) What are the uses of immobilized enzymes?
(26) What is artificial enzyme?
(27) What is ribozyme?
(28) What is a biosensor?

9
Healthcare Biotechnology

Introduction

The medical and scientific approaches to human health have two main aspects: the curative and the preventive. Infectious diseases have been approached through these two aspects. Prevention of infectious disease seeks the reduction of their occurance through immunization, isolation, disinfection and disinfestation of the population. In the case of genetically determined diseases, prevention is made through genetic screening, antenatal counselling and gene therapy. In developing countries like India the development of substances related to the prevention of human diseases through the new biotechnological methodology is of great social importance. The methods and findings of recombinant DNA have interfused with the practice of clinical medicine at an amazingly rapid pace and this has had having a major impact on the field of health.

Human insulin, growth hormone, tissue plasminogen activator, streptokinase and a couple of interferon species are commercial products with many more in the pipeline. A host of diagnostics based on a variety of immunochemical techniques for the detection of cancers and other genetic disorders, as well as infectious diseases are slowly flooding the market. At least half a dozen diagnostics developed in our country are more or less ready for commercial exploitation.

One of the major medical applications of gene cloning is the diagnosis of genetic diseases in foetuses. In future, it may also be possible to treat some genetic diseases by transplanting normal genes into the cells of genetically sick people. Sickle cell anaemia, muscular dystrophy, and cystic fibrosis are just three of the over 500 known genetic diseases that result from recessive mutations in single genes. Biotechnology offers some interesting possibilities to diagnose and treat diseases.

9.1 Production of Rare Biological Molecules

Rare biological molecules which have the potential for immediate clinical application are those peptide hormones and proteins, present in normal individuals as blood products. Once the genes for these products are cloned and the protein overexpressed, intravenous administration should adequately supplement the levels of the polypetide which is deficient in the patient. Examples of products suitable for replacement therapy in this way are hormones such as the growth hormone and insulin, blood clotting factors (i.e factor vii, ix, VWF), factors important for erythropoiesis (erythropoieten), those involved in blood clot inhibition or breakdown (e.g. antithrombin III, tissue plasminogen activator) and humoral factors involved in mediating the immune response (e.g. interferons α, *β*, γ and the interleukins).

9.1.1 Steps Involved

The initial step in producing a rare biological molecule for the purpose of clinical application is the isolation of the gene. It is the genetic engineer's job to isolate the gene wl1ich codes for a protein of potential clinical use, while it is up to the physician to realize the potential value of obtaining a rare protein in a pure form and implementing its use judiciously.

To clone a gene for a rare biological molecule, one must first determine the tissue in which that gene is maximally expressed since it should contain the highest levels of messenger RNA and thus will increase the chances of its cloning. Cultured cells from this tissue, or from a large tissue source expressing the gene, such as blood or tumour, are used as the starting material. Total RNA is isolated from these cells. Since the majority of RNA is ribosomal RNA, the purified total RNA is passed over a poly-dT column and the polyadenylated RNA is purified. The mRNA for a particular protein may be further purified by isolating mRNA of a particular size or by immunoprecipitation of polyribosomes. This purified mRNA is converted into cDNA and cloned into an expression vector which will allow proper expression and regulation in either *E. coli,* yeast, or mammalian cells in culture. The cloned DNA fragment of interest may be isolated by identifying those cells producing a molecule with the correct biological activities.

An alternate approach may be used if some primary structural information (amino acid sequence) is available for the protein. This information can be used to synthesize oligonucleotides as probes to isolate the gene for that protein. There is a way in which *in vitro* synthesized oligonucleotides may be used finally in genetic engineering, i.e. if the protein has a small molecular weight, the entire gene can be synthesized.

A method of isolation which requires no gene or protein structural information is the *λ*. gtll cloning system. In this system one utilizes an expression vector and an antibody to the protein whose gene is to be cloned. A lambda *λ*. gtll cDNA library is constructed by isolating total poly A mRNA, converting it to cDNA, and then adding EcoRI linkers and ligating it to EcoRI digested lambda *λ*. gtll phage DNA. After *in vitro* packaging of recombinant phage DNA, a specific *E. coli* strain of cells is transfected and the phage plaques are probed with a labelled antibody against the protein whose gene is to be isolated and cloned. If a portion of the gene has been cloned in the phage vector, it expresses a beta-galactosidase fusion protein from a *lacz* gene within the lambda *λ* gtll DNA. If the hybrid protein produced from the recombinant phage/cDNA clone contains the epitope which the antibody recognizes, then a plaque formed from infection with that specific recombinant will bind the antibody. This phage recombinant is purified and amplified and the cDNA portion is utilized either to obtain the genomic copy or isolate a full length cDNA.

Most genes isolated for the purpose of purifying a rare biological product have been expressed in *E. coli.* For expression of a cloned eukaryotic gene in a prokaryotic system, the expression vector must contain proper prokaryotic transcriptional and translational initiation signals. The better the RNA polymerase binding site, the stronger the promoter, which improves the likelihood of high level exprcssion of the gene product.

9.1.2 Biological Molecules

One of the rare biological molecules already available for clinical use is insulin, which is needed by diabetic patients. Human insulin has the advantage over the previously used porcine and bovine insulins in that it has no variant amino acids and as a result it is less antigenic. Growth hormone helps in growth of tissues. Somatostatin blocks growth and releases hormone. Interferons act as antiviral and antitumour agents. Relaxin facilitates parturition. Renin increases erythrocyte production. Antihemophilic factor VIII controls hemophilia. Antihemophilic factor IX is useful against Christmas disease. Antithrombin III is used to remove blood clotting, Interleukins enhance immune responses. Plasminogen activator helps in lysis of clots in mycocardial infarction. Superoxide dismutase helps to prevent post-ischemic free-radical induced cellular destruction. Tumour necrosis factor acts as an antitumour agent.

9.2 Antibiotics, Vaccines, and Steroid Hormones

The introduction of penicillin and a host of new antibiotics has lifted the scourge of many infectious diseases and saved millions of lives,

9.2.1 Antibiotics

Antibiotics are antimicrobial compounds produced by living microorganisms and are therapeutically and sometimes prophylactically used in the control of infectious diseases. Today there are about 100 different antibiotics available for use on humans, This is only a small fraction of the 5000 or so compounds isolated from microbes which have been shown to kill or disable other microbes. A large number of antibiotics that are not used in medicine are rejected either due to harmful side effects or to the high expenses involved during manufacture on a large scale or due to lack of specificity. The four major classes of antibiotics—the penicillins, the tetracyclin, cephalosporins and erythromycin—are worth over US $ 4 billion in bulk sales each year, and all are superb examples of the art of biotechnology.

In 1928, Fleming reported the lethal effects of *Penicillium diffusate* on gram positive pathogens. Later on, large scale productions were carried out to fight gram positive pathogens. In 1945 Guiseppe Brotzu found a species of *Cephalosporium* producing a substance that killed a wide range of bacteria. Later on it was found that this organism manufactured cephalosporin antibiotic. Cephalosporin was developed to tackle pneumonia and other types of bacterial infection. Both penicillin and cephalosporin are members of the group of antibiotics known as beta-lactams, after a characteristic type of chemical ring structure they possess. They operate by preventing certain bacteria from building proper cell walls.

Then next useful antibiotic to be discovered was streptomycin. This was discovered by Selman Waksman and his colleagues, in 1944. Streptomycin is produced by the filamentous bacterium *Streptomyces griseus*. Streptomycin belongs to the group of antibiotics known as aminoglycosides. They block bacterial protein synthesis and impair membrane function as a result of their binding to ribosomes. Streptomycin proved particularly valuable because it attacks microbes which are unharmed by penicillin and cephalosporin. In particular, it revolutionized the treatment of tuberculosis. Some commercially important antibiotics are: actinomycin D, ampicillin, bacitracin, cephalosporin, chloramphenicol, erythromycin, gentamycin, nitamycin, penicillin G, Rifamycin, Steptomycin and tetracycline

Genetic engineering could be used to create modified antibiotics. If antibiotic-producing cells could be induced to employ their methyltransferases to tack on methyl units to their antibiotic molecules, a new antibiotic would be produced with different and perhaps even more useful properties. Genetic engineering attempts to produce strains of microbes which can produce high amounts or novel types of antibiotic by introducing specific genes into the microbes. Cell fusion techniques are also used today to produce better strains for the production of novel antibiotics.

9.2.2 Vaccines

Vaccines are biological preparations utilized for prevention of diseases . The most efficient way to prevent infectious diseases is active immunization through vaccination programmes. The basic principle of immunological protection through vaccination is the modified antigen that loses its pathogenic characteristics but still retains the capacity to induce antibodies that neutralize the native antigen. In 1967, over 10 million people were infected with small pox and the disease was endemic in more than thirty countries. Today this affliction has been wiped off the map through mass vaccination programmes.

Many other vaccines to fight viral infections such as polio, yellow fever, rabies, rubella (German measles) and hepatitis B have been successfully used.

The recombinant DNA approach to the preparation of vaccines is very similar to the isolation of rare biological molecules. First we identify the DNA sequence that code for pathogenicity determinants e.g. production of toxin.

By removing those specific sequences, we can transform the microorganism into an attenuated variant that retains all other characteristics and can be used as an immunizing agent. This is the approach in the production of vaccines against typhoid fever, and diarrheas caused by enterotoxigenic strains of *E. coli.*

Another approach is to identify the specific surface antigens of an infectious agent. The genes that code for the protective antigen protein are located, cloned and allowed to overexpress. The purified protein is then inoculated into an individual by a standard vaccination protocol and the individual mounts an immune response to the recombinant protein. If successful, the vaccinated individual will then be able to effectively overcome a subsequent encounter with the infectious agent. This approach is further refined if one can determine the region of the immunodominant surface antigen protein which is the protective antigenic determinant. Small peptides may be synthesized, conjugated to a carrier molecule, and utilized as the sole antigen source for eliciting a protective immune response.

Another approach is the utilization of monoclonal antibodies to identify a protein antigen in a given organism. This approach has yielded remarkable results when applied to the development of an antimalarial vaccine. The causative agent is the *Plasmodium* species of parasites. Sporozoite is the stage of the *Plasmodium* life cycle which is inoculated into the bloodstream by the bite of the female Anopheles mosquito while she takes a blood meal to feed her eggs. This stage expresses a major surface antigen which elicits an immune response. The gene for this antigen was cloned using monoclonal antibodies to screen a recombinant *DNA E. coli* expression library. This plasmid DNA library contained *Plasmodium* cDNA isolated using sporozoite mRNA, fused to an *E. coli* promoter. When the fusion gene expressing the cDNA which encodes the sporozoite surface antigen was isolated, the plasmid was subjected to Tn 5 mutagenesis and the immunodominant surface antigen epitope was delineated. The nucleotide sequence of this isolated recombinant cDNA clone enabled the synthesis of peptides which mimicked the immunodominant epitope.

Still another approach to vaccine development involves the use of a recombinant vaccina virus genome. In this method, DNA for surface antigen epitopes from viruses such as Hepatitis B or Influenza A or from parasites such as *Plasmodium* are cloned into the vaccinia viral genome. These cloned genes are expressed from a vaccinia viral promoter. Inoculation of an individual with the recombinant vaccinia virus produces a local infection and virus reproduction with the expression of gene products from the recombinant genome. In the process the host is exposed to the vaccinia derived and recombinant antigens and, hopefully, the host mounts a protective immune response to them. This yields a polyvalent vaccine. Inoculation with one recombinant vaccine containing these cloned epitopes will render the host immune to vaccinia, hepatitis B, Influenza and *Plasmodium*. Table 9.1 gives a list of vaccines under production by recombinant DNA methods.

Table 9.1
Vaccines under production by recombinant DNA methods

	Organism	Cloned gene
(a)	**Virus**	
	Hepatitis B	Hepatitis B surface antigen (Hbs Ag)
	Influenza	Hemaglutin in/Neuraminidase
	Herpes	Various coat subunits
	Foot and Mouth	VPI capsid protein
	HIV (HTL VIII, LA V)	Surface antigen
(b)	**Parasites**	
	Plasmodium (Malaria)	Sporozoite surface antigen
	Trypanasoma (Sleeping Sickness)	Merozoite surface antigen
	(Chagas Disease)	Surface antigen
	Schistosoma (Bilharzia)	Surface antigen
	Trichinella (Trichinosis)	Surface antigen
	Filaria	Surface antigen

9.2.3 Steroid Hormones

Hormones are the body's chemical messengers. They are complex organic molecules with varying chemical composition, secreted by ductless glands (endocrine glands). Hormones transfer all sorts of information from one group of cells to another distant tissue. The production of steroid hormones is a combination of chemical and microbiological processes. Microbiological modification of molecules in an otherwise chemical reaction is valuable when chemical modification produces two or more isomers, only one of which is active. Or the chemical reaction may have a mixture of compounds as the product, whereas the microbial product is one pure compound. Examples of enzymic or microbial transformations range from the simple conversion of glucose to sorbitol or gluconic acid, to the specific conversions of steroid and prostaglandin molecules.

Many hormones are steroids. Cortisone and hydrocortisone were known as adrenal hormones since 1930, but in 1950 it was shown that they suppressed the inflammation of rheumatoid arthritis. The sudden increased demand could not be met by the existing source (the extraction from adrenal glands of slaughtered animals). Chemical conversion of relatively cheap sources of sterols, i.e. bile acids, lanosterol from wool, ergosterol from yeast or various plant sterol glycosides, was difficult, complicated and therefore expensive. Also the number of reaction steps involved made semi-synthetic hormones prohibitively expensive (US $ 200 per gram).

Therefore the realization that microbial enzymes mediated the addition or removal of specific groups, with no significant side reactions, was a major advance in the production of steroid hormones. Cortisone was first commercially produced in 1952. Chemists found out that thirty seven separate chemical reactions were involved in the production of cortisone. Just then it was found that the bread mould *Rhizopus arrhizus,* could convert another steroid, progesterone, into a compound from which cortisone could be produced much more easily. The price of cortisone dropped to US $ 6 per gram and by 1980 further improvements had reduced the cost to US$ 0.46 per gram. Many different manipulations are performed now as a result of extensive search in a wide range of microorganisms for enzymic ability to modify sterol\ structure. Microorganisms are genetically manipulated to alter the efficacy of their enzyme systems.

9.3 Diagnostic Tests

Diagnostic tools are important guides to medical practice. Quick and accurate diagnosis is the first and crucial step in combating disease. Sometimes a patient's symptoms are so clear and characteristic of a particular disease that doctors have little trouble in making the correct diagnosis. In other cases, a certain set of symptoms could have a number of different causes; identifying the disease will depend upon a battery of other tests. Modern medicine depends on laboratory tests as aids in the diagnosis of many diseases. Biotechnology methods allow for the production of highly specific diagnostic tests.

In the area of infectious disease, diagnosis in many cases depends. on isolation and identification of a specific pathogen, whether bacterium, virus or parasite. One of the characteristics being used for the identification of viruses, bacteria or other agents is their surface structure. Antisera prepared against surface components can be utilized in the serological typing of such organisms. With regard to bacterial diseases, the identification procedure requires the investigation of a large number of characteristics: colony morphology, biochemical tests such as sugar fermentation, amino acids and enzyme production, serological typing, arid production of virulence factors, for instance, toxins.

Non-identification of the microorganism can bring about several serious consequences, such as the administration of wrong antibacterial drugs. The development of diagnostic test to identify microorganisms by biotechnological techniques enables rapid and specific diagnosis.

The production of monoclonal antibodies by hybridoma technique against specific antigenic determinants of the cellular surface provides an efficient method for the accurate identification of several microorganisms. These monoclonal antibodies are effective in recognizing several parasitic infections such as schistosomiasis, malaria and trypanosomiasis. They may also be used for identification of some viral infections such as poliomyelitis.

Among the bacterial diseases, the infectious diarrheas have been studied more extensively with regard to the development of new identification techniques, mainly those caused by enterotoxigenic *E. coli.* This bacterium is a major cause of diarrhea illness in adults and children in the developing countries. Its virulence is mainly due to the production of two enterotoxins (LT and ST) that are active in the small intestine promoting alterations in hydrosaline metabolism with consequent diarrhea.

Biotechnological techniques have contributed to the development of alternative assays for the detection of enterotoxigenic *E. coli*. These assays employ a simple method that can be used routinely by clinical laboratories. Genes that encode both LT and ST enterotoxins have been isolated and characterized using recombinant DNA techniques. These sequences, when labelled, *in vitro* with 32P, can be used as a probe for detection of homologous DNA sequences, by colony hybridization. This method detects the gene that encode the enterotoxins.

Development of organism-specific DNA sequences which act as probes would be more sensitive if they could detect suitable specific repetitive DNA sequences from an organism. Short pieces of DNA called probes can be designed to stick very specifically to certain other pieces of DNA. They can be used, for example, to find out if a patient's blood contains the DNA of a particular bacterium, and thus provide a diagnostic clue. It is possible to design probes which can be used to look for almost any type of DNA that interests the scientists or doctors. Not only can all types of microbial infections be identified but probes can also indicate genetic defects, detect contamination in donated blood, help in matching organs for transplantation and even assist seed suppliers to test the quality of their seeds.

The technique depends on the fact that two strands of DNA which have 'complementary' sequences of bases will stick together. To check if a sample contains a particular type of DNA (say, from a microbe) a biotechnologist will mix a DNA probe into the sample. The probe is designed in such a way that it is complementary to some part of the DNA which is being sought. If the probe finds its opposite number the two link together. If the 'target' DNA is absent then the test gives a negative result.

There are several tests like VDRL (Venereal Disease Research Laboratory), RPR (Rapid Plasma Reagin) ART (Automated Reagin Test) and STS (Standard Test for Syphilis) to identify syphilis. They depend on the use of non-treponemal derived substances to precipitate antibody in the host. Two other tests FTA-ABS, (Flourescent Treponema Antibody Absorbed Test) and MHA-TP (Micro hemagluttination-Treponema pallidum) use antigen derived from *T. pallidum* to precipitate host antibody. These tests are of no value when attempting to establish the diagnosis of syphilis in a new born due to the fact that the passive transfer of the maternal antibody will produce many false positives.

Using recombinant DNA methods, an antibody specific to *T. pallidum* could readily be isolated for use in a diagnostic laboratory test. One would first isolate DNA from *T. pallidum* and use this to construct a lambda λ. gtll genomic library. After packaging the recombinant *T. pallidum* phage library and infecting the appropriate bacterial strain, the phage plaques are screened using sera from a patient who tested positive for syphilis. Once the *T. pallidum* monoclonal antigens are isolated using the patient's polyclonal sera, individual phage recombinants are harvested and grown. The *T. pallidum* DNA sequences are overexpressed. Purification of the recombinant protein is readily performed by virtue of the fact that the hybrid contains a portion of the beta-galactosidase protein. An affinity column with anti-beta-galactosidase antibody is used to isolate the recombinant beta-galactosidase *T. pallidum* antigen proteins. The isolation yields specific *T. pallidum* surface antigen proteins which can be used to inoculate animals and isolate monoclonal or polyclonal antibodies. Then the antibodies can be used in a specific diagnostic laboratory test for detection of the presence of *T. pallidum*.

In the area of oncology recent evidence has demonstrated that most, if not all, human tumours are associated with the altered expression of oncogenes. Present prognostic indicators for cancer patients depend on clinical staging of the cancer, which is useful for anticipating future problems during the course of the illness. Tumour diagnosis based on the degree of expression of an altered oncogene, or on cytogenetic markers, may be a more accurate means of prognosticating as well as providing a rational molecular approach to intervention.

In 1993, scientists at the National Institute for Medical Research (NIMR) in London have found a. novel means of stopping cancer cells from producing tumours using heat shock proteins. These are molecules produced by cells when they are exposed to a stressful environment and which have profound effects on other molecules in the cell. The NIMR team transferred genetic material, coding for a heat shock protein from a bacterium into tumour cells. The protein had two effects. The cancer cells became incapable of producing tumours and their new impotency enabled their use to immunize against ordinary cancer cells because the immune system .was now able to recognize and eliminate the cancerous cells before they could produce tumours.

Enzyme linked immunosorbent assay (ELISA) is the most rapid and highly efficient method employed for diagnostic purpose. It is a sensitive serological test for detection and quantification of viruses, proteins and small molecules such as hormones, formed on a microtiter plate. The most wi dely used form of ELISA test uses the double antibody sandwich technique. A more sensitive technique called immuno-PCR using marker DNA is employed in clinical diagnosis.

9.3.1 Prenatal Diagnosis

The number of human diseases described as genetically determined is about 2500. For most of these diseases, only the symptoms are known and for genetic diseases such as phenylketonuria, hemophilia, and diabetes only a palliative treatment is applied. In some other cases the carrier will never have a normal life and so diagnosis and therapeutic abortion remains the only option. Nearly 40 different recessive diseases have been diagnosed prenatally, to date.

Elucidation of the molecular struc;ture of human genes has been possible by the application of recombinant DNA technology. Human genes and highly polymorphic unique anonymous DNA segments from man have continued to be isolated at a logarithmic rate. The eventual goal of mapping the entire human genome will bring with it the realization of a molecular understanding for many disease processes and also the ability to predict an individual's susceptibility to a disease. These cloned human genes can be used as probes in association with RFLP to prenatally diagnose a number of genetic diseases.

RFLPs are variations in size of DNA fragments generated due to differences (base pair changes) in the DNA segments in different individuals. They are visualized as different fingerprint patterns on a southern blot using specific DNA probes. RFLPs reflect polymorphisms in normal DNA and are inherited according to Mendelian principles. The physical basis for an RFLP is the difference in the DNA sequence of different individuals. The difference may be as little as a single base pair change, which destroys or creates a new restriction endonuclease recognition site at that point, or the diference may be due to a deletion or insertion of chromosomal DNA, which has occurred around the probe hybridization site. These mutations lead to a mobility change in the place of DNA detected with the specific probe when run at agarose gel due to altered DNA cutting (or size) and thus yield distinct patterns in Southern blotting. An RFLP linked to a given genetic disease may be found using a cloned gene as a probe or it may be associated with a linked anonymous DNA segment marker.

To perform prenatal diagnosis of an inherited disease when a probe is available, cells are isolated from the amniotic fluid during routine amniocentesis in the first trimester of pregnancy and are cultured in the laboratory. DNA is isolated from the cultured amniotic cells, digested with restriction enzymes, run on an agarosegel, and transferred to nitrocellulose by the method of southern blotting. The southern blots are probed using parental DNA, isolated from the peripheral lymphocytes for comparison. The procedure can be performed earlier in pregnancy if cells from a chorionic villus biopsy rather than cultured amniotic fluid are used for analysis.

Using the actual cloned locus as a probe in prenatal diagnosis has an advantage over using an RFLP in that, due to the possibility of recombination occurring between the linked RFLP and the disease loci, the diagnostic accuracy is not 100 per cent. The ultimate test in terms of predictive value occurs when a given mutation responsible for a genetic disease is due to a base pair change which occurs within the sequence of a specific restriction site. This occurs in sickle cell anemia where an Mstll restriction site is lost as a result of an A > T transversion which is responsible for valine substitution for glutamic acid in the β chain of the haemoglobin molecule. This leads to sickle cell phenotype. In some instances oligonucleotide probes have been used to directly analyse a mutation. However most genetic disease are heterogeneous at the genotypic level. DNA analysis is applicable to families where given genetic disease is known to occur. It is of limited value in diseases due to new mutations because one cannot anticipate the occurrence of such mutations. When some defects in chromosomes are identified through prenatal diagnosis, then it is possible to give genetic counseling to parents and help them to psychologically be prepared to make right decisions.

9.3.2 β-Thalassemias

The inherited disorders of haemoglobin synthesis, the thalassemias, have been the most extensively studied at the DNA level. Thalassemia is the name given to a condition in which there is a low level of, or sometimes a complete lack of, synthesis of one of the globin polypeptides. A defect in the rate of synthesis of a given protein could theoretically be due to an aberration in any one of the many steps in the pathway of gene expression: transcription, RNA processing, mRNA stability, or translation. Such aberrations may be due to point mutations leading to frameshift or nonsense mutations or to deletions of all or part of the gene itself. Each of these types of defects has been found in naturally occurring β-thalassemias.

β-thalassemia, in which there is a complete absence of β-globin synthesis, has been found to be caused by a point mutation either in amino acid codon 17 or in amino acid codon 39. In both cases, the mutation gives rise to a translation-termination codon. Other types of β-thalassemias have been found to be due to deletions or insertions in the β-globin coding sequence; these have resulted in a shift in the reading frame.

Only two naturally occurring β-thalassemias that are due to mutations affecting transcription have been identified. One is a nucleotide substitution at –87 relative to the mRNA cap site; the other is in the Tata box – 30 position.

Perhaps the most interesting class of β-thalassemias that has been discovered is the one due to aberrant splicing of β-globin transcripts. The dinucleotide sequence GT is always found at the 5′ (the donor) splice junction. Two different β^0-thalassemias in which this GT has been changed to AT have been identified. This leads to an incorrectly spliced (and untranslatable) mRNA.

9.3.3 Sickle-Cell Anaemia

Sickle-cell anaemia results from a mutation that changes a glutamic acid residue, coded by the triplet GTG, for a valine residue, coded by GTG at position 6 in the β-globin chain of haemoglobin. As a result, sickle haemoglobin tends to crystallize in red blood cells; the cells become less flexible and are removed by the spleen; and anaemia results. The mutation of A to T in the base sequence of the β-globin gene eliminates a restriction site for the enzyme *Dde I*. The sickle haemoglobin mutation can, therefore, be detected by digesting sickle-cell and normal DNA with *Dde I* and performing Southern blot hybridization. Normal DNA will generate two *Dde I* fragments of 201 and 175 base pairs, whereas sickle-cell DNA will generate only one fragment of 376 base pairs.

Although the restriction enzyme *Dde I* can be used to detect the sickle-cell mutation, it is not ideal for routine hospital screening procedures because there are too many *Dde I* restriction sites in the β-globin gene. Another convenient enzyme. *Mst III* has been of greater use sinc it cuts at the sequence CCTNAGG and generates 1.3 kilobase fragments which are much longer than *Dde I* generated fragments.

9.3.4 AIDS

AIDS (Acquired Immune Deficiency Syndrome) is causing intense concern among doctors and the general public. When AIDS was first discovered in 1981 by Dr. Luc Montagnier, it was restricted almost entirely to a few specific groups, notably male homosexuals, intravenous drug users, haemophiliacs and Haitians. The effects of AIDS vary but the most common effect is a drastic reduction in the patient's ability to fight infections thus leading to a slow death. The debilitating effects of AIDS often lead to a previously rare type of cancer known as Kaposi's sarcoma, and to very severe pneumonia. Once the disease has taken a hold, the chances of recovery from AIDS are very slim.

AIDS is caused by human immuno deficiency virus (HIV). It is also termed as LAV or HTLV III. The two HIV viruses—HIV-1 and HIV-2—have more in common with the simian viruses—SIV—than with each other. Of the two, HIV-2 is less virulent, causing AIDS in 10 per cent cases or less, while HIV-1 causes AIDS in 90 per cent of the cases.

In infected people, the virus is present in blood and other body fluids as semen, vaginal secretions, (not saliva) etc. It can be transmitted by infected needles, blood transfusion, unsafe sex etc. When the virus gets into the body, it works in the body's immune system and destroys a white blood cell called CD_4. Due to this, it looses the capacity to fight infections.

Doctors and scientists have yet to find effective ways of treating or preventing AIDS, but two biotechnological approaches are receiving great attention. Since most haemophiliacs are prone to AIDS due to receiving contaminated blood proteins, genetically engineered anti-haemophilia proteins have been made by cloning the genes for Factors VIII and IX and the small scale production of the proteins by bacteria. Secondly genetically engineered vaccines are being developed using the protein coat of the AIDS virus.

One diagnostic test that has been developed by Dr. Abraham Karpas to detect AIDS is described below. Cells derived from a specific line obtained from a leukaemia patient, are inoculated with the AIDS virus and introduced into the wells in a microscope slide containing 30 wells coated in Teflon. The specific cell line taken from the leukaemia patient is selected for its ability to host the AIDs virus and encourage viral replication. Detection of AIDS antibodies in blood is possible since the cells, which host the virus, become highly antigenic. Acetone is used to fix the cells, break open their membranes and free the virus.

To perform the test, a sample drop of blood serum is placed in one of the wells in the slide, incubated for an hour arid washed in saline to remove excess antibody. In an AIDS positive test, the antibody binds to the virus at the base of the wells. This is confirmed by the addition of a protein-peroxidase conjugate which binds to the antibody-virus complex. This is then incubated for 30 minutes and washed to remove excess peroxidase. The result is made visible by a colour change when aminoethylcarbazol is added and reacts with the bound peroxidase. If the membranes and cytoplasm of the cells are stained when seen under the microscope, then the test is positive for AIDS.

Recently (1993) a team of scientists from Harvard had reported that using a combination of two marketed drugs AZT (ZIDOVUDINE) and DOL with either of the two experimental ones, pyridinone and nevirapine, blocked the virus HIV from growing and spreading by attacking an enzyme that makes the copies. Later the same team reported that HIV had developed resistance by mutation.

9.4 Gene Replacement Therapy

Broadly speaking, gene therapy is the genetic modification of the cells of a patient in order to combat disease. Gene therapy simply means the introduction of normal genes to the cell of a patient in order to replace defective genes, which do not produce an essential protein. It is a process in which scientists take cells by adding healthy genes, and then replace the cells back into the patient. Alternately, the healthy genes are inserted into a carrier such as a retrovirus and placed into tissues of the patient. Retroviruses have the ability to encode DNA using their RNA as a model and insert the DNA into human chromosomes. In doing so, the retroviruses carry the new genes into the cell. The new genes then provide the genetic codes for proteins, which the patient lacks.

In other words gene therapy is a process for producing proteins in the body by inserting into cells the genes that encode for such proteins. These proteins could be useful for correcting deficiencies that lead to genetic disease, for enhancing body resistance to disease or for generally improving the quality of life. The idea behind gene therapy is very simple. If disease is caused by faulty genes, then let us replace the bad genes with good ones by adding a few good genes into cells. Although conceptually simple, the process of gene therapy involves biochemical problems of gene delivery, gene control and duration of gene action.

The genetic material may be transferred directly into the cells within a patient (*in vivo* gene therapy), or cells may be removed from the patient and the genetic material inserted into them *in vitro*, prior to replacing the cells in the patient (*ex vivo* gene therapy).

There are several necessary criteria for gene replacement to be implemented as a form of medical therapy. These include: (i) high efficiency of gene transfer, (ii) stable replication of the introduced gene as either an integrated transgene or as an extrachromosomal element; (iii) effective expression of the gene product in the target tissue, and (iv) adequate safety during the gene transfer period and throughout the life of the patient undergoing replacement therapy.

Vectors for Gene Therapy

Gene therapy is performed with non-reproductive cells, generally known as somatic cells such as blood cells, skin cells, bone marrow cells, intestinal cells, or any other cell except sperm or egg cell. The use of somatic cells ensures that there is no carryover of the inserted genes to the next generation. Most of the gene therapy attempts are exclusively somatic gene therapy. When sperm, egg and zygote is used for gene therapy it is called germline gene therapy.

A carrier molecule called a vector from the Latin word *vehere* (meaning to carry) is used to deliver genes into somatic cells. The vector can be a plasmid, or a cosmid or a virus. Retrovirus, a type of virus, is the most often used vector in gene therapy experiments. A retrovirus is a RNA virus that penetrates a host cell and uses its reverse transcriptase function to encode a DNA molecule that can integrate with the DNA of the cell.

A retrovirus contains RNA. The RNA is used as a template to synthesize DNA after the retrovirus enters the host cell. Then the DNA gets incorporated into the DNA of the genome of the host cell. The retrovirus is called a *provirus* in its DNA form. Usually a provirus causes no harm to the cell but some retroviruses like the human immunodeficiency virus (HIV) causes Acquired Immune Deficiency Syndrome (AIDS). Retroviruses are very efficient at transferring DNA into cells and integration of viral DNA occurs usually at a single chromosomal site. The integrated DNA can be stably propagated offering the possibility of a permanent cure for a disease.

In order to use a retrovirus as a vector, sophisticated biochemical methods must be used to remove the genes that might make the virus harmful. For example, a retrovirus can be made harmless by removing the genes that encode for its pathogenecity. Once retrovirus is altered, scientists can insert human genes into the body for therapy. Because the retrovirus is an RNA virus, the human genes are inserted in their complementary RNA form and not in the usual DNA form. Because vector viruses lack genes for synthesizing certain essential parts, the vector viruses cannot replicate in cells; thus, they have only a one-way passage into the cell. Once they deliver their genetic material, they can never leave the cell. In the retrovirus group, the most popular tool to be used as a vector is a strain of murine leukemia virus. This virus causes a form of leukemia, cancer of the white blood cells, in mice. The envelope protein of the virus attaches itself easily with a cell surface protein of the humans because of close similarity. Murine leukemia virus can only infect dividing cells. It can accommodate inserts upto 8 kb.

Adenoviruses are also used as vectors. Adenoviruses are DNA viruses that produce infections of the upper respiratory tract and have a natural tropism for respiratory epithelium, the cornea and the gastro-intestinal tract. Unlike retroviruses, adenoviruses can infect a wide variety of cell types. Entry into cells occurs by receptor-mediated endocytosis. It is efficient but the inserted DNA does not appear to integrate and hence the expression of inserted genes can only be sustained over short periods. Adenovirus vectors accept insert sizes up to 7-8 kb.

Herpes simplex virus can also be used as vector. Herpes simplex virus vectors are tropic for the central nervous system and can establish lifelong latent infections in neurons. They are non-integrating and so long-term expression of transferred genes is not possible. Their major applications are expected to be delivering genes into neurons for the treatment of neurological diseases, such as

Parkinson's disease and for treating central nervous system tumors. They have a comparatively large insert size capacity (>20 kb).

Adeno-associated viruses also can be used as vectors. Adeno-associated viruses are a group of small, single-stranded DNA viruses, which cannot usually undergo productive infection without co-infection by a helper virus. Helper virus is a virus that provides certain viral functions which are essential for productive infection such as viral DNA replication, viral assembly, e.g. adenovirus, Herpes simplex virus.

Adeno-associated virus integrates into cell's chromosomal DNA at specific site. Subsequent super-infection with an adenovirus (Helper virus) activates the integrated virus DNA. Adeno-associated virus vectors can only accommodate inserts up to 4.5 kb. They have the advantage of providing long-term gene expression with a high degree of safety.

Some concern has been expressed regarding the safety of viral vector systems, since there is a remote possibility of introduced viruses recombining with endogenous retroviruses. Some non-virus vectors are also available.

Vectors other than viruses

A vector of a completely different type is the human artificial chromosome. It is a vector DNA molecule synthetically produced with qualities of a human chromosome. This vector carries human genes that are too long to fit a virus or plasmid, and it encodes a protein more consistent with human protein than do the other vectors. The human artificial chromosome behaves like a natural human chromosome and passes from cell to cell during mitosis. It is a fully synthetic, self-replicating human 'micro-chromosome' about one-fifth to one-tenth the size of a normal human chromosome.

In some cases, DNA can be injected directly with a syringe and needle into a specific tissue. This is a direct injection method. An alternative direct injection approach uses particle bombardment technique where the DNA is coated on to metal pellets (e.g. gold bullet) and fired into cells with a special helium pressurized gun.

Receptor-mediated endocytosis is another method. In this method, the DNA is coupled to a targeting molecule that can bind to a specific cell surface receptor, inducing endocytosis and transfer of the DNA into cells with a special helium pressurized gun. Coupling is normally achieved by covalently linking polylysine to the receptor molecule and then arranging for binding of the negatively charged DNA to the positively charged polylysine component. Even though gene transfer efficiency is high this method is not designed to allow integration of the transferred genes.

A liposome is a microscopic spherical vesicle containing fat molecules. Coated with genes, the liposome is absorbed through the fat-based cell membrane into the cell cytoplasm, where the genes are released. The lipid coating allows the DNA to survive *in vivo*, bind to cells and be endocytosed into the cells. The efficiency of gene transfer is low and the introduced DNA is not designed to integrate into chromosomal DNA of the cell.

Retrotransposon is a small DNA segment from a cell that copies and inserts itself outside a gene. Retrotransposons are known to exist in human cells. They can also be used as vectors.

General Gene Therapy Strategies

Different strategies are used for gene therapy:

Gene augmentation therapy: For diseases caused by loss of function of a gene, introducing extra copies of the normal gene may increase the amount of normal gene product to a level when the normal phenotype is restored. As a result gene augmentation therapy is targeted at clinical disorders where the pathogenesis is reversible. This has been particularly applied to autosomal recessive disorders where even modest expression levels of an introduced gene can make a substantial difference.

Targeted killing of specific cells: Genes are directed to the target cells and then expressed so as to cause cell killing. This approach is popular in cancer gene therapies. Direct cell killing is possible if the inserted genes are expressed to produce a lethal toxin (suicide gene), or a gene encoding a prodrug is inserted, conferring susceptibility to killing by a subsequently administered drug. Indirect cell killing uses immunostimulatory genes to provoke or enhance an immune response against the target cell. The idea of modifying a patient's own tumor cells for use as a vaccine (adoptive immunotherapy) has been used to treat a wide variety of cancers. Here we immunize the patients specifically against their own tumors by genetically modifying the tumor with one of a variety of genes that are expected to increase the host immune reactivity to the tumor. Subcutaneous injection of genetically modified fibroblasts is also used in adoptive immunotherapy.

Targeted mutation correction: If an inherited mutation produces a dominant-negative effect, it can be corrected at the gene level by gene targeting methods based on homologous recombination or at the RNA transcript level by using particular types of therapeutic ribozymes or therapeutic RNA editing.

Targeted inhibition of gene expression: If disease cells display a novel gene product or inappropriate expression of a gene (as in the case of many cancers, infectious diseases, etc.), a variety of different systems can be used specifically to block the expression of a single gene at the DNA, RNA or protein levels. The basis of the therapy is to knock out the expression of specific gene which is responsible for cancer or infection or allergy or inflammation, without interfering with normal cell function. In some cases allelo-specific inhibition of expression may be possible.

Therapy by selective inhibition of gene expression is technically possible at all three expression levels: i) triple helix therapeutics (involves binding of gene-specific oligonucleotides to double-stranded DNA in order to inhibit transcription of a gene); ii) antisense therapeutics (involves binding of gene specific oligonucleotides or polynucleotides to the RNA; in some cases, the binding agent may be a specifically engineered ribozyme, a catalytic RNA molecule that can cleave the RNA transcript); iii) use of intracellular antibodies (intrabodies) and oligonucleotide aptamers (involves the construction of antibodies that can be directed to specific locations within cells in order to bind a specific protein, or oligonucleotide aptamers, which can bind specifically to a selected polypeptide).

Applications

Adenosine deaminase is an enzyme that breaks down certain by-products of a cell's nucleic acid metabolism. When adenosine deaminase gene is defective it produces a disease of the immune system called server combined immunodeficiency disease (SCID). If adenosine deaminase enzyme is not present in a T-lymphocyte, an enzyme called kinase converts one of the metabolic by-products to a toxin, and the toxin destroys the T-lymphocyte. T-lymphocytes are essential cells of the body's immune system. They not only participate in immune responses directly, but they also influence indirectly, by controlling the activity of B-lymphocytes, the cells that produce antibodies.

Thus adenosine deaminase deficiency causes the body to lose the protection of both kinds of lymphocytes, and without that protection, the patient cannot mount a defense against infectious disease and soon the patient will die. The gene for adenosine deaminase is located on chromosome 20 and has 32,000 base pairs and 12 exons.

In 1990, R. Michael Blaese and W. Fresch Anderson applied gene therapy to treat adenosine deaminase deficiency. They removed lymphocytes from the patient (Ashanti) and exposed them to billions of retroviruses carrying the genes for adenosine deaminase production. After the genes were inserted into the chromosomes of the lymphocytes, the lymphocytes were returned to the patient. The amount of adenosine deaminase produced by the gene-altered lymphocytes increased with time and the patient's ability to produce antibodies had also increased substantially.

In 1995, Blaese identified three fetuses with adenosine deaminase deficiency, obtained blood stem cells from umbilical cord when the babies were delivered, and successfully added adenosine deaminase genes to those stem cells. Four days after birth, the infants received the cells with adenosine deaminase genes which started producing a permanent population of adenosine deaminase producing cells.

Alternative treatments for adenosine deaminase deficiency do exist. For example, bone marrow transplantation from a perfectly HLA-matched sibling donor, which provides a cure in about 80% of cases or enzyme replacement therapy, consisting of weekly intramuscular injections of adenosine deaminase combined to polyethylene glycol.

Gene therapy for Cancer was done by Steven Rosenberg and W French Anderson. They used tumor-infiltrating lymphocytes (TIL), special cells of the immune system. Under normal conditions, TILs are stimulated by cancer cells and TILs enter tumors and destroy anticancer agent called tumor necrosis factor (TNF). TNF is a protein product of macrophages, the amoeba-like cells that provide defense against cancer cells. The TNF protein can be produced by genetic engineering techniques and it can be used to enhance the cancer-fighting ability of tumor – infiltrating lymphocytes.

Rosenberg and his colleagues treated patients having advanced malignant melanoma, a virulent form of skin cancer that normally fails to respond to treatment. They removed a piece of tumor tissue from the patient and isolated a number of TILs from the patient's blood. They cultivated the TILs with cells from the tumor tissue to stimulate the TILs and enhance their selectability for the patient's melanoma cells. They included in the mixture of substance called interleukin-2, which is a naturally occurring lymphocyte protein, to encourage rapid multiplication of TILs. Then they mixed the stimulated TILs together with retroviral vectors carrying the genetic code for TNF. The viruses invaded the cytoplasm of the TILs and carried the TNF gene into the chromosomes. The genetically altered TILs were cultivated for sometime to produce a colony of TNF-producing tumor-infiltrating lymphocytes.

As a next step, Blaese and his colleagues infused the TNF producing TILs into the patient's circulation. With their enhanced ability to destroy cancer cells and their selectivity for melanoma cells, the TILs attacked the cancer cells and delivered their anticancer TNF. Healthy parts of the body were avoided because TILs were selectively stimulated to seek out melanoma cells.

Again in 1993 Michael Blaese and Kenneth Culver introduced into brain tumor cells the gene that encodes the enzyme thymidine kinase. Thymidine kinase is used by certain microorganisms in the synthesis of DNA during cell division. Its activity can be interrupted by the drug ganciclovir. The enzyme thymidine kinase acts by combining phosphate groups with nucleosides to form nucleotides. The drug ganciclovir bears a close structural resemblance to certain nucleosides, and the thymidine kinase mistakenly takes up the ganciclovir to form a false nucleotide. During cell division, another enzyme called DNA polymerase attaches the false nucleotide onto a developing DNA molecule during DNA synthesis. Since the false nucleotide lacks an attachment point for the next nucleotide, the elongation of the DNA molecule comes to an abrupt halt. Because DNA synthesis ends, the cells cannot undergo division,

Inserting a gene for thymidine kinase to a cell would make the cell sensitive to ganciclovir activity. Tumor cells take the thymidine kinase gene, become dependent on thymidine kinase activity during cell division and develop sensitivity to ganciclovir which when injected, inhibits cell division and kills the tumor cell. A retrovirus altered with genes for thymidine kinase production from herpes simplex virus was used as vector.

Gene therapy has been attempted for cystic fibrosis also. Cystic fibrosis is a genetic disease in which sticky, dehydrated mucus accumulates in the airways and other ducts and makes breathing difficult. A major problem in patients with cystic fibrosis is the buildup of chloride ions within cells lining the body's organs and vessels. The ions normally pass out of cells through a channel-shaped, tunnel-like protein called cystic transmembrane conductance regulator (CTCR) protein. In persons with cystic fibrosis, the CTCR protein is

Table 9.2
Examples of some gene therapy trials

Disorders	Cells altered	Gene therapy strategy
1. Adenosine deaminase deficiency	T-Cells and homopoietic stem cells	*Ex vivo* gene augmentation therapy using recombinant retroviruses containing an adenosine deaminase gene.
2. Cystic fibrosis	*Respiratory epithelium*	*In vivo gene augmentation therapy using recombinant adenoviruses or liposomes to deliver the CFTR gene*
Contd…		
3. Familial hypercholesterolemia	Liver cells	*Ex vivo* gene augmentation therapy using retrovirus to deliver the lipoprotein receptor gene
4. Gaucher's disease	Hemopoeitic stem cells	*Ex vivo* gene augmentation therapy using retrovirus to deliver the glucocerebrosidase gene
5. Brain tumor	Tumor cells *in vivo* Tumor cells *ex vivo*	Implanting of murine fibroblasts containing recombinant retroviruses to infect brain cells and ultimately deliver HSV-tk gene
6. Breast cancer	Fibroblasts *ex vivo*	Retroviruses to deliver MDRI gene
7. Ovarian cancer	Tumor cells *in vivo*	Retroviruses to deliver wild type TP53 gene
	Tumor cells *ex vivo*	Retroviruses to deliver HSV-tk gene.

not produced because of a gene defect, and the ions concentrate in the cells. There they draw water into the cells and leave a dehydrated, sticky mucus in the body's passageways, especially its airways conditions such as these are conducive for infection. Adenovirus was used as vector. Gene-altered adenoviruses were sprayed into the patient's nasal passage, lungs and nose. Successful insertions to both nasal passage and lung cells were reported.

Gene therapy may also be used to treat acquired immune deficiency syndrome (AIDS), familial hypercholesterolemia (a genetic disease accompanied by a higher than normal level of cholesterol in the blood owing to the absence of cholesterol receptors), sickle cell anemia (a genetic disease in which the hemoglobin is formed incorrectly and the red blood cells collapse and assume a sickle shape) Lesch-Nyhon disease (a genetic disease in which the absence of a certain enzyme interferes with guanine and hypoxanthine metabolism, resulting in a build up of uric acid), peripheral artery disease (blocking of arteries in the legs), Gaucher's disease (an inherited disease of the central nervous system accompanied by enlarged spleen and liver, erosion of the long bones and yellowing of the skin in adults), hemophilia B (a form of hemophilia in which the patients fail to produce an adequate blood clot because of the absence of an essential clotting factor) and baldness.

Gene therapy may be the long-term answer to the problem of genetic disease. For successful therapy, the gene causing the disease must be isolated and reproduced; enough copies of the gene must be inserted into tissues that make the gene product; the genes must express themselves approximately, and the gene must be harmless to the patient.

9.5 Nanomedicine

Scientists have now developed tiny delivery vehicles that can carry anticancer therapeutic agents directly into infected cells, using strands of genetic material constructed through nanotechnology. These delivery agents are called nanoparticles, and are assembled from three short pieces of ribonucleic acid.

The microscopic particles are designed in such a way that they possess both the right size to gain entry into cells and also the right structure to carry other therapeutic strands of RNA inside with them, where they are able to halt viral growth or cancer's progress.

The nanoparticles have been created by linking together different kinds of RNA, after the successful manipulation of these stringy molecules into different shapes, including rods, triangles and arrays.

The particles pass through cell membranes into the cell's interior and the tiny triangles fit and interrupt the growth of cancer cells. Nanomedicine offers a potential wealth of new treatments for chronic diseases.

Nanomedicine may be broadly defined as the comprehensive monitoring, control, construction, repair, defense, and improvement of all human biological systems, working from the molecular level, using engineered nanodevices and nanostructures.

Nanomedicine, an offshoot of nanotechnology, refers to highly specific medical intervention at the molecular scale for curing disease or repairing damaged tissues, such as bone, muscle, or nerve. A nanometer is one-billionth of a meter, too small to be seen with a conventional lab microscope. It is at this size scale – about 100 nanometers or less – that biological molecules and structures inside living cells operate.

Nanotechnology involves the creation and use of materials and devices at the level of molecules and atoms. Research in nanotechnology began with applications outside of medicine and is based on discoveries in physics and chemistry. This is because it is essential to understand the physical and chemical properties of molecules or complexes of molecules in order to control them. The same holds true for the molecules and structures inside living tissues. Researchers have developed powerful tools to extensively categorize the parts of cells in vivid detail, and we know a great deal about how these intracellular structures operate. Yet, scientists have still not been able to answer questions such as, "How many?" "How big?" and "How fast?" These questions must be addressed in order to build "nano" structures or "nano" machines that are compatible with living tissues and can safely operate inside the body. Once these questions are answered, we will design better diagnostic tools and engineer structures for more specific treatments of disease and repair of tissues.

Research directed toward gathering extensive information about the physical properties of intracellular structures will inform us about how biology's molecular machines are built.

As this catalogue of the interactions between molecules and larger structures develops, patterns will emerge, and we will have a greater understanding of the intricate operations of molecular structures, processes, and networks inside living cells. Mapping these networks and understanding how they change over time is crucial to help us understand nature's rules of biological design that, in turn, will enable researchers to use this information to correct biological defects in unhealthy cells. This knowledge will lead to the development of new tools that will work at the "nano" scale and allow scientists to build synthetic biological devices, such as tiny sensors to scan for the presence of infectious agents or metabolic imbalances that could spell trouble for the body, and miniature devices to destroy the infectious agents or fix the "broken" parts in the cells.

Study Outline

Production of Rare Biological Molecules

Peptide hormones and proteins present in normal individuals as blood products are some of the rare biological molecules which have potential and immediate clinical application. By cloning these gnes, we can produce these proteins in bulk and use them for treatment. Products such as growth hormone, insulin blood clotting factors, erythropoietin, antithrombin, tissue plasminogen activator and interferon are some examples.

Antibiotics, Vaccines and Steroid Hormones

There are about 100 different antibiotics available today for human use. The four major classes of antibiotics—the penicillins, the tetracyclins, the cephalosporins and erythromycin—are superb examples of the art of biotechnology. Genetic engineering is also used to create modified antibiotics, by introducing new genes into microbes.

The most efficient way to prevent infectious diseases is active immunization through vaccination programmes. The recombinant DNA approach to prepare vaccines is very similar to the isolation of rare biological molecules. Various approaches are available such as, (i) identifying the DNA sequences that code for pathogenicity and transforming the microorganism into an attenuated variant (ii) identifying the specific surface antigens of the infectious agent, cloning it to produce in large amount (iii) using monoclonal antibodies to identify a protein antigen in a given organism, (iv) using recombinant vaccinia virus genome. Different kinds of vaccines have been produced.

A combination of chemical and microbiological processes are used in the production of steroid hormones. Chemical methods alone make the products very costly. Microorganisms are genetically manipulated to alter the efficacy of their enzyme systems and thus help in bulk production of steroids.

Diagnostic Tests

Since quick and accurate diagnosis is the first and crucial step in combating diseases, biotechnological methods allow for the production of highly specific diagnostic tests. In the area of infectious disease, diagnosis depends on the isolation and identification of the specific pathogen and its surface structure. The production of monoclonal antibodies by hydridoma technique against specific antigenic determinants of the cellular surface provides an efficient method for the accurate identification of several microorganisms. Organism specific DNA sequences which act as probes are also used.

Prenatal diagnosis using amniotic fluid is helpful to diagnose diseases caused by recessive genes. The cloned human genes can be used to prenatally diagnose a number of genetic diseases. AIDS is caused by human immuno-deficiency virus (HIV) and many biotechnological procedures have been developed to diagnose the disease.

Gene Therapy

Gene therapy aims at replacing a defective gene in an individual, thereby curing that person of the genetic disease. Retroviral vectors are one of the tools used in this procedure. Recombinant retroviruses are constructed by placing a cDNA copy of the gene of interest in a plasmid DNA vector. Since gene therapy is concerned with healing a whole individual consisting of billions of semi-independent cells, it is not an easy task. Gene replacement therapy can only be attempted in a very few selective genetic diseases. These include single gene defects in which the molecular details of the affected gene are well understood.

Questions

(1) Name some of the rare biological molecules produced by biotechnological methods.
(2) What are the steps involved in the production of biological molecules?
(3) What are antibiotics? How can we produce novel antibiotics?
(4) What are the methods of producing vaccines using biotechnological techniques?
(5) Give some of the names of vaccines produced biotechnologically.
(6) How is biotechnology helpful in the production of steroid hormones?
(7) What are the techniques used to produce diagnostic tests?
(8) In what ways is prenatal diagnosis helpful?
(9) What is the causative organism of AIDS? How do you diagnose?
(10) What is gene replacement therapy? How is it carried out?
(11) What is the use of ELISA?

10
Environmental Biotechnology

Introduction

Environmental biotechnology deals with the use of biotechnological tools to protect and conserve the environment. Two important areas of environmental biotechnology are waste treatment and bioenergy production. The anticipated increase in human population by the turn of the century would naturally imply augmentation of our energy resources so that productivity is maintained for sustained growth.

The world's oil resources are shrinking at a fast rate and production costs in the utilisation of fossil fuels are increasing. Hence, recycling and utilization of agricultural and animal wastes over the last decade and a half has gained ground, contributing not only to increased food production, but also to a variety of valuable commodities and energy. Waste can be used to produce energy with subsequent valorization of biomass and the curtailment of environmental pollution.

10.1 Waste Treatment

In terms of volume, the treatment of sewage and waste water from domestic and industrial sources is the largest biotechnological industry. Although the technology of sewage treatment is relatively new, the art of sanitation is several thousand years old. The most famous pre-historic sewerage systems are those of: (a) the Akkadian city of Eshnunna, situated close to what is now Baghdad (b) the city of Mohenjo-Daro in Pakistan and (c) the Aegean civilization of Minos equipped with flushing toilets, on the Island of Crete. Initially the treatment of sewage was aimed both at improving the environment and utilizing the manurial value of the sewage on the land. Treatments were done by filtration with the use of filters (upflow filters, brush wood filters, biofilters), and mechanical aeration systems (oxidation, activated sludge).

Wastes and by-products of activities in agriculture, forestry and food industry can be used for various purposes, particularly to produce energy. They can also be degraded into fermentative compounds by microorganisms or transformed into proteins in the same way as saturated aliphatic hydrocarbons, n-paraffins (by-products of oil refining), methane or methanol.

The cultivation of algae on waste water, which has been markedly developed and improved, contributes to the purification of this water and provides a biomass high in proteins and trace elements.

10.1.1 Treatment Systems

Many types of wastes are suitable for biological treatment and some may even yield useful products. For example, wastes from intensive cattle rearing may be fermented anaerobically to produce methane as a fuel. SCP for animal feed purposes may be produced from the waste streams of food processing plants and paper and pulp mills. Other wastes may be more problematic: e.g. oily water discharges from petrochemical industries and distillery wastes with a high COD and a high concentration of salts including Cu and S require special treatment, the latter often being discharged onto waste land. Wastes which are especially toxic or of very high COD are often treated in specialized plants within the chemical works producing them; wastes of lower toxicity or with only a moderate COD are dealt with in municipal treatment plants. Some chemicals may resist biodegradation and this may be especially true for those of man-made orgin (xenobiotics).

Dry disposal of wastes involves compacting material into layers alternating with soil and finally covering with soil. Such landfills are limited by the availability of suitable sites. This is used extensively by municipal authorities. The decomposition occurs slowly and anaerobically with methane being the expected product. Some preliminary treatment is required for most wastes in order to remove large particulate materials and to allow some suspended solids to settle down.

10.1.2 Anaerobic Waste Treatment

Many anaerobic digesters consist essentially of closed containers with some provision for gas collection and occasional mixing (Fig. 10.1). Recent innovations include film reactors employing immobilized microorganisms. Biogas is the product of the anaerobic decomposition of organic material and the most important component produced is methane. Methane is very insoluble and separates readily from a fermentation system and is easily collected and pressurised or liquified for storage. In addition, it is readily combustible and as such is a valuable energy source. The composition of biogas varies with the nature and concentration of substrates and the temperature of incubation. The methane content would usually be in the range of 60-75 per cent with CO_2 accounting for 25-30 per cent and the remainder being H_2 and N_2.

The overall production of methane from organic wastes is a complex fermentation involving a number of groups of micro organisms which vary in numbers and composition depending upon the effluent composition and other environmental parameters. Growth is slow, but based on a 7-14 day throughput, anaerobic digesters reduce COD typically by about 75 per cent. The initial step involves the breakdown of polymeric materials, carbohydrates, proteins, fats, etc. These are carried out by facultative anaerobes as well as anaerobes and form end products such as ethanol and lower fatty acids (acetic, propionic, and butyric acids) together with H_2 and CO_2. This process lowers the molecular weight of the wastes and in sewage treatment it is often called sludge liquifaction.

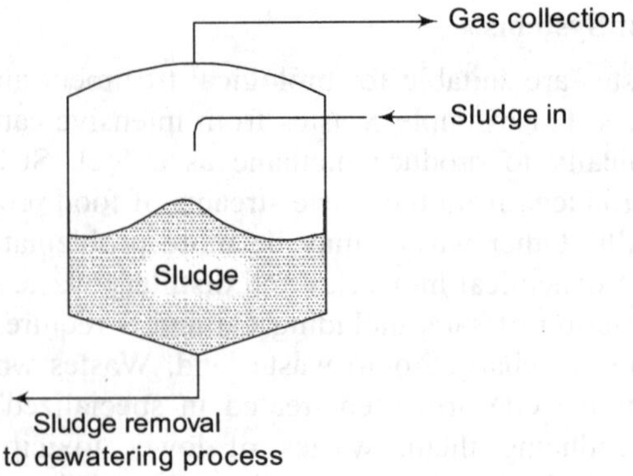

Figure 10.1

Simplified anaerobic sludge digester.
(***Source:*** *Brown, C.M.; Campbell, I.; Priest, F.G. Introduction to Biotechnology. © 1987 Oxford, Blackwell Scientific Publications. Reprinted by permission.*)

The methane producing bacteria (methanogens) are members of the Archaebacteria and are restricted to highly anaerobic environments such as the rumen of cattle and organically enriched sediments. For methane production, they utilise only a restricted range of substrates, including H_2 and CO_2, acetate, methanol and formate. Methanogens from the genera *Methanococcus, Methanobacterium* and *Methanospirillum* have been isolated from anaerobic treatment plants.

10.1.3 Aerobic Waste Treatment

Aerobic systems are the most common and range in complexity from the percolating filter, through the various types of activated sludge plants to the most modern inventions, which often use oxygen sparging to produce high rates of microbial activity.

Aerobic digestion requires a large population of actively metabolizing microorganisms able to degrade both colloidal and soluble organics and with a high rate of conversion to CO_2 and water. The most common aerobic systems are the trickling (percolating) filters (Fig. 10.2) and the activated sludge (Fig. 10.3) fermenters. The latter depends upon organisms growing in flocs which are kept in suspension by mechanical agitation or sparging with compressed air. The flocs contain a large number of bacteria including *Zoogloea ramigera* (thought to be responsible for the production of the extracellular polymers which are characteristic of the flocs) and species of *Pseudomonas, Alcaligenes, Achromobacter* and *Brevibacterium.* Ciliated protozoa, such as *Vorticella* sp. are also present and are thought to prey on the bacteria, exerting a control on their numbers and therefore aiding floc stability.

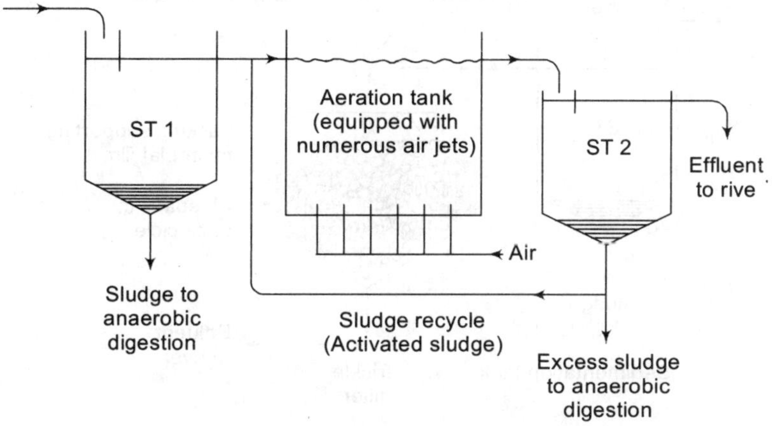

Figure 10.2

Simple system of effluent treatment by trickle filter (percolating filter) The weir at point of effluent input is necessary to maintain still conditions in the sedimentation tank.
(***Source:*** *Brown, C.M.; Campbell, I.; Priest, F.G. Introduction to Biotechnology. © 1987 Oxford Blackwell Scientific Publications. Reprinted by permission.*)

Activated sludge plants are the largest application of continuous or semi-continuous fermentation, with fresh effluent being added and sludge removed in order to maintain a (roughly) constant population of organisms. The sludge removed is passed to some form of settlement or other dewatering system prior to disposal. In addition to this problem of sludge disposal, the activated sludge process is also expensive in terms of the power requirements for agitation and aeration. The low solubility of oxygen is usually considered to limit the size of the microbial population and hence the overall rate of oxidation. This low efficiency of oxygen transfer of the traditional activated sludge systems and the large ground area required for their installation has led to developments of new fermentation systems.

While lowering of COD is a prime objective of waste treatment, some effluents also contain high concentrations of nitrogen and phosphorous which, if allowed into water courses would encourage eutrophication. The removal of both elements may be achieved by alternating aerobic and anaerobic treatment strategies. The degradation of nitrogen containing compounds gives rise to ammonia as a principal product. This ammonia is oxidized to nitrate by chemolithotrophic nitrifying bacteria in an aerobic reactor. The next step is anaerobic and relies on the action of denitrifying bacteria which use nitrate and nitrite as electron acceptors and convert these to nitrogen gas which is discharged. The removal of phosphorous involves release into the liquid waste in an anaerobic stage followed by assimilation into bacteria in an aerobic stage. This assimilation appears to involve *Acinetobacter* sp. which accumulates polyphosphate in intracellular granules. The bacterial mass is removed as a part of the sludge.

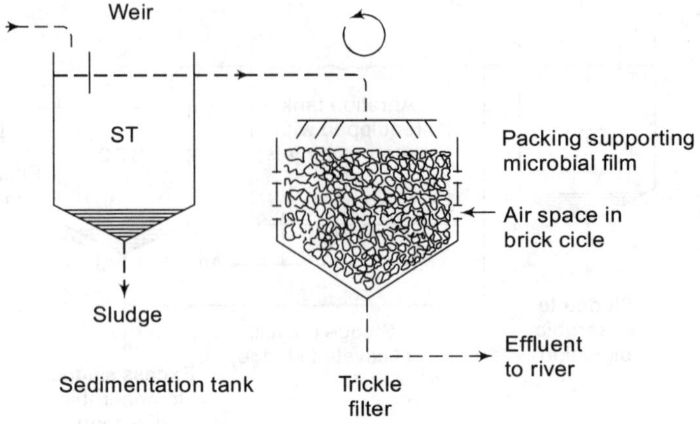

Figure 10.3

Aerated effluent treatment (activated sludge process). STl and ST2 are sedimentation tanks. (***Source:*** *Brown, C.M.; Campbell, I.; Priest, F.G. Introduction to Biotechnology. © 1987 Oxford, Blackwell Scientific Publications. Reprinted by permission.*)

10.1.4 Biodegradation

Biodegradation is the process by which waste materials such as oil spill, herbicides, pesticides etc., are degraded by the action of microbial systems. Organic compounds may be biodegradable (transformed by biological mechanisms which might lead to complete mineralization), persistent (fail to undergo biodegradation in a particular environment or under specific set of experimental conditions) or recalcitrant (inherently resistant to biodegradation). Most naturally occurring (or biogenic) compounds are biodegradable while man-made (or xenobiotic) compounds may be biodegradable, persistent or recalcitrant.

Table 10.1 lists some microorganisms which have been reported to be metabolically able to carry out the biodegradation of some of these compounds.

Biodegradation in a particular environment requires the presence of suitable microorganisms. This may involve a complex microbial community. The environment must also be suitable both for the growth of these organisms and for any chemical transformation reaction to proceed at a significant rate. Important factors include the concentration of the toxic chemicals (which most probably will be toxic to the microorganisms carrying out the transformation), the presence of other substrates and nutrients, temperature, pH, oxygen concentration, etc. In addition, the physical nature of the toxic material is of significance, for example, aerobic transformation of a water insoluble compound will proceed faster in a well-mixed and aerated environment (such as surface seawater) than if the same compound is coated on to fine sediment particles in an undersea dumpsite.

Table 10.1

Microorganisms able to degrade some toxic chemicals

Organisms	Toxic Chemicals
Pseudomonas spp	4-alkylbenzoates, alkylammonium, alkylaminoxides, anthracene, benzene, hydrocarbons, malathion, naphthalene, methyl naphthalenes, organophosphates, PCBs, p-xylene, p-cymene, parathion, phenanthrene, phenoxyacetates, phenylureas, polycyclic aromatics, rubber, secondary alkylbenzenes, toluene, phenolics, oleaginous materials, pulp byproducts.
Alcaligenes spp.	halogenated hydrocarbons, linear alkyl benzene, sulphonates, polycyclic aromatic PCBs
Arthrobacter spp.	benzene, hydrocarbons, pentachlorophenol, phenoxyacetates, polycyclic aromatics.
Bacillus spp.	aromatics, long chain alkanes, phenylureas.
Corynebacterium spp.	halogenated hydrocarbons, phenoxyacetates.
Mycobacterium spp.	aromatics, branched hydrocarbons, benzene, cycloparaffins.
Nocardia spp.	hydrocarbons, alkylbenzenes, naphthalene, phenoxyacetates, polycyclic aromatics
Streptomyces spp.	diazinon, phenoxyacetates, halogenated-hydrocarbons
Xanthomonas spp.	hydrocarbons, polycyclic hydrocarbons
Candida tropicalis	PCBs
Cunninghamella elegans	PCBs, polycyclic aromatics
Fusarium solani	propanil.

(***Source:*** *Brown, CM.; Campbell, I.; Priest, F.G. Introduction to Biotecbnology.* @ 1987 *Oxford, Blackwell Scientific Publications. Reprinted by permission.)*

Xenobiotic chemicals, because they are man-made and have been developed quite recently, are present in the environment for comparatively short periods of time from a geological point of view. This in turn means that the microbial communities present in these environments may not have evolved specific mechanisms for their degradation. A number of possible mechanisms exist, however, which may lead to active biodegradation. Some enzymes can bind analogues of their natural substrates which contain xenobiotic functional groups. If these do not greatly alter the charge of the active site, it is possible for the enzyme to catalyze a particular reaction with the xenobiotic as substrate. The success of this metabolism as a biodegradation mechanism depends on other factors also, such as the ability of the xenobiotic to act as an inducer and the nature of the product formed.

Table 10.2

Examples of Cometabolism

Organism	Growth substrate	Cometabolic substrate*	Products
Methylomonas	methane	ethane	ethanol, acetaldehyde, acetic acid
Nocardia	hexadecane	toluene	2,3 dihydroxybenzoic acid
	hexadecane	ethylbenzene	phenylacetic acid
Achromobacter	benzoic acid	3-chlorobenzoate	4-chlorocatechol, salicylic acid
Corynebacterium	hexadecane	naphthalene	2-hydroxy, 3-napthoic acid
glucose	anthracene	3-naphthoic acid	

*Cometabolism is the transformation of a non-growth substrate in the obligate presence of a growth substrate or another transformable compound.
(***Source:*** *Brown, C.M.; Campbell, I.; Priest, F.G. Introduction to Biotechnology. © 1987 Oxford, Blackwell Scientific Publications. Reprinted by permission*.)

A further mechanism which involves the gratuitous use of existing enzyme systems is cometabolism. A cometabolite does not support the growth of the organism concerned and the products of the transformation are accumulated stoichiometrically. The transformation does not require energy consumption of the organism and this is usually measured as an increased uptake of oxygen by the culture. A number of examples of cometabolism are listed in Table 10.2.

The degradation of a range of compounds, however, has been shown to proceed more readily with a mixed culture of organisms and the utilization of some compounds may not proceed at all in monocultures. A list of examples is given in Table 10.3.

While most of the functions essential for the growth of a bacterial cell are encoded in chromosomal genes, the presence of plasmids gives the host cell a survival or growth advantage under some conditions. Gene coding for some enzymes essential for the biodegradation of a number of organic compounds are plasmid borne (Table 10.4) and organisms have been constructed to degrade difficult waste. For example a patented process has been developed with a strain of *Pseudomonas putida* constructed to contain plasmids coding for the breakdown of octane, xylene, metaxylene and camphor. This organism is claimed to be useful in the cleansing of oily water discharges and oil spills.

There is also a clear potential for the use of recombinant DNA technology to construct strains with special degradative capacities. For example, using genetic engineering techniques, Anand Chakrabarty and his co-workers produced a multiplasmid *Pseudomonas* which was able to clear up oil spills. Recombinant bacteria containing plasmids such as cam plasmid for biodegradation of compounds have been generated.

Table 10.3

Some compounds degraded by synergistic microbial communities.

dalapon	Lontrel
chlorfobenzoate	4.4-dichloro-biphenyl
parathion	polychlorinated-biphenyls
isopropyl thiocarbamatc	cyclohexane
benzoate	linear alkylbenzoate sulphonates
nitrosamines	diazinon
2 -(2 -methoxy,4-chloro)phenoxy	propionic acid
alkylphenol ethoxylates	styrene
3,4- dichloropropionanilide	isopropyl phenylcarbamate

(***Source:*** *Brown, C.M.; Campbell, I.; Priest, F.G. Introduction to Biotechnology. © 1987 Oxford, Blackwell Scientific Publications. Reprinted by permission.*)

10.1.4.1 *In situ* leaching

Conventional mining involves removing rock from the ground, breaking it up and treating it to remove the minerals being sought.

In situ leaching (ISL), also known as solution mining, involves leaving the ore where it is in the ground, and using liquids which are pumped through it to recover the minerals out of the ore by leaching. Consequently there is little surface disturbance and no tailings or waste rock generated. However, the orebody needs to be permeable to the liquids used, and located so that they do not contaminate ground water away from the orebody.

In situ leaching mining was first tried on an experimental basis in Wyoming during the early 1960s. The first commercial mine began operating in 1974. Today a few projects are licensed to operate in the USA, (in Wyoming, Nebraska and Texas) and most of the operating mines date from the 1990s. They are small (under 1000 t/yr) but they supply most of the US uranium production. About 21% of world uranium production is by ISL (including all Kazakhstan and Uzbekistan output). *In situ* leaching can also be applied to other minerals such as copper and gold.

There are two operating regimes for *in situ* leaching, determined by the geology and groundwater. If there is significant calcium in the orebody (as limestone or gypsum), alkaline (carbonate) leaching must be used. Otherwise, acid (sulfate) leaching is generally better.

Techniques for *in situ* leaching have evolved to the point where it is a controllable, safe, and environmentally benign method of mining which can operate under strict environmental controls and which often has cost advantages.

10.1.5 Microorganisms in Pollution Control

The purification of sewage and the elimination of an important proportion of the organic matter contained in residual effluents, are carried out by aerobic and anaerobic microorganisms. For example, spectacular results were obtained in the processing of effluents from yeast, oil and cider works, from milk and cheese dairies, and potato starch works, by an anaerobic process in which the active biological compound is recycled. This produces less residual sludge, prevents to a great extent the escape of foul smells, and produces a little methane, which is used to fuel the boilers of the processing facilities.

Table 10.4

Some plasmids concerned in biodegradation

Chemical species	Plasmid	Chemicals transformed
Alkanes	OCT	octane, decane
aromatic and	TOL (pWWO)	xylenes, toluene
polyaromatic		
hydrocarbons and	NAH	naphthalene
metabolic products	SAL	salicylate, benzoate
terpenes	CAM	camphor
alkaloids	NIC	nicotine, nicotinate
chlorinated	pPl	2.4 D
hydrocarbons	pAC21	3-p-chlorobiphenyl
		3-chlorobenzoate
		chlorobenzoate

(***Source:*** *Brown, C.M.; Campbell, I.; Priest, F.G.* Introduction *to Biotechnology. © 1987 Oxford, Blackwell Scientific Publications. Reprinted by permission*.)

Microbial strains can be isolated in order to control various forms of chemical pollution, for instance to decompose biocides, (the biodegradation of which is difficult to achieve), detergents, plastic materials or hydrocarbons. Thus, bacteria belonging to the genus *Pseudomonas* have oxidoreduction or hydroxylation enzymes capable of degrading a large number of hydrocarbon molecules or aromatic compounds that are often highly toxic. Certain microbes can modify a molecule that will then be degraded by others. This cometabolism phenomenon takes place, for instance, in the decomposition of a powerful, highly polluting insecticide, parathion. Often, detoxification, rather than a complete degradation of the toxic molecule is the consequence of a chemical conversion of this molecule: e.g. phosphorylation, methylation, acetylation, etc. The enzymes that catalyze these detoxification reactions are often specified by genes borne by plasmids. Genetic recombination techniques should make it possible to achieve such a result and it would then be possible to envisage the construction of microbial strains capable of decomposing and assimilating numerous compounds, most often non-biodegradable (xenobiotics) produced by the chemical industry in particular.

10.1.6 Bioremediation

Bioremediation is defined as the use of biological treatment systems to destroy, or reduce the concentrations of hazardous wastes from contaminated sites. Bioremediation can be done on site; it keeps site disruption to the minimum; it eliminates transportation costs and liabilities; it eliminates long-term liability; it uses biological systems, often inexpensive; it can be coupled with other treatment techniques.

Different bioremediation treatment technologies are available such as bioaugmentation (addition of bacterial cultures to a contaminated medium), biofilters (using microbial stripping columns), biostimulation (simulating microbial populations), bioreactors (using reactors), bioventing (supplying oxygen), composting and land farming.

10.1.7 Biological Bleaching

Production of paper and cardboard requires great amount of pulp from wood. The pulp needs to be bleached. Formerly chemicals were used for bleaching. Now oxidative enzymes from white-rot fungi are used. These enzymes depolymerize and mineralize lignin and other high molecular weight pollutants.

10.2 Biomass Production

Energy is defined as the ability to work. It is obtained in different forms such as nuclear energy, fossil fuel energy (coal, oil and gas), and non-fossil and non-nuclear energy such as solar energy, wind energy and tidal energy. Solar energy is expected to contribute in a considerable way towards the production of heat, electricity and synthetic fuels using crops such as sugar-cane and algae.

The conservation of existing energy resources as well as the exploration of alternate resources has been engaging the attention of the world scientific community. With the rapid depletion of fossil fuels which have so far played a vital role in agriculture and industrial development, greater attention is now being paid to vegetable and animal matters as the main sources of energy in many regions of the developing world.

Forests make up about 68 per cent of terrestrial biomass, grass ecosystems about 16 per cent, and cultivated lands only 8 per cent. The earth's plant cover is equivalent to over 1,800 billion tonnes of dry matter corresponding to the known reserves of 'fossil' energy. This considerable energy potential of biomass is exploited for energy consumption. In the case of dry matter, the simplest method for the conversion of biomass into energy is combustion, which provides heat, which in turn is converted into mechanical or electric power. On the other hand, the conversion into biogas (methane) represents the oldest and the most efficient conversion method as regards wet matter.

Biofuels

Biofuels are fuels generated from the conversion of biomass; bioethanol, biomethane, biobutanol and biodiesel are some of the examples. Biofuels are considered as substitutes for the rapidly depleting, non-renewable and increasingly expensive fossil fuels. Biofuel will provide fuel security, improve rural income, promote eco-friendly mechanisms and reduce atmospheric pollution.

10.2.1 Biomass as Source of Energy

Using photosynthetic pigments such as chlorophyll a, chlorophyll b, chlorophyll c, xanthophylls and carotenoids, plants utilize solar energy for the production of food. During photosynthesis in plant cells, in the presence of chlorophyll, CO_2 is converted into complex carbohydrates with the evolution of oxygen; solar energy is trapped by light harvesting molecules in the chloroplasts and conversion of CO_2 into carbohydrates, fats and proteins occurs. These are referred to as primary products. Later these become biomass. The biomass consists of all forms of matter derived from biological activities and present on the surface of soil or at different depths of vast bodies of water, lakes, rivers, seas and oceans. Biomass includes wood, crops, herbaceous plants, residues from agricultural and forest products, manure, fresh water and marine plants and microorganisms as well. Besides plant material, biomass also includes all animal waste, manure, etc. because in essence, the latter are basically plant based. Different types of biomass of various sources are given in Table 10.5.

Plant cell wall is made up of mainly six components: (a) cellulose (b) hemicellulose (c) lignin (d) water soluble sugars, amino acids and aliphatic acids (e) ether and alcohol soluble constituents (e.g. fats, oils, waxes, resin and many pigments), and (f) proteins. These components build up plant biomass. Cellulose constitutes the major portion of plant cell wall, the fundamental unit of which is glucose. From each glucose unit, one molecule of water is removed to yield an anhydrous glucose. The anhydrous glucose units are linked end to end with β 1-4 linkage to form the long chain polymer of cellulose. Hemicellulose is also constituted by sugar (xylans) which comprises of 20-25 per cent plant biomass on a dry weight basis. In addition, it also contains glucose and several other hexoses (galactose and mannose) and pentoses (xylose and arabinose). Lignin is a complex high molecular weight polymer. It is formed by de-hydrogenation of P-hydroxy-cinnamyl alcohols such as P-coumaryl (1), coniferyl (11) and sinapyl (111) alcohols. Presence of these alcohols differs in different plant groups. For example, gymnosperm lignin is formed from coniferyl alcohols, angiosperm lignin is formed from the mixture of coniferyl and sinapyl alcohols, and grass lignin from mixture of coniferyl, sinapyl and coumaryl alcohols.

Table 10.5
Biomass as the source of energy (after Dubey, R.C, 1993)

Source of Biomass	Forms of Biomass	Conversion Process	Forms of Energy
Sylviculture (energy plantation)	Fire wood Fuel wood	Combustion Destructive distillation	Heat (fire) Charcoal
Agriculture (energy crops)	Carbohydrates Hydrocarbon	Fermentation Fermentation	Ethanol Fuel Oil
Aquatic biomass	Aquaculture	Fermentation	Methanol
Weeds	Whole plant body	Fermentation	Methane
Rural/urban/ industrial wastes	Wastes	Combustion Pyrolysis Fermentation	Fire/fuel Fuel oil Methane and Ethanol
Forestry wastes	Wastes	Combustion Pyrolysis Gasification Fermentation	Fire/fuel oil gas gas Methane, ethanol
Agricultural Wastes	Wastes	Fermentation	Methane
Weeds and aquatic biomass	Wastes	Fermentation Combustion	Methane Fire/fuel
Cattle dung	Wastes	Fermentation	Methane (biogas)

10.2.2 Wastes as Renewable Sources of Energy

Waste is the spoilage, loss or destruction of either matter or energy in a way that is not useful to human beings. Based on the chemical nature, material wastes are of various types:

(a) inorganic wastes (those generated by metallurgical and chemical industries, coal mines, etc.)

(b) organic wastes (agricultural products, dairy and milk products, slaughter houses, sewage, foresty etc)

(c) mixed wastes (those discharged from industries dealing with textiles dyes, gas, plastic, wool, leather, petroleum, etc.). The inorganic wastes may be recovered by chemical/mechanical treatment, whereas organic and mixed wastes require biological as well as chemical treatments. The organic wastes and residues are sources of renewable energy in multifarious ways.

Industries such as paper mills, chemical and pharmaceutical factories, oil refineries, cotton mills, food processing units, dairy, and sugar mills generate various types of wastes/by products which contain sufficient amount of energy. Agriculture also produces a huge amount of residues/wastes which are thrown away due to the non-availability of technologies for utilization.

10.2.3 Biomass Conversion

Biomass can be converted into energy using the non-biological process and the biological process. There are different non-biological routes for biomass conversion into energy viz., direct combustion, gasification, pyrolysis and liquifaction. Direct combustion involves the direct burning of biomass of plant or animal origin for cooking and other purposes. In recent years hog fuel technology has been developed for the generation of electricity in U.S.A. The mixture of wood and bark waste is burnt directly in a boiler. Pyrolysis is the destructive distillation or decomposition of organic matter, for example, solid residues, wastes (saw dust, wood chips, wood pieces) in an oxygen-deficient atmosphere or in the absence of oxygen at a high temperature (200-500°C or rarely 900°C). Products of pyrolysis are gases, organic liquids and chars, depending on the pyrolysis process and temperature. Gasification is a process of thermal degradation of carbonaceous material under controlled amount of air or pure oxygen, and high temperature up to around 1000°C to produce gas. Liquifaction involves the production of oils for energy from wood, or agriculture and carbon residues in combination with carbon monoxide and water/steam at high pressure (4000 lb/in2) and temperature 350-400°C) in the presence of catalysts.

The biological process is also called bioconversion. Bioconversion involves the conversion of organic materials into energy, fertilizers, food, and chemicals through biological energy. Bioconversion takes place enzymatically, anaerobically and aerobically. Enzymatic digestion involves the conversion of cellulosic and lignocellulose materials into alcohols, acids and animal feeds by using microbial enzyme e.g. cellulase, hemicellulase, amylase, pectinase, etc. Anaerobic digestion is a partial conversion of organic substrates into gases by microorganisms in the absence of air. Anaerobic digestion is accomplished in three stages: solublization, fermentation and methanogenesis. Aerobic digestion involves the conversion of utilizable forms in the presence of air to produce gases, single cell protein, fertilizers, etc.

10.2.3.1 Production of Ethanol

Ethanol is a high grade fuel as well as an excellent raw material for chemical and plastic industries. The production of ethanol from plant biomass includes the extraction and hydrolysis of storage carbohydrates followed by their microbial fermentation into alcohol. The chemical synthesis of ethanol is carried out from ethylene (derived from petroleum or natural gas), which is converted at a high temperature in the presence of water and catalysts. Among the alcohol producing plants that are already being exploited or that could be cultivated with a view to producing ethanol, cassava, cereals (maize), potatoes and Jerusalem artichokes must be mentioned. Sugar-cane, pineapple, sugar-beet and sweet sorghum are also used, their main carbohydrate being sucrose.

Ethanol is a solvent, an extractant and .an antifreeze; it is also a substrate for the synthesis of many other solvents such as dyes, pharmaceuticals, lubricants, adhesives, detergents, pesticides, plasticizers, explosives and resins for the manufacture of synthetic fibres. Using ethanol as a fuel in internal combustion engines can be done either in the form of anhydrous ethanol mixed with petrol up to a 20 per cent ratio, or else in the form of hydrated ethanol (94 per cent) not blended with petrol.

In sugarcane factories, the cane is crushed and the cellulose (bagasse) is separated from the sweet juices. Bagasse is dried, then burnt to generate the energy required. The sweet juices are then concentrated, sterilized and then fermented. Ethanol is separated from the fermentation solids and from the eight to ten per cent alcohol solution by distillation.

In 1975, the Brazilian Government decided to mass produce alcohol from sugar-cane or cassava as a petrol substitute. This decision was made following a rise in the price of oil and also, to a lesser extent, a drop in the price of sugar in the world market. Cassava seemed to be highly preferred for this since one tonne of cassava produced 80 litres of alcohol in contrast to one tonne of sugar-cane yielding only 65 litres of alcohol. In America gasohol—a mixture of six to nine parts of petrol for one part of ethanol was advocated for fuel use. Many other countries also use different raw materials to produce ethanol.

10.2.3.2 Production of Biogas

Methane fermentation or biomethanogenesis, is an ancient process for the conversion of biomass into energy. It was discovered in 1776 by Volta, who demonstrated the presence of methane in marsh gas. The biogas produced by this process is in fact a mixture of 65 per cent methane, 30 per cent carbon dioxide, one per cent hydrogen sulphide, traces of nitrogen, oxygen, hydrogen and carbon monoxide. It is odourless and burns with a blue flame without smoke.

Biomethanogenesis takes place in three stages: solubilization and hydrolysis of the organic components, acidogenesis and methanogenesis. The first stage is never completed in the methanization of wastes, because it is too long. Three groups of bacteria are involved in this process: the first convert complex substrates into butyric, propionic and lactic acids; the second, acetogenic bacteria, convert these organic acids into acetic acid, hydrogen and carbon dioxide; the methanogenic bacteria reduce carbon dioxide to methane and consume the hydrogen which otherwise would inhibit the acetogenic bacteria. Acetogenic and methanogenic microorganisms form a symbiotic association.

From a biochemical point of view, methane fermentation is in fact a type of anaerobic respiration in which electrons from organic substrates are finally transferred to carbon dioxide which is then reduced to methane. In addition to various organic substrates (such as acetate), hydrogen, which is produced in the soil by several types of anaerobic bacteria serves as a donor of electrons for the methanobacteria. Methane can also be derived from aromatic compounds under conditions of strict anaerobiosis. This process is probably widespread in nature, particularly in the treatment of sewage and effluents, as well as in the conversion of certain biocides. Methanobacteria are, under natural conditions, closely associated with hydrogen producing bacteria; this is a trophic association, profitable to both type of bacteria. The former utilize the gaseous hydrogen produced by the latter and prevent it from reaching concentrations that would be toxic for them.

The methane fermentation takes place in a water-tight cylindrical digester with a side opening into which the fermentative material is introduced; above the digester, there is a steel cylindrical container that is used to collect the gas and which hovers like a bell over the mixture during fermentation so as to prevent any air from getting in, because the whole process has to be strictly anaerobic. Most often the gas bell is fitted with a pipe for retrieving the biogas. Digesters are made of claybricks, concrete or steel; the bell used to collect the gas can be made of nylon and is easily adapted to the digester, which is made of rigid plastic material. The gas produced inflates the nylon bag which is linked to a compressor in order to increase the pressure of the gas.

In the case of household refuse or liquid manure, the ratio between solids and water must be 1:1. The mixture of fermentative matters is generally seeded with acetogenic and methanogenic bacteria or else with sludge from another digester. A low pH inhibits the growth of methanogenic bacteria and slows down the production of biogas, as does overloading the digester. Acidity can be lowered by adding lime. Optimum digestion takes place between pH 6 and 8. The maximum temperature of the process depends on the mesophilic and thermophilic properties of the microorganisms (30-40°C or 50-60°C). Sudden changes in temperature are rather unfavourable. The digesters are usually buried in order to benefit from the insulation which the soil provides; in cold climates, the digester can be heated by the installations provided for the composting of agricultural wastes.

It is advised to stir the suspension of fermentative substances so as to prevent stratification that inhibits fermentation. Solids must be fragmented in order to avoid the formation of large aggregates that hinder the production of methane. The standard duration of the digestion of cattle dung ranges from between two and four weeks; liquid manures from a pig sty requires about ten days' fermentation; manure from cattle dung and poultry droppings need about twenty days.

Production of biogas in rural areas has been a priority in the energy policy of India. The production of biogas from the methane 'fermentation' of wastes and residues available locally is one of the solutions to the problem of meeting the energy needs of most rural areas in developing countries. In fact, experience shows that successful popularization programmes and the involvement of decision makers are sufficient to gain the support of the populations concerned with these programmes These programmes have a two fold advantage of meeting the energy needs and of protecting the environment.

10.2.4 Production of Hydrocarbons

Recent investigations have shown that many plants contain hydrocarbons and other substances similar to petroleum in their composition. Hydrocarbon producing plants grow in abundance in Asia and the pacific region. Some species of plants transform the CO_2 taken by them all the way down to the hydrocarbon stage, which contains no O_2 This eliminates the use for any external processes for converting CO_2 to hydrocarbon. These plants mostly belong to the Euphorbiaceae family. It must be emphasized that more than a thousand species of Euphorbiaceae are known which secrete latex containing an emulsion of about 30 per cent hydrocarbon in water. *Hevea brasiliensis,* the rubber tree latex has a molecular weight of one million and in many other Euphorbiaceae species the molecular weight of latex is around 10,000 and they have the potential for cracking into gasoline fractions. Such plants are selected and grown for energy purposes either for direct use or as feedstock for more convenient liquid fuel or other energy chemicals. These plants can be used either to get diesel fuel, or after their conversion, high quality liquid fuel.

Thevetia neriifolia, Calotropis procera, Argemone mexicana, Givortia rottaliiformis, Vitis quadrangularis, Aloe vera, Euphorbia antiquorum, Euphorbia nervifolia, Jatropha curas, Wrightia tomentosa, Plumeria alba, Allamanda cathartica, Calotropis gigantea, Daemia extensa, Cryptostegia grandiflora, Artocarpus integrifolia, Bassia latifolia, Cereopegia tuberosa, Pedalium murex, Agave americana, Euphorbia hirta, Euphorbia royleana, Pedilanthus tithymaloides, Tabernaemontana cornaria, Plumeria acutifolia, Nerium odorum, Asclepias curassavicca, Calotropis procera, Stapelia grandiflora, Artocarpus incisca, Mimusops elengi are some of the plants that can be used for the production of hydrocarbons. *Jatropha curcus* trees are reported to yield two kg of seed oil per plant per year and oil from this plant is expected to replace the conventional diesel in agricultural machinery.

A species of unicellular alga, *Botryococcus brauni* seems to have hydrocarbons of 15 to 75 per cent of the weight of its dry matter. This fresh or brackish water alga is found in temperate and in tropical zones where its proliferation in bodies of water can be spectacular. It comes in two forms, distinguishable by their pigmentation (green and red) and by the structure of the hydrocarbons synthesized. The green alga contains linear hydrocarbons with an odd number of carbon atoms (25 to 31) low in double bonds; the red alga contains hydrocarbons with 34 to 38 carbon. atoms and several double bonds. Hydrocarbons get accumulated in cell walls and their synthesis is a metabolic activity of the alga in its growth phase. This suggests the possibility of extracting hydrocarbons by centrifugation, without having to break the cells, which could be replaced in the culture medium after the hydrocarbons have been recovered.

The composition of the hydrocarbons produced by *B. braunii* is such that they can be used as a source of energy or as raw materials for petrochemicals (either directly or after a slight cracking).

10.2.5 Hydrogen Fuel

Hydrogen is the simplest molecule present in the universe. The production and use of hydrogen represents a potential alternate source of fuel. It can be easily collected, stored and transported. More importantly, after the use, hydrogen does not pollute the environment. For the production of hydrogen, water serves as a source of raw material. The bond between hydrogen and oxygen in water can be broken by providing necessary energy by heat, electricity or light photons. Based on the types of energy used the following modes of splitting water are used: (a) electrolysis (splitting of water using electricity) (b) thermolysis (splitting of water using heat) (c) thermochemical lysis (splitting of water using both heat and chemical catalysts) (d) photolysis (splitting of water using light).

Biophotolysis refers to the break down of water and production of oxygen and hydrogen by biological process. In the early 1960s, production of hydrogen was demonstrated by using chloroplasts isolated from spinach (*Spinacia oleracea*) in the presence of artificial electron donors and bacterial extracts containing hydrogenase. Electron donors (organic compounds) transferred electrons to photosystem 1 of the chloroplast from where electrons were received by electron carriers (e.g. ferredoxin). Hydrogenase accepted the electrons from the electron carrier. In the visible light, hydrogenase separated high energy electrons from ferredoxin and facilitated their transfer to H^+. Ultimately H_2 was evolved.

Hydrogenase is restricted to a variety of bacteria, cyanobacteria and other green algae. Those plants which produce carbohydrates lack hydrogenase. Research works are being carried out on the production of hydrogen from organic waste by using many anoxygenic phototrophic bacteria, water using cyanobacteria or green algae grown under conditions of light.

10.3 Biodiversity

Biodiversity is the variety and differences among living organisms from all sources, including terrestrial, atmospheric, marine, and other aquatic ecosystems and the ecological complexes of which they are a part. This includes genetic diversity within and between species and of ecosystems. Thus, in essence, biodiversity represents all life. India is one of the mega biodiversity centres in the world and has two of the world's 18 'biodiversity hotspots' located in the Western Ghats and in the Eastern Himalayas. The forest cover in these areas is very dense and diverse and of pristine beauty, and incredible biodiversity.
According to an MoEF Report (1999), the country is estimated to have over 49,219 plant species and 81,251 animal species representing 12.5% of the world's flora and 6.6% of its fauna.

The sacred groves of India are some of the areas in the country where the richness of biodiversity has been well preserved. The Thar Desert and the Himalayas are two regions rich in biodiversity in India. There are 89 national parks and 504 wildlife sanctuaries in the country, the Chilika Lake being one of them. This lake is also an important wetland area.

Over the last century, a great deal of damage has been done to the biodiversity existing on the earth. Increasing human population, increasing consumption levels, and decreasing efficiency of use of our resources are some of the causes that have led to overexploitation and manipulation of ecosystems. Trade in wildlife, such as rhino horn, has led to the extinction of species. Consequences of biodiversity loss can be great as any disturbance to one species gives rise to imbalance in others. In this the exotic species have a role to play.

To prevent such loss, the Government of India is setting up biosphere reserves in different parts of the country. These are multipurpose protected areas to preserve the genetic diversity in different ecosystems. Some examples are Nilgiri, Nandadevi, Nakrek, Great Nicobar, Gulf of Mannar, Manas, Sunderbans, Similipal, and Dibru Saikhowa. A number of NGOs are being involved in the programme to create awareness. But legal protection is provided only to national parks and sanctuaries, which cover about 4.5% of India's land area.

Agricultural biodiversity refers to the variety and variability of animals, plants and micro-organisms used directly or indirectly for food and agriculture (including, in the FAO definition, crops, livestock, forestry and fisheries). It comprises the diversity of genetic resources (varieties, breeds, etc.) and species used for food, fodder, fibre, fuel and pharmaceuticals. It also includes the diversity of non-harvested species that support production (e.g. soil micro-organisms, predators, pollinators and so on) and those in the wider environment that support agro-ecosystems (agricultural, pastoral, forest and aquatic), as well as the diversity of the agro-ecosystems themselves. Globally, however, biodiversity is under siege. The 2000 IUCN (World Conservation Union) Red List of Threatened Species indicates that species extinction is on an increasing spiral. Since the last assessment of globally threatened species in 1996, the number of Critically Endangered primates has increased from 13 to 19. While the 1996 IUCN Red List of Threatened Animals, listed 169 Critically Endangered (CR) and 315 Endangered mammals, the 2000 analysis lists 180 CR and 340 Endangered mammals.

Similarly, for birds there is an increase from 168 to 182 CR and from 235 to 321 Endangered species. As many as one in four of mammal species and one in eight bird species are threatened and the number of threatened animal species has increased from 5,201 to 5,435. Approximately, 25% of reptiles, 20% of amphibians and 30% of fishes (mainly freshwater) are listed as threatened. The number of Critically Endangered Reptiles has increased from 10 to 24 and Endangered from 28 to 47 species. Turtles and tortoises in particular are greatly threatened. The number of Critically Endangered species among freshwater turtles went from 10 in the 1996 IUCN assessment to 24 in the 2000 IUCN assessment, and this can be ascribed to unregulated harvests for food and medicines. Trends suggest that the trade in turtles after depleting populations in Southeast Asia is shifting to the Indian subcontinent and even to the Americas and Africa.

Biodiversity is the foundation for many biotechnological programmes. If biodiversity is not preserved, it will lead to genetic erosion which is the loss of genetic diversity, including the loss of individual genes, and the loss of particular combinations of genes (i.e. of gene-complexes) such as those manifested in locally adapted landraces.

Bioprospecting

Bioprospecting is the search for new chemicals in living things that will have some medical or commercial use. While it is a high risk area for investors, it can have massive returns. Of the world's 25 top-selling pharmaceuticals, 10 were originally sourced from animals, plants or micro-organisms.

Indigenous peoples of the world possess a vast store of knowledge about the properties of many native plants. Pharmaceutical companies and agribusiness use indigenous knowledge as a precursor to screening, and this is happening with little regard for the protection of indigenous intellectual property and with no equitable sharing of profits.

Study Outline

Waste Treatment

This deals with the use of biotechnological tools to protect and conserve the environment. Waste treatment and bioenergy, production are two important areas. Waste treatment is done aerobically and anaerobically. Biogas is a useful product of anaerobic decomposition.

Types of Treatment System

Activated sludge and percolating filters are the most commonly used aerobic treatment systems.

Biodegradation

It is another process where waste materials are digested by microorganisms. This involves the complex microbial community, as suitable environment for the growth of the organism and chemical transformations favour biodegradation. Enzymes are also employed for this purpose. A further mechanism which involves the gratuitous use of existing enzyme systems is cometabolism.

In Situ Leaching

In situ leaching (also known as solution leaching) involves leaving the ore wjere ot os om the ground, and using liquids which are pumped through it to recover the minerals out of the ore by leaching Geology and groundwater determine the operating regimes.

Microorganisms in Pollution Control

Microorganisms are also useful agents in pollution control. These are employed to decompose biocides, plastic materials, detergents and hydrocarbons. The bacteria belonging to the genus *Pseudomonas* have hydroxylation enzymes capable of degrading a great number of hydrocarbon molecules or aromatic compounds that are often highly toxic. A phenomenon known as cometabolism takes place during the decomposition of a powerful insecticide parathion. The enzymes responsible for the detoxification are situated in the plasmid region of the microorganism. Biotechnology aims at the construction of microbial strains capable of assimilating or decomposing numerous compounds especially nonbiodegradable substances.

Energy Production

Environmental biotechnology also deals with various energy sources. Biomass is the converted energy by combustion and fossil energy is yet another source. Ethanol is formed from various sources, such as cassava, cereals, potato, sugarcane, pine apple, sugarbeet etc. It is a solvent and also a substrate for the synthesis of many other solvents and dyes. Biogas formation and methanogenesis are although ancient forms: to-day they are in great demand. Methane fermentation is widely practised and is one of the easily available sources of. energy. Agricultural wastes and farm yard wastes are efficiently used for this purpose. Production of biogas in rural areas has been a priority in the energy policy of India.

Biodiversity and Bioprospecting

Biodiversity is the variety and differences among living organisms from all sources, including terrestrial, atmospheric, marine and other aquatic ecosystems and the ecological complexes of which they are a part. Biodiversity is under great threat. Agricultural biodiversity refers to the variety and variability of animals, plants and microorganisms used directly or indirectly for food and agriculture. Genetic erosion refers to the loss of genetic diversity. Bioprospecting is the search for new chemicals in living things that will have some medical or commercial use.

Questions

(1) Define BOD and COD.
(2) What are Xenobiotics. State the reason why they resist biodegradation?
(3) What are different types of waste treatments?
(4) Name the biological organism involved in anaerobic digestion.
(5) What is the role played by micro organisms in pollution control?
(6) What is biomethanogenesis? What is its role in biogas formation?
(7) Explain the method of ethanol production.
(8) Explain plant biomass. How do you convert biomass into energy?
(9) How are plants useful in hydrocarbon production?
(10) What is hydrogen fuel?
(11) What is bioremediation?
(12) What is biological bleaching?
(13) Define biodiversity.
(14) What is Bioprospecting?
(15) What is *in situ* leaching?

11
Bioinformatics

Bioinformatics is defined in various ways. Some of the definitions are as follows:

(i) Bioinformatics is the use of computer in solving information problems in life sciences; mainly it involves the creation of extensive electronic database on genomes and protein sequences. Secondarily it involves techniques such as the three-dimensional modeling of biomolecules and biological systems.

(ii) Bioinformatics is a computational management of all kinds of biological informations, including genes and their products, whole organisms or even ecological systems.

(iii) Bioinformatics is an integration of mathematical, statistical and computational methods to analyse biological, biochemical and biophysical data. It deals with methods of storing, retrieving and analyzing biological data, such as nucleic acid and protein sequences, structures, functions, pathways and genetic interactions.

(iv) Bioinformatics is the storage, manipulation and analysis of biological information via computer science. Bioinformatics is an essential infrastructure underpinning biological research.

In its broadest sense, the term bioinformatics can be considered to mean information technology applied to the management and analysis of biological data. From 1950 onwards, large amount of sequence data related to various living organisms have been collected and stored in databases. Since it is not very convenient to compare the sequences of several hundred nucleotides and amino acids by hand, several computational techniques were developed. Where data can be amassed faster than they can be analyzed and utilized, there is a great need for professionals who can use software to digest this ever-growing mass of information.

11.1. Important Contributions

Hereunder we are giving a chronological list of developments that contributed to the emergence of bioinformatics

1866 – Gregor Mendel published the results on his investigations of the inheritance of 'factors' in pea plants.

1928 – Erwin Schrodinger proposed that this factor is of 1000 angstroms.

1933 – Tiselius introduced a new technique known as electrophoresis for separating proteins in solution.

1951 – Pauling and Corey proposed the structure for the alpha helix and beta-sheet of polypeptide chain of protein.

1952 – Rosalind and Wilkins used X-ray crystallography to reveal repeating structure of DNA

1953 – Watson and Crick proposed the double helix model for DNA

1954 – Perutz's group developed heavy atom methods to solve the phase problem in protein crystallography.

1955 – F. Sanger announced the sequence of bovine insulin

1957 – Arthur Kornberg produced DNA in a test tube

1968 – Werner Arber, Hamilton Smith and Daniel Nath described uses of restriction enzyme

1969 – Linking computers at Stanford and UCLA created the APRANET

1970 – The details of the Needleman Wunsch algorithm for sequence comparison were published.

1972 – Paul Berg made the first recombinant DNA molecule using ligase enzyme

- Stanley Cohen, Annie Chang and Herbert Boyer produced the first recombinant DNA organism

1973 – Joseph Sambrook and his team refined DNA electrophoresis technique using agarose gel

- Stanley Cohen cloned DNA
- Brookhaven Protein Data Bank was announced

1975 – P.H.O'Farrell announced two-dimensional SDS polyacrylamide gel electrophoresis

- E.M. Southern published experimental details for Southern Blot analysis.
- Bill Gates and Paul Allen found Microsoft Corporation.

1976 – Prosite database was reported by Bairoch *et al.*

1977 – Fredrick Sanger, Allen Maxam and Walter Gilbert pioneered DNA sequencing.

1980 – Mark Skolnick, Ray White, David Botstein and Ronald Davis created RFLP marker map of human genome.

- The first complete gene sequence for an organism (FX 174) was published.
- Wuthrich *et al.* published a paper detailing the use of multidimensional NMR for protein structure determination.
- IntelliGenetics Inc. was founded in California. Their primary product was the IntelliGenetics Suite of programs for DNA and protein sequence analysis.
- The Smith – Waterman algorithm for sequence alignment was published.
- US Supreme Court holds that genetically – modified bacteria are patentable.

1981 – IBM introduced its personal computer to the market

- Human mitochondria DNA was sequenced

1982 – First recombinant DNA – based drug was marketed

- Genetics Computer Group (GCG) was created as a part of the University of Wisconsin at Wisconsin Biotechnology Center.

1983 – The Compact Disk (CD) was launched

1984 – Jon Postel's Domain Name System (DNS) was placed on-line. Apple computer announced the Macintosh.

1985 – Kary Mullis invented PCR

- FASTP algorithm was published
- Robert Sinsheimer made the first proposal for Human Genome Project

1986 – Thomas Roderick coined the term Genomics to describe the scientific discipline of mapping, sequencing and analyzing genes.

- Amoco Technology Corporation acquired IntelliGenetics. The Swiss-PROT database was created by the Department of Medical Biochemistry of the University of Geneva and the European Molecular Biology Laboratory (EMBL)

- Leroy Hood and Lloyd Smith automated DNA sequencing.

- Charles DeLisi convened a meeting to discuss the possibility of determining the nucleotide sequence of human genome.

1987 – United States Department of Environment (US DoE) officially began human genome project.

- The physical map of *E. coli* is published by Y. Kohara *et al.*

- The use of yeast artificial Chromosome (YAC) is described by David T. Burke *et al.*

1988 – United States National Institute of Health (US NIH) took over genomic project with James Watson at the helm.

- Pearson and Lipman published the FASTA algorithm

1989 – NIH established National Centre for Human Genome Research.

- The Genetics Computer group became a private company

- Oxford Molecular Group Ltd (OMG) founded in Oxford, UK, created products such as Anaconda, Asp, Cameleon and other (molecular modeling, drug design, and protein design) products.

1990 – The BLAST programme to align DNA sequences was developed by Altschul *et al.*

1991 – CERN, Geneva announced the creation of the protocols which make up the World Wide Web.

- Craig Venter invented expressed sequence tag (EST) technology

- Incyte Pharmaceuticals, a genomics company was formed in California.

- Myriad Genetics Inc. was founded in Utah with a goal of discovering major common disease genes and their related pathways.

1992 – Human Genome systems, Maryland was formed by William Haseltin

- Craig Venter established the Institute for Genomic Research (TIGR).

- Mel Simon and coworkers (Cal Tech) invented BACs, crucial for clone by clone gene assembly.

- Wellcome Trust joined human genome project

1993 – Francis Collins took over Human Genome project. Sanger Center is opened in UK. Other nations joined in the effort. 2005 was projected as completion year.

1994 – Netscape Communications Corporation was founded and it released Navigator.

- Attwood and Beck published the PRINTS database of protein motifs.

1995 – Researchers at the Institute for Genomic Research published the first genome sequence of free-living organism: *Haemophilus influenzae*.

- Patrick Brown and Stanford university colleagues invented DNA micro-array technology.

1996 – The genome of *Saccharomyces cerevisiae* was sequenced.

- International Human Genome project consortium established 'Bermuda rules' for public data release.

1997 – The genome for *E. coli* was published

- Oxofed Molecular Group acquired the Genetics Computer Group.
- LION bioscience AG was founded.

1998 – The genomes for *Caenorhabditis elegans* and baker's yeast were published

- Graig Venter forms Celera in Maryland
- Inphamatica, a new Genomics and Bioinformatics company was established by the University College, London.
- Gene Formatics, a company dedicated to the analysis and prediction of protein structure and function was formed in San Diego.
- The Swiss Institute of Bioinformatics was established as a non-profit foundation
- NIH began SNP project to reveal human genetic variation.
- Celera Genomics proposed to sequence human genome faster and cheaper than consortium.

1999 – Wellcome Trust formed SNP consortium

- First Human Chromosome sequence was published.

2000 – The genomes of *Pseudonomas aeruginosa, Arabidopsis thaliana* and *Drosophila melanogaster* were sequenced.

- Pharmacopeia acquired Oxford Molecular Group.

2001 – Science and Nature published annotations and analysis of human genome by mid February.

2002 – More genome sequences of other organisms were published.

All the above mentioned developments have contributed significantly to the growth of bioinformatics in one way or another.

11.2 Sequencing Development

Before 1945, there was not even a single quantitative analytical method available for any one protein. However, significant progress with chromatographic and labeling techniques over the next decade eventually led to the elucidation of the first complete sequence, that of the peptide hormone insulin. The sequence of the first enzyme ribonuclease was complete by 1960. By 1965, around 20 proteins with more than 100 residues had been sequenced, and by 1980, the number was estimated to be around 1500. Today more than 3,00,000 sequences are available.

Initially a majority of protein sequences were obtained by the manual process of sequential Edman degradation – dansylation. A very important step towards the rapid increase in the number of sequenced proteins was the development of automated sequences which, by 1980, offered a 10^4 fold increase in the sensitivity compared to the procedure implemented by Edman and Begg in 1967.

The first complete protein sequence assignment using mass spectrometry was achieved in 1979. This technique played a vital role in the discovery of the amino acid γ-carboxyglutamic acid, and its location in the N-terminal region of prothrombin.

During 1960s and 1970s scientists were finding it difficult to develop methods to sequence nucleic acids. When the techniques were available, the first techniques to emerge were applicable only to RNA (ribonucleic acid), especially transfer – RNAs (tRNA). tRNAs were ideal materials for this early work, because they are short (typically 74-95 nucleotides in length), and because it is possible to purify individual molecules.

DNA (deoxyribonucleic acid) consists of thousands of nucleotides and assembling the complete nucleotide sequence of an entire chromosomal DNA molecule is a very big task. With the advent of gene cloning and PCR, it became possible to purify defined fragments of chromosomal DNA. This paved the way for the development of fast and efficient DNA sequencing techniques. By 1977, two sequencing methods had emerged, using chain termination and chemical degradation approaches. These techniques with some minor modifications laid the foundation for the sequence revolution of the 1980s and 1990s and the subsequent birth of bioinformatics.

The polymerase chain reaction (PCR) due to its sensitivity, specificity and potential for automation, is considered the front-line analytical method for analyzing genomic DNA samples and constructing genetic maps. Over the years, incremental improvements in basic PCR technology have enhanced the power and practice of the technique. Since the introduction of the first-semi-automated sequence in 1987, coupled with the development of PCR in 1990 and fluorescent labeling of DNA fragments generated by the Sanger dideoxy chain termination method, there have been large-scale sequencing efforts which have contributed greatly. Technologies for capturing sequence information have also become advanced over a period of time. In the early 1980s, researchers could use digitizer pens to manually read DNA sequences from gels. Then came image-capture devices, which were cameras that digitized the information on gels. In 1987 Steven Krawetz, helped to develop the first DNA sequencing software for automated film readers. In the early 1990s, J. Craig Venter and his colleagues devised a new method to fine genes. Rather than taking the single base chromosomal DNA, Venter's group isolated messenger RNA molecules, copied these mRNA molecules into DNA molecules and then sequenced a part of the DNA molecule to create expressed sequence tags or ESTs. These ESTs cold be used as handles to isolate the entire gene. The EST approach also has generated enormous databases of nucleotide sequences and the development of the EST technique is considered to have demonstrated the feasibility of high-throughput gene discovery, as well as provided a key impetus for the growth of the genomics industry.

At the start of 1998, more than 3,00,000 protein sequences have been deposited in publicly available non-redundant data bases, and the number of partial sequences in public and proprietary Expressed Sequence Tag (EST) databases was expected to run into millions. By contrast, the number of 3D structures in the Protein Data Bank (PDB) is still less than 2000.

The United States Department of Energy (DoE) initiated a number of projects in 1980s to construct detailed genetic and physical maps of the human genome. Their aim was to determine the complete nucleotide sequence of human genome and to localize the estimated 30,000 genes. Work of such a great dimension required the development of new computational methods for analyzing genetic map and DNA sequence data, and demanded the design of new techniques and instrumentation for detecting and analyzing DNA. To benefit the public most effectively, the projects also necessitated the use of advanced means of information dissemination in order to make the results available as rapidly as possible to scientists and physicians. The international effort arising from this vast initiative became known as the Human Genome Project (HGP).

A very useful guide can be found in the website: http://www.ornl.gov/ TechResources/ Human_Genome/

Overview of the role, history and achievements of the US Department of Energy in the HGP can be found in the website: http://ornl.gov/techResources/ Human_Genome/ publicat/tko/index.html

Genome Annotation Consortium (GAC) provides comprehensive sequence-based views of a variety of genomes in the form of an illustrated guide, with progress charts, etc., and it can be found in the website: http://compbio.ornl.gov/gac/index.shtml.

Mapping and sequencing the genomes of a variety of organisms have been taken up and this can be found in the website: http://www-fp.mcs.anl.gov/~gaasterland/ genomes.html.

In understanding the meaning of sequences, two distinct analytical themes have emerged: i, in the first approach, pattern recognition techniques are used to detect similarity between sequences and hence to infer related structures and functions and ii, *ab initio* prediction methods are used to deduce 3D structures and ultimately to infer function directly from the linear sequence. The direct prediction of protein three-dimensional structure from the linear amino acid sequence is the objective of bioinformatics.

11.3 Aims and Tasks of Bioinformatics

The underlying principle of bioinformatics is that, biological polymers such as nucleic acid molecule and proteins, can be transformed into sequences of digital symbols. Besides, only limited numbers of alphabets are required to represent the nucleotide and amino acid monomers. This flexibility of analyzing the biomolecules with the help of limited alphabets resulted in the flourishing of bioinformatics. The growth and performance of bioinformatics rely on the developments in computer hardware and software. The simplest tasks used in bioinformatics concern the creation and maintenance of databases of biological information.

The aims of bioinformatics are as follows:

(i) To organize data in a way that allows researchers to access existing information and to submit new entries as they are produced.
(ii) To develop tools and resources that aid in the analysis of data.
(iii) To use these tools to analyze the data and interpret the results in a biologically meaningful manner.

The tasks in bioinformatics involve the analysis of sequence information. This process involves:

– identifying the genes in the DNA sequences from various organisms.

– Developing methods to study the structure and/or function of newly identified sequences and corresponding structural RNA sequences.

– Identifying families of related sequences and the development of models.

– Aligning similar sequences and generating phylogenetic trees to examine evolutionary relationships.

11.4 Application of Bioinformatics

Biocomputing has found its application in many areas. Apart from providing the theoretical background and practical tools for scientists to explore proteins and DNA, it also helps in many other ways.

11.4.1 Sequence Homology Analysis

One of the driving forces behind bioinformatics is the search for similarities between different biomolecules. Apart from enabling systematic organization of data, identification of protein homologues has some direct practical uses. Theoretical models of proteins are usually based on experimentally solved structures of close homologues. Wherever biochemical or structural data are lacking, studies could be carried out in yeast like lower organisms and the results can be applied to homologues in higher organisms such as humans. It also simplifies the problem of understanding complex genomes by analyzing simple organisms first and then applying the same principles to more complicated ones.

This would result in identifying potential drug targets by checking homologues of essential microbial proteins.

11.4.2 Drug Design

The adoption of a bioinformatics-based approach to drug discovery provides an important advantage. With bioinformatics, genotypes associated with pathophysiologic conditions could be defined, which might lead to the identification of potential molecular targets. Given the nucleotide sequence, the probable amino acid sequence of the encoded protein can be determined using translation software.Sequence research techniques could then be used to find homologues in model organisms; and based on sequence similarity it is possible to model the structure of the specific protein on experimentally characterized structures. Finally, docking algorithms could design molecules that could bind to the model structure, leading the way for biochemical assays to test their biological activity on the actual protein.

11.4.3 Predictive Functions

Through large-scale screening of data, one can address a number of evolutionary, biochemical and biophysical questions. We can identify a) specific protein folds associated with certain phylogenetic groups, b) commonality between different folds within particular organisms, c) the degree of folds shared between related organisms, d) the extent of relatedness derived from traditional evolutionary trees, and e) the diversity of metabolic pathways in different organisms. Once can also integrate data on protein functions, given the fact that particular protein folds are often related to specific biochemical functions. Combining expression information structural and functional classifications of proteins, one can predict the occurrence of a protein fold in a genome, which is indicative of high expression levels. IN conjuciton with structural data, one can compile a map of all protein-protein interactions in an organism.

11.4.4 Medical Areas

Applications in medical sciences have centered on gene expression analysis. This usually involves compiling expression data for cells affected by different diseases and comparing the measurements against normal expression levels. Identification of genes that are expressed differently in affected cells provides a basis for explaining the causes of illness and highlights potential drug targets. With this one would design compounds that bind to the expressed protein. Given a lead compound, microarray experiments can be sued to evaluate responses to pharmacological intervention; it can also help in providing early tasks to detect or predict the toxicity of trial drugs.

If bioinformatics is combined with experimental genomics, a lot of advances could be made to revolutionize the future healthcare programs. This involves postnatal genotyping to assess susceptibility or immunity from specific diseases and pathogens; prescription of a unique combination of vaccines; minimizing the healthcare costs of unnecessary treatments and anticipating the onslaught of diseases later in life, which could lead to guidance for nutrition intake and early detections of any illness. In addition, drug-based treatments cold be tailored specifically to the patient and disease, this providing the most effective course of medication with minimal side effects. Human genome project will benefit forensic sciences, pharma industries, discovery of beneficial and harmful genes, contribute to a better understand of human evolution, diagnosis of disease and disease risks, genetics of response to therapy and customized treatment, identification of drug targets and gene therapy.

11.4.5 Intellectual Property Rights

Intellectual Property Rights (IPR) are essential part of today's business. IPRs are the means to protect any intangible asset. Examples of IPR are Patent, Copyright, Trademark, Geographical Indication and Trade Secret. A patent is an exclusive monopoly granted by the Government to an inventor over his inventin for limited period of time.

Major areas of bioinformatics which need intellectual property protection are a) analytical and information management tools (e.g. modeling techniques, databases, algorithms, software and b) genomics and proteomics and c) drug discovery/ design.

Innovations

Majority of bioinformatics innovation involves applications of computer-implemented protocols or software in collecting and/or processing biological data. These inventions fall within the general category of computer related inventions called inventions implemented in a computer and inventions employing computer readable media. These inventions have two aspects (a) software and b) hardware.

For example, a computer based system for indentifying new nucleotide sequence clusgters from a given set of nucleotide sequences based on sequence similarity may comprise an input device, a memory and a processor as hardware components of the system and a data set or method of operating instructions stored in the memory and operable by the processor as a software for the system. Patent protections would be invaluable in protecting methods, which use computational power, such as sequence alignments, homology searches and metabolic pathways modeling.

Genomics and Proteomics

Genomics involves isolation and characterization of gene and assigning a function or use to the gene sequence, i.e., either expression of a particular protein or identification of the gene as a marker for a particular disease. This work involves a great deal of laboratory experiments as well as computational techniques. These techniques can also be protected under IPR.

Proteomics involves purification and characterization of proteins using technologies like 2D-electrophoresis, multidimensional chromatography and mass spectroscopy. The application of these techniques to characterization and funding relation of the protein, i.e. marker with a particular disease is challenging, time consuming and needs heavy investment.

Drug design by modeling which involves computer and computation can also be protected under IPR. Table 11.1. gives some examples of patents in bioinformatics.

Table 11.1

Some examples of patents in bioinformatics

Code Number	Specific title
1. US 6,355,423	Methods and devices devices for measuring differential gene expression
2. US 6,334,099	Methods for normalization of experimental data
3. US 5,579,250	Method of rational drug design based on ab initio computer simulation of conformational features of peptides
4. WO 98/15652	DNA sequencing and RNA sequencing using sequencing enzyme
5. EPI 108779	Spatial structures of at least one polypeptide
6. EPO 807687	Recombinant protease purification and computer program for use in drug design.

11.5 Challenges and opportunities

There are numerous challenges:

(i) We must be able to deal with increasingly complex data and to integrate data sources into a single system.
(ii) Diverse types of data must be handled simultaneously to provide a better understanding of what genes do.
(iii) Data have to be annotated, filtered and visualized better.
(iv) Genomics and gene expression data have to be integrated more effectively.
(v) Better methods have to be evolved to predict structures of protein from sequences.
(vi) Better methods have to be designed to identify drug candidates.

There are numerous opportunities as well:

(i) Trained and skilled bioinformaticists are needed by many bioinformatics and drug companies.
(ii) Research and academic institutions are looking for trained people.
(iii) Trained people will be useful in the identification of useful genes leading to the development of new gene products.
(iv) Skilled bioinfomraticists will contribute greatly in genomics and proteomics research.
(v) Bioinformaticists will help in rvolutinazing drug development and gene therapy.
(vi) Bioinformaticists will be able to analyze the patterns of gene expression with computer algorithms.
(vii) Bioinformaticists will help to understand toxic responses and top predict toxicity.

11.6 Drug Discovery

A drug is a molecule that interacts with a target biological molecule in the body and through such interaction triggers a physiological effect. The target molecules are usually proteins. Drugs can be beneficial or harmful depending on their effect. The aim of pharmaceutical industry is to discover drugs with specific beneficial effects to treat diseases especially humans.

A chemical compound to qualify as a drug should have the following characteristic: It should be safe, effective, stable (both chemically and metabolically), deliverable (should be absorbed and make its way to its site of action), available (by isolation from natural sources or by synthesis) and novel (patentable).

11.6.1 Discovering a Drug

Discovering a drug can be arrived at by two methods: the empirical and the rational. The empirical method is a blind hit or lose method; it is also called black box method. Thousands of chemical compounds are tested on the disease without even knowing the target on which the drug acts and the mechanism of action. Occasionally a serendipitous discovery like the discovery of Penicillin may come up. Usually thousands of chemical compounds are tested for drug action. One out of 10,000 may hit the target. In this type of approach, no one knows initially which target the drug attacks and the mechanism involved in the attack. Rational approach starts from the clear knowledge of the target as well as the mechanism by which it is to be attacked. Drug discovery involves finding the target and arriving at the lead. Target refers to the causal agent of the disease and lead refers to the active molecule which will interact with the causal agent.

When diseases are treated with drugs they interact with targets that contribute to the disease and try to control their contribution thus producing positive effects. The disease target may be endogenous (a protein synthesized by the individual to whom the drug is administered) or, in the case of infectious diseases, may be produced by a pathogenic organism. Drugs act either by stimulating or blocking the activity of the target protein.

11.6.2 Target Identification and Validation

Developing a drug is not that easy. It is a complex, lengthy and expensive process. Drug development begins with the identification of a potentially suitable disease target. This process is called target identification. One has to study what is known about diseases, possible causes, its symptoms, its genetics, its epidemiology, its relationship to other diseases – human and animal – and all known treatments. The biology of the disease (cause of illness, the spread of the disease in the population, the development of the disease inside the patient, the biochemical and physiological changes in the patients, etc.) has to be ascertained. In the past, target identification was based largely on medical need. Presently, target identification depends not only on medical need but also on factors such as the success of existing therapies, the activity of competing drug companies and commercial opportunities.

The targets for the drugs are usually the biomolecules, such as enzymes, receptors or ion channels. The validity of the enzyme as a target depends upon how much important it is for the survival of the pathogen. If it is less significant, then the target has no value. If the drug target is located inside the human system, the fluctuation of the target activity must correspond to the fluctuation of the disease severity. Only when we are able to establish a high level of significance in the regulation of the target for effective disease control, the target will have relevance to the disease. Once the target is confirmed, we can identify the modulators of the target. There are positive modulators and negative modulators (Table 11.2).

Table 11.2

List of positive and negative modulators

Biomolecules	Positive modulators	Negative modulators
Enzymes	Activators	Inhibitors
Receptors	Agonists	Antagonists
Ion Channels	Openers	Blockers

Once the target is identified, it has to be validated. This process is called target validation. It involves extensive testing of the target molecule's therapeutic potential. Validation may include the creation of animal disease models, and the analysis of gene and protein expression data. By comparing the levels of gene expression in normal and disease states, novel drug targets can be identified *in silico.* Micro array technique can be used in this. Once the gene which is 'up or down regulated' (expressed in higher or lower level than in normal tissue) in a disease state is identified, its nature can be identified using bioinformatic tools. Similar genes or proteins can be traced using BLAST from the sequence database. Similar genes and proteins will help to deduce the function of the up or down regulated gene. If the target happens to be one of a highly tractable structure class (such as receptors, enzymes or ion channels), the drug designing will be easier. A valid target must have a high therapeutic index, that is, a significant therapeutic gain must be predicted through the use of such a drug. If a known protein is the target, binding can be measured directly. A potential anti-bacterial drug can be tested by its effect on growth of the pathogen. Some compounds might be tested for effects on eukaryotic cells grown in tissue culture. If a laboratory animal is susceptible to the disease, compounds can be tested on animals.

If the target happens to be an enzyme, the following characters are studied: the active site, the amino acids associated in the formation of active site, presence or absence of metal component, number of hydrogen donors and acceptors present in the active site, the topology of the active site, and the details about hydrophobic and hydrophilic amino acids present in the active site. If the target happens to be a biochemical substance or a substrate of an enzyme, the following details are collected: size of the molecule, chemical nature, groups that show hydrogen donor or acceptor capacity, its metabolic byproducts and how this compound can be modified chemically.

1.6.1.2 Identifying the Lead Compound

Once a target has been validated, the search begins for drugs that interact with the target. This process is called lead discovery, and involves the search for lead compounds, that is, substances with some of the desired biological activity of the ideal drug. A lead molecule should have the following desirable qualities: a) the potency (able to modulate the target effectively), b) solubility (it should be easily soluble in water for quicker action), c) a milder lipophilicity (ability to penetrate plasma membrane), d) metabolic stability (should not get destroyed quickly inside the body; a longer shelf life is desirable), e) bioavailability (quicker absorpotion into the body and at the same time retained for longer time for sustained activity), f) specific protein binding, g) less toxic or not at all toxic. Lead compounds can be found using some of the following ways:

(i) serendipity – through chance observations (discovery of penicillin by Alexander Fleming).
(ii) Survey of natural sources – from traditional medicines (quinine from *Chincona* bark).
(iii) Study of what is known about substrates or ligands or inhibitors and the mechanism of action of the target protein, and select potentially active compounds from these properties.
(iv) Trying drugs effective against similar diseases
(v) Large-scale screening of related compounds
(vi) Occasionally from side effects of existing drugs.
(vii) Screening of thousands of compounds.
(viii) Computer screening and *ab initio* computer design.

11.6.1.3 Optimization of Lead Compound

Once a lead compound is found, it must be optimized. Lead optimization involves the modification of lead compounds to produce derivatives which are called candidate drugs with better therapeutic profiles. For example, deliverability of a drug to a target within the body requires the capacity to be absorbed and transmitted. It requires metabolic stability. It requires the proper solubility profile – a drug must be suf7ficiently water – soluble to be absorbed, but not so soluble that it is excreted immediately; it must be sufficiently lipid-soluble to get across membranes, but not so lipid-soluble that it is merely taken up by fat stores. Once this is done the candidate drugs are assessed for quality, taking into account factors such as the ease of synthesis and formulation. After this, they are registered as an investigational new drug and submitted for clinical trials. This is the lengthiest and most expensive part of the drug development process. Due to this most projects are abandoned before this stage. Clinical trials are designed to determine safety and tolerance levels in humans, and to discover how the drug is metabolized. Trials are divided into several stages.

Pre-clinical phase:	- Studies using animals
Phase I:	- Normal (healthy) human volunteers
Phase II:	- Evaluation of safety and efficacy in patients, and selection of dose regimen
Phase III:	- Large patient number study with placebo or comparator; at this stage regulatory approval is sought and a commercial launch decision is taken
Phase IV:	- Long-term monitoring for adverse reactions reported by pharmacists and doctors.

Drug development has been benefiting much from genomics, proteomics, combinational chemistry and high-throughput screening. Genomics and proteomics have revolutionized the way target molecules are identified and validated. Traditionally, drug targets have been characterized on an individual basis and lead compounds have been sought with specific clinical effects. With the advent of genomics, particularly the availability of the entire human genome sequence and its annotations, thousands of potential new targets can now be identified by sequence, structure and function. Bioinformatics is important not only because of its role in the analysis of sequences and structures, but also in the development of algorithms for the modeling of target protein interactions with drug molecules. This allows rational drug design, in which protein structural data is used to predict the type of ligands that will interact with a given target, and thus form the basis of lead discovery.

Of late systematic methods are used to identify lead compounds. These methods are based on high throughput screening in which lead discovery is accelerated through the use of highly parallel assay formats, such as 96-well plates. In turn, this requires the assembly of large chemical libraries for testing. This has been made possible by combinational chemistry approaches, in which large numbers of different compounds can be made by pooling and dividing materials between reaction steps.

11.7 Pharmainformatics

The term pharmainformatics is often used to describe the mix of biology, chemistry, mathematics and information technology required for data processing and analysis in the pharmaceutical industry. The scope of pharmainformatics is summarized in Table 11.3.

Table 11.3

Areas of biology and chemistry where informatics plays a vital role in the drug discovery pipeline.

Application	Role of Bioinformatics
Biology	
Genomics proteomics (human genome project	Target identification, validation in the human genome
Characterization of human genes and proteins	Cataloguing single nucleotide polymorphisms, and association with drug response patterns (pharmacogenomics)
Genomics, proteomics (human pathogen genome projects).	Target identification, validation in pathogens
Characterization of the genes and proteins of organisms that are pathogenic to human	
Functional genomics (protein structure)	Prediction of drug/ target interactions
Analysis of protein structures (human and their pathogens)	Rational drug design
Functional genomics (expression profiling)	Gene classification based on drug responses
Determining gene expression patterns in disease and health	Pathway reconstruction
Functional genomics (genome-wide mutagnesis)	Databases of animal models
Determining the mutant phenotypes for all genes in the genome	Target identification, validation

Contd…

Table 11.3 Contd…

Application	Role of Bioinformatics
Functional genomics (protein interactions)	Characterization of protein interactions
Determining interactions among all proteins	Reconstruction of pathways Prediction of binding sites.
Chemistry	
High throughput screening	Storing, trecking and analyzing data
Highly parallel assay formats for lead identification	
Combinational chemistry	Cataloguing chemical libraries.
Synthesis of large number of chemical compounds	Assessing library quality, diversity Predicting drug, target interactions

11.7.1 Chemical Libraries and Search Programs

High throughput screening in drug discovery depends on the availability of diverse chemical libraries, such as those generated by combinational chemistry, since these maximize the chances of finding molecules that interact with a particular target protein. It is not easy to quantify chemical diversity. Attempts have been made to understand this based on the concept of 'chemical space'. In essence, chemical space encompasses molecules with all possible chemical properties in all possible molecular positions. A diverse library would have broad coverage of chemical space, leaving no gaps and having no clusters of similar molecules.

Usually library diversity is quantified using measures that compare the properties of different molecules based on descriptors such as atomic position, charge and potential to form different types of chemical bond. We can compare two molecules using the Tanimoto coefficient (Tc), which evaluates the similarity of fragments of each molecule. The coefficient is calculated by the formula $Tc=c/(a+b-c)$, where a is the number of fragment –based descriptors in compound A, b is the number of fragment-descriptors in compound B, ad c is the number of shared fragment-based descriptors. Hence, for identical molecules, $Tc=1$, while for molecules with no descriptors in common, $Tc=0$. In a chemical library of ideal diversity, most-pairwise comparisons would generate a Tanimoto coefficient near to zero.

When we do not know much about the binding specificity of the target protein, diverse libraries will be useful for lead discovery. When only some form of sequence or structural information is available for the target, this can be used to design focused libraries that concentrate on one region of chemical space. For example, if the sequence of a particular target protein is known, then database homology searching will often find a related protein whose structure has been solved and whose interactions with small molecules have been characterized. In these cases, it is possible to design a chemical library based on particular molecular scaffold, which preserves a framework of sites present in a known ligand, but which can be modified with diverse functional groups. Some of these groups may have previously been shown to be important for drug binding. Such sites are known as pharmacophores. Many tools and resources are available for the design of combinatorial libraries and the assessment of chemical diversity. A program called Selectors, available from Tripos, allows the user to design very diverse libraries or libraries focused on a particular molecular skeleton. Chem-x, developed by the Oxford Molecular Group, allows the chemical diversity in a collection of compounds to be measured and identifies all the pharmacophore. ComibiLibMaker, another Tripos program, allows a virtual target.

11.8 Search Programs

Before starting laboratory-based screening experiments, it is always better to generate as much information as possible about potential drug/ target interactions. The computational screening of chemical databases, using a target molecule of known structure, is one way in which such information can be obtained. Alternatively, the solved structure of a close homology may be used, or the structure may be predicted using a threading algorithm. Algorithms can be used to identify potential interacting ligands based on goodness of fit, if the structure of a target protein is known, thus allowing rational drug design.

Already many docking algorithms have been developed which attempt to fit small molecules into binding sites using information on steric constraints and bond energies (Table 11.4).

One of the most established docking algorithms is autodock. Another widely used program is DOCK. Another program is CombiDOCK. In DOCK, the arrangement of atoms at the binding site is converted into a set of spheres called

Table 11.4

Chemical docking software available over the internet freely

URL	R/F	Description	Availability
http://www.scripts.edu/pub/olson-web/dock.autodock/index.html	F	Autodock	Download for UNIX/LINUX
http://swift.embl-heidelberg.de/lignin/	R	LIGIN, a robust ligand-protein interaction prediction limited to small ligands	Download for UNIX or as apart of the WHATIF package
http://www.bmm.icnet.uk/docking/	R	FTDock and associated programs. RPScore and mMultiDock, can deal with protein-protein interactions. Ralies on a Forier transform library	Download for UNIX/LINUX
http://reco3.musc.edu/gramm/	R	GRAMM (Global Range Molecular Matching) an empirical method based on tables of inter-bond angles. GRAMM has the merit of coping with low-quality structures.	Download for UNIX or Windows
http://cartan.gmd.de/flex-bin/FlexX	F	FlexX, which calculates favorable molecular complexes consisting of the ligand bound to the active site of the protein, and ranks the output.	Apply on-line for FlexX Workspace on the server

Note: R means Rigid; F means Flexible; they indicate whether the program regards the ligand as a rigid or flexible molecule.

site points. The distances between the spheres are used to calculate the exact dimensions of the binding site, and this is compared to a database of chemical compounds. Matches between the binding site and a potential ligand are given a confidence score, and ligands are then ranked according to their total scores. In combiDOCK, each potential ligand is considered as a scaffold decorated with functional groups. Only spheres on the scaffold are initially used in the docking prediction and then individual functional groups are tested using a variety of bond torsions. Finally it is bumped before a final score is presented.

Chemical databases can be screened not only with binding site (searching for complementary molecular interactions) but also with another ligand (searching for identical molecular interactions). Several available algorithms can compare two-dimensional or three-dimensional structures and build a profile of similar molecules.

The three dimensional structure (3D) of the target is a prerequisite (X-ray Crystallography, nuclear magnetic resonance imaging) for designing a compound that can bind or act on it. The compound is chosen from existing chemical compound library by the combinatorial structure docking. The lead compounds from the library are docked or tried by complementary fixing onto the active site of the target molecule. This intitial *in silico* fixing reduces the number of compounds that have to be synthesized and tested in vitro, since the databases contain the chemical property and method of synthesis of the compounds.

By studying the active site of the target molecule carefully, the lead compound is built piece-by-piece using computer software. The surface of the target molecule to be interacted by lead may have various chemical environment such as hydrophobicity, hydrogen bonding or catalytic zone. To this field, fragments of a hypothetical compound is placed. The orientation of the fragments provide a clue about the final form of the lead compound. GRID, GREEN, HISTE, HINT and BUCKTS are some of the softwares used for this kind of active site analysis. Sometimes the entire molecule is fit into the receptor site or active site. DOCK is a software that uses 'shape fitting' approach (Fig. 9.1). It searches all possible ways of fitting a ligand into the receptor site. The binding site of the receptor or enzyme molecule contains hydrogen bonding regions and hydrophobic regions. Initially a prototype molecule is positioned inside the active site to satisfy a few of the bonding energy. Additional building blocks are fitted in stepwise manner till all the bonding energies are satisfied. CLIX is a software that creates the active site points and then searches for chemical structure database that would satisfy the active site. In drug development, lead compounds are optimized by decorating the molecular skeleton with different functional groups and testing each derivative for its biological activity. If there are several open positions on the lead molecule that can be substituted, the total number of molecules that need to be tested in a comprehensive screen would be very large. The synthesis and screening of all these molecules would be time-consuming and laborious, especially since most would have no useful activity. In order to select those molecules most likely to have a useful activity and thus guide in chemical synthesis, QUSAR can be used. QSAR is Quantitative Structure –Activity Relationship, a mathematical relationship used to determine how the structural features of a molecule are related to biological activity.

Here, essentially, the molecules are treated as groups of molecular properties (descriptors), which are arranged in a table. The QSAR mines these data and attempts to find consistent relationships between particular descriptors and biological activities, thus identifying a set of rules that can be used to score new molecules for potential activity. A QSAR is usually expressed in the form of a linear equation:

$$\text{Biological activity} = \text{constant} + \sum_{i=1}^{i=n} CiPi$$

P_1-P_N are parameters (molecular properties) established for each molecule in the series and C1-CN are coefficients calculated by fitting variations in the parameters to their biological activities. Once the lead molecules are identified, they have to be optimized for potency, selectivity and pharmacokinetic properties. Four qualities such as the H bond donors <5, the hydrogen acceptors <10, the relative molecular weight <500 and lipophilicity <5 are recommended for high bioavailability (intestinal absorption). The drugs targeted on Central Nervous System should have the penetrability of Blood – Brain Barrier (BBB).

Some useful websites are given below:
http://www.netsci.org/science/compchem/feature19.html
http://clogp.pomona.edu/medchem/chem./master/search.html
http://chemfinder.cambridgesoft.com
http://www.cas.org/casdb.html
http://www.mdli.com
http://www .daylight.com/dayhtml/smiles/smiles-into.html#TOC

Bioinformatics

Bioinformatics is the storage, retrieval, manipulation and analysis of biological data using computational tools. Many important discoveries such as sequencing developments have contributed to the growth.

Aims and Tasks

The aims of Bioinformatics are to organize data to access existing information and to submit new entries, to develop tools and resources that aid in the analysis of data and to use these tools to analyze the data and interpret the result of meaningfully.

Application of Bioinformatics

One of the driving forces behind Bioinformatics is the search for similarities between different biomolecules. It is helpful in sequence homology analysis. It is also useful in drug design. Through large-scale screening of data one can address a number of evolutionary, biochemical and biophysical questions. It is also useful in medical areas. Many innovations in Bioinformatics lead to intellectual property rights.

Challenges and Opportunities

We must be able to deal with increasingly complex data and integrate them. Data have to be annotated, filtered and visualized better. Better methods have to be designed to identify drug candidates. There are many opportunities for jobs in companies and universities.

Drug Discovery

A drug is a molecule that interacts with a target biological molecule in the body and through such interaction triggers a physiological effect. The aim of pharmaceutical industry is to discover drugs with specific beneficial effects to treat diseases. Drugs discovery involves finding the target and arriving at the lead. Target refers to the causal agent of the disease and lead refers to the active molecule which will interact with the casual agent.

Pharmainformatics

The term pharmainformatics is often used to describe the mix of biology, chemistry, mathematics and analysis in the pharmaceutical industry. High throughput screening in drug discovery depends on the availability of diverse chemical libraries since they maximize the chances of finding molecules that interact with a particular target protein. When we do not know much about the binding specificity of the target protein, diverse libraries will be useful for lead discovery. Many search programs are useful in this.

Questions

(1) What is bioinformatics?
(2) What is the contribution of Rosalind and Wilkins?
(3) Who produced the first recombinant DNA organism?
(4) When was Compact Disk (CD) launched?
(5) Who developed BLAST program?
(6) Who published PRINTS database?
(7) In which year the human genome annotations were published?
(8) Write a short history on sequencing.
(9) What are the aims of bioinformatics?
(10) What are the tasks in bioinformatics?
(11) What are the various applications of bioinformatics.

12
Biotechnology and Ethics

Introduction

Biotechnology is the most controversial scientific discovery of the recent times and hit the headlines of newspapers throughout the world because of its good and bad effects on the ethical and social aspects of the present-day civilized society. There are innumerable biotechnical, agricultural, industrial and medical applications such as the acceleration of breeding techniques; improvement of quality of meat, adjustment of new pharamacodynamic agents, construction of new organisms with useful qualities (e.g. bacteria capable of absorbing atmospheric nitrogen), the rapid and economical synthesis of natural products such as insulin and interferons, the biological solution of energy related problems and the clinical applications to control diseases etc. Growth hormones, and monoclonal antibodies are also available for treatment and diagnosis.

Gene therapy helps in the betterment of certain human characteristics by diagnosing the genetic defects and replacing the faulty genes with good ones. As long as recombinant DNA technology is helpful for good and beneficial things, it is acceptable. However, when it is a matter of interventions that are not strictly therapeutic, aiming, for example, at the improvement of the human biological condition, then it becomes arbitrary and unjust. If it reduces life to a thing and injures a person's dignity by exposing it to the whims of others then it is unacceptable. In spite of all the beneficial discoveries, there seems to be a real possibility that there are some discoveries leading to unethical and uncontrolled proliferation of strongly pathogenic new viruses, introduction of some terrible toxin or tumour forming genes into bacteria and using them as instruments of effective and deadly bacteriological warfare, or treating a human being as a laboratory animal or an object. Let us now look into various aspects of biotechnology and locate areas where there are specific problems with regard to their ethical orientation and the best way that the scientists could avoid the pitfalls.

12.1 Medical and Chemical Biotechnology

From the medical point of view, biotechnology has revolutionized the scene by providing new and efficient tools to combat diseases. Production of new biomolecules therapeutic reagents, diagnostic kits and other advanced treatment systems have added a new dimension to medical treatment.

Scientists have succeeded in producing an insulin called humulin. They have also produced a class of regulatory proteins of the immune system called inferferons which has played a significant role in combating diseases. Scientists have also succeeded in producing a large quantity of vaccines and antibodies in pure state to act against viral diseases. They have also succeeded in producing monosex fertility pills to act on pituitary hormones called inhibin. Scientists have also succeeded in discovering more sensitive and quicker methods for detecting and treating Hepatitis B, venereal diseases, viral infections, cancer, AIDS etc. Using monoclonal antibodies, scientists are trying to develop specific types of reagents to combat diseases.

From the chemical point of view, the transformation of substances by biocatalysts offers new routes to products that are difficult or expensive to produce by chemical transformations and can give rise to new products such as biopolymers. Activities range from improving or engineering raw materials such as oil seeds; processing waste into fuel or potential intermediates such as industrial feedstock; generating new antibiotics or producing alternate structural materials to plastics.

Biotechnologists have triumphed in producing some speciality chemicals such as amino acids, vitamins, enzymes which are so essential for normal biological functions.

In spite of all these, commercial biotechnology, if left alone, will seek profit to the detriment of the public well being and pharmaceutical companies will direct their research toward treating profitable diseases, i.e. diseases that already have been contracted and therfore represent an immediate market.

Three international experts on AIDS, Dr. John Seale from London, Dr. Robert Strecker from California and Dr.Jacob Segal from West Berlin claimed in 1987 that the AIDS virus was artificially created by American Scientists during laboratory experiments when they were trying to discover a cure for cancer by combining parts of Maedi-visna virus found in the sheep and Human T-cell leukaemia virus type 1 (HTLVY1). They argued that the scientists or anybody else in the laboratory could have been infected with the new virus through a minute cut or even by inhaling.

12.2 Agriculture and Food

Biotechnologists have contributed a great deal to the field of agriculture and food. Agricultural applications range from the improvement of plant and animal stock to pest control and animal food stuff. The food processing industry has a constant demand for acceptable additives such as colourants, sweeteners and sauces, including sóy sauce, or for bulk protein, novel catalysts and preservatives. The incorporation of novel fungi into milk also increases the monetary value of products such as yoghurt and cheese.

Biotechnologists have given a great boost to increased food production by the introduction of plants with increased and improved primary products. Single cell proteins are regarded as wholesome food in many respects. Scientists have also succeeded in producing sun-bean, a hybrid of sun flower and French bean using biotechnological methods. They have developed plants resistant to pollution, insects, pests, and even pesticides. Biotechnologists are trying to transfer the genes of neem tree for resistance. To some extent, scientists have been trying and have even succeeded slightly in transferring nitrogen fixing genes into non-leguminous plants. Using biotechnological methods, they have succeeded in enhancing the production of secondary products like wood, leaves, resins and also improving other products like fatty acids, organic acids, vanilla, pigments, etc. Production of monoclones is another advancement towards creating disease resistant plants.

Human beings have always been trying to produce sturdy and better animals. Biotechnology has helped in this. Scientists have been able to produce animals which could yield more milk to meet the demands of a large population; they have also succeeded in increasing the meat yield; they have increased the fertility and reproductive efficiency of animals. They have evolved ways and means to efficiently increase the conversion potential of food and feed efficiency. Many newer methods have been evolved to fertilize and make the animals deliver more offsprings.

The use of animals like pigs, cattle, monkeys and others is problematic as regards animals rights as also the utility of transfer of such knowledge to humans. Cows and cattle developed artificially as milk machines with enormous heavy udders and as meat factories are a pathetic sight and almost an abomination to friends of animals.

12.3 Energy and Environment

As we all know, plants are the most efficient energy stores. So biotechnologists have been trying to produce a diesel like fuel directly from plants. They have efficiently produced alcohol from bagasse. They have genetically engineered bacteria which are able to release oil from rocks. They have been trying to produce oil-eating bacteria to fight oil slicks and oil spills from refineries for cleaning up the sea and sea resorts and have succeeded to some extent. Biotechnologists have been trying to produce microbes to release metal from ores. Waste treatment has improved essentially as a large scale fermentation industry requiring new catalysts and improved reactors to treat toxic wastes. The energy industries have provided new fuel sources and have improved the efficiency of energy recovery from existing ones. Biocatalysts act as biological fuel cells.

There is every possibility of disturbing global symbiosis and bio-equilibrium due to pragmatic (profit) and anthropocentric motives that are involved in biotechnological endeavours, e.g., using microbes for biologicai warfare. With regard to *Escherichia coli,* a bacterium that inhabits the colon of humans, which is greatly used as an easy experimental material in many biotechnological endeavours because; it has been genetically explored to a great extent, there is a real danger of some of their mutant entering humans. If bacteria with cellulose degrading genes inhabit the intestines, we can imagine the uncontrollable diarrhea that will be caused. Some of these *E. coli* mutant strains are also resistant to antibiotics. There is also a danger of oil eating bacteria *(Pseudomonas sp.,* first patented animals) spreading to oil wells and creating havoc.

Growing apprehensions about the possible military use of genetic engineering and other new biotechnologies are threatening to undermine the international ban on biological weapons. The issue is the use of biology, previously like chemistry and physics, to produce new weapons of mass destruction.

The possibility that recombinant DNA technology could be used to produce biological warfare agents by creating new pathogens or modifying natural ones always has bothered many people.

The biological weapons convention of 1972 prohibits the development and possession of biological and toxin weapons; their use was previously outlawed by the Geneva protocol of 1925. The convention now has 103 signatories, including all the major nations outside the middle East. The convention permits the development and possession of biological agents and toxin of types and in quantities that are justified for prophylactic, protective or other peaceful purposes including defence. This is the loophole in the treaty that is arousing worldwide suspicions and concern that defensive programmes, which are usually carried out in secret, might be used to mask the development of designer weapons that could evade opposing defences.

A variety of previously unimaginable biological weapons can now be conceived. New toxin or antibiotic resistance genes can be inserted into naturally infectious agents, thereby making them more dangerous and more resistant to treatment. Moreover, by altering surface antigens, pathogens can be rendered insensitive to standard vaccines and to the immunological defences of the host. Antigen alternation can also interface with diagnosis and identification of the agent. The stability of an agent, in principle, can be increased by splicing in genes for resistance to inactivation by ultraviolet light, drying, acrosol formation, and other stresses encountered in use as a weapon.

The very existence of a new pathogen would be a threat to life, because no degree of security can fully guarantee against its eventual escape or release by careless or irrational individuals or terrorists, nor can logic assure that, if an unreliable weapon is in hand, hazards such as the possibility of mutation after release will not be ignored some day in the heat of battle.

12.4 Humans

Innumerable discoveries have helped human beings to lead a better and healthy life. Biotechnology has taken great strides in recent times and has considerably enhanced the capacity to allay human sufferings and prevent and cure diseases. At the same time, it can also cause immense harm to the life and health of people if it is not practised properly.

12.4.1 Artificial Insemination (AI)

Artificial insemination technique, which is widely used now, has been developed in an effort to overcome infertility. Here the husband's sperm or the donor's sperm (when the husband cannot produce it himself) is placed in the genital tract of his wife by artifical means and thus conception is made possible.

Artificial insemination is usually resorted to when conception through natural sexual intercourse is not possible for physiological or emotional reasons. Children are the fruits of the mutual love between husband and wife and every couple naturally longs for at least one or two children. Lack of children can adversely affect the happiness of the couple, their sense of fulfilment and even their mutual fidelity and commitment. In this context, AI is considered a great boon to such suffering couples.

Artificial insemination may lead to many complications and problems particularly when the sperm is not from the husband but from some other male. It may lead to adultery under the present law. There is an unwarranted interference with a natural process. The husband may claim at a later stage that he is not the legal father of the child. The child may be declared "illegitimate". The children born to the donors will never know who their real father was. There will be other psychological consequences on the parents and on the child leading to frustration, self reproach, blame, uneasiness, anxiety etc. The child is denied the opportunity to be born into an atmosphere of filial relationship based on a genetic bond and a stable family. Proper growth and development of the child is affected; they in turn bring about unhealthy and damaging consequences for the society.

12.4.2 *In vitro* Fertilization (VF) and Embryo Transplants (ET)

Test tube baby is the popular media expression. *In vitro* is a Latin phrase meaning literally in glass and refers to a situation in which a woman's ovum is fertilized by a male sperm in a glass dish or a test tube and then implanted in her womb. This technique is used to overcome female infertility. This is resorted to when the union of ovum and sperm and consequent fertilization is not possible within the body of the woman for certain reasons, especially damage or block in the fallopian tubes. Another off-shoot of this technique is the introduction of baby-hatcheries which will completely eliminate the problems of a woman having to bear a child. Using this technique it is possible for a woman to collect an egg and a sperm from germ cell banks, have them fertilized *in vitro,* hand the embryo over to the hatchery, visit the hatchery frequently to see how the baby is growing and collect the baby at the end of nine months.

As far as we know, the first test tube baby, Louise Brown, was born in 1978 in Oldham, a town in Northwestern England. Louise was hailed as the miracle child, the baby of the century and so on. Due compliments were paid also to Patrick Steptoc and Robert Edwards, the renowned gynaecologist and the reputed physiologist respectively, who steered this venturesome process to successful completion. At the same time, warnings were also sounded by jurists, theologians and even scientists regarding the legal, ethical and social implications of the new achievement.

There are many ethical problems raised with regard to IVF and ET. Some people object to the very principle of external fertilization on anthropological grounds. There are doubts about the origin and procurement of sperm both in relation to the methods used as well as the concomitant risks. Some raise doubts about the eventual risks for the further development of the embryo. The problem of surplus eggs and embryos is quite genuine, since there is a danger of discarding them or using them for experimentation. This implies that tbe rights of an embryo to develop and form into a human being will be denied. Discarding the surplus embryo will amount to murder of potential human beings. Baby hatcheries bring in their own complications. Marriages will not be necessary leading to a breakdown of society, family and so on. This technique also poses many problems. Who is the mother? Of what nature will that baby be? What would be its feelings and affiliation towards the woman who collects it? What about the personality of the baby? What kind of bondage will be there between the baby and the parents? This dehumanisation and the incidental erosion of the tested institutions of marriage, family and filial relationship is certainly not a development to be wished for.

12.4.3 Surrogate Motherhood and Womb Leasing

This technique also is an extension of *in vitro* fertilization. Some women are not only unable to conceive but are also unwilling or unable to carry their embryos in the womb. In such cases, the embryo which is formed by *in vitro* fertilization, is transferred into the uterus of a volunteer woman who agrees to serve as a foster mother, or a surrogate, for the duration of the pregnancy, and to hand over the child after delivery to the biological parents. A variant of this procedure occurs in what is called womb leasing or lending. Here a second woman has the already fertilized ovum placed in her womb and she then carries it until the birth of the child. She literally leases her womb. Another form of surrogacy has appeared on the scene. Unmarried women wishing to satisfy their maternal instincts resort to embryo transfer.

Surrogate motherhood is done for a fee Rich childless couples are willing to pay large sums to a surrogate mother who relieves them of the ordeals of child bearing. Instances have occurred in recent years where surrogate mothers have refused to part with the child, after getting attached to it by bearing it for nine months. As a consequence, the natural parents institute legal proceedings for the recovery of the child.

The problems arising out of womb leasing or lending are fairly complicated. We shall soon be called upon to distinguish legal fathers and mothers from biological fathers and mothers; children born our of surrogate motherhood can pose difficult legal problems cutting across laws of inheritance, adoption, vestings, rights etc. The sanctity of marriage and its vows, the integrity of the family and the identity of the child are all affected. Above all these, the psychological and emotional difficulties encountered by various parties concerned are too complicated to be solved. Substitute motherhood reduces pregnancy to a simple function of production, fabrication and makes it lose any symbolic value. Some other problems like the refusal to give up the child by the woman who bore it or refusal to accept the child by the parents who demanded this service, death of the parents etc., are likely to arise.

12.4.4 Freezing Germ Cells and Human Embryos

As a result of artificial insemination techniques, scientists developed the idea of storing germ cells for future use. This type of storage was referred to as germ cell banks; from these banks, a sperm and an egg can be drawn, fertilized and, grown. An offshoot of *in vitro* fertilization, is the possibility of storing human embryos in a frozen state. When women opt for *in vitro* fertilization a number of eggs are collected from them although only one may be needed for producing a child; the unused eggs can be stored.

This means that the surplus germ cells and embryos may be thrown away or preserved in a deep freeze for future use or research purposes etc. This too leads to many problems such as denying the human rights to the tiny child, or belittling human dignity.

12.4.5 Stem cells and cloning

Stem cells are undifferentiated cells that have the unique ability to give rise to many different cell types. Adult stem cells are derived from somatic cells. Embryonic stem cells are derived from embryos.

Ethically there are strong objections from various religious leaders and many countries with regard to embryonic stem cell research since they consider embryos as potential human beings and destroying embryos is equivalent to destroying life. However some countries have permitted embryonic stem cell research for therapeutic purposes. Human cloning refers to the possible production of human beings using somatic cell nuclear transfer technique as was done by Ian Wilmut and his group or embryo transfer technique with cloned embryos as was done by Woo Suk Hevang and his group.

There is strong opposition to human cloning experiments due to known risks of abnormalities in the cloned babies, chances of still births and miscarriages, wastage of innumerable potential human beings. Many countries have banned human cloning. In March 1997, WHO released a statement condemning human cloning as ethically unacceptable. Many religious leaders considered it a serious threat to human dignity. The European parliament has stated that cloning of human beings cannot be justified or tolerated. UNESCO has also disapproved reproductive human cloning. United Nations has totally banned human cloning in 2005. However there are a few countries which are advocating human cloning for therapeutic purposes.

Cloning is a clear case of manipulation of human genetic endowment. It will also tend to undermine marriage and the family by severing the bond between marital love and procreation; it would render the male unnecessary as far as procreation is concerned and give rise to serious problems about personal identity and individuality. Furthermore cloning will produce a monotonous world of identical individuals. It will also diminish the chances of natural selection and genetic variability which are the very foundations of species diversity.

12.4.6 Grafts and Transplants

Organ transplants (heart, kidney, liver, brain) are another application of the discoveries of biotechnology which help to prolong the life of an individual with a non-functioning kidney, liver, heart or brain. This in itself is a noble act. But, the crisis that has developed is that far too many people need replacement of organs and far too few donors are available and it appears that the gap can never be bridged. There is room for exploitation and malpractices. Suppose, a doctor has two patients, one rich and the other poor, both needing kidneys of the same cellular type, and there is only one such kidney available what will be the criteria used to select the recipient? Bidding for organs will become rampant and immoral avenues will be pursued just to live longer.

12.4.7 Pre-natal Diagnosis

The aim is to provide accurate information on the state of health of the infant yet to be born. To achieve this purpose various methods like amniocentesis, echography, blood tests, sex determination etc., are used. At as early as 90 days of pregnancy, it is possible to extract a sample of amniotic fluid from a pregnant woman. This fluid contains exudate cells and excretory products discharged by the foetus. The cells, some of which are alive, may be centrifuged and cultured with a view to determining the chromosomal status of the foetus. Such a procedure enables the determination of the sex of the foetus and also of any chromosomal abnormality which it may carry.

The main ethical problem here is that of the possible direct or indirect link between prenatal diagnosis and abortion in the case of anomalies, deformation or undesired sex of the child. In many countries amniocentesis is being used merely to determine the sex of the foetus in order that abortion may be resorted to if the foetus is not of the desired sex. Particularly in India where sons are preferred, female foetus is likely to be aborted in large numbers.

12.4.8 Therapeutical Procedures for Sustaining Life

This involves not only merely extending the length of our life but also tries to ensure that youth and all the faculties are maintained longer. Attempts are being made to extend the length of life through drugs. To achieve this, medical measures are taken.

Sometimes this leads to the continuation of certain hard, painful and expensive treatment without any result, other than the protraction of an inescapable death-struggle. When death is knocking at the door, it is unreasonable to deny its imminence and inhuman to delay its appearance. The parody of life thus protracted is a cruel dehumanising trial for the patient and his relatives. Therapeutic procedures for sustaining life are a deviation from the medical spirit; in part at least, it is the expression of a certain enslavement of medical and paramedical professions by technological means.

12.4.9 Euthanasia

Etymologically the word euthanasia is derived from two greek words *eu* (good, well) and *thanatos* (death) thus meaning good death, happy death, comfortable or easy death without severe pain and suffering. Today, however, the word has acquired different connotations. It is construed as some medical intervention whereby the sufferings of sickness or of final agony are reduced even with the risk of suppressing life prematurely. The word euthanasia is also used in a more particular sense to mean mercy killing, for the purpose of putting an end to extreme suffering, or putting an end to abnormal babies. The mentally ill, or the incurably sick from the prolongation of a miserable life, could impose too heavy a burden on their families or on society.

Human life is not merely a physical and biological reality but essentially an ethical and religious reality, characterized by the union of body and soul both destined for eternal life.

Killing oneself or another innocent person implies a violation of divine law, an offence against the dignity of human persons, a crime against life and an attack on humanity.

The prohibition of euthanasia is based on an instinctive appreciation and profound reverence for human life, and on man's eternal destiny. If is based on the perception that life which is created and preserved by God, possesses an inherent right which is totally independent of its social utility.

12.4.10 Gene Therapy

This is a procedure that aims to help parents and potential parents to arrive at an accurate estimate of any special extra risks of disease, malformation or handicap in any children they might have. It provides a genetic profile of the unborn child indicating whether or not it is normal and can also show whether potential parents are likely to produce deformed offspring. Such a therapy also gives the parents accurate information about any particular handicap and how to cope with it. Gene therapy helps in correcting the disorders in the gene.

Gene therapy is a beneficial facility with an important role in the welfare of the society. However, if it is merely a preliminary to the abortion of the foetus, then it is morally not acceptable. Genetic screening gives information about the genetic profile of an individual. Here again there are possibilities for abuses and dishonest exploitation of karyotypic profiles in relation to contracts of employment, insurance policies, abortions etc. Gene therapy at the progeny level is problematic morally, legally, socially and aesthetically since it may lead to eugenics.

Adding genes to a person's blood or liver cells as in somatic cell therapy does not pose much of a problem. It will affect only that person and will not be carried to the progeny. But, gene therapy on germ cells is another story altogether. No geneticist is currently planning to transfer genes to human germ cells. The reasons are both practical and ethical. Besides the fact that viral vectors have been unsuccessful at depositing their genitic cargo in sex cells, the risks involved in germ cell therapy are not known. Yet some day, sex cell manipulation will become technically possible. This is the fear of critics of genetic engineering. If biologists can change the course of heredity, they can try to play God and influence human destiny.

Though scientists have been rearranging germ lines of crops and farm animals to suit their needs, researchers do not advocate extending such genetic tinkering to humans. Gene therapy to cure hereditary disease and relieve human suffering seems reasonable but any attempt to produce some sort of a super man would destroy humanity's rich genetic heritage.

In the U.S., scientists who wish to apply gene therapy to humans have to first obtain the approval of local ethics committee attached to their research institution. They then have to submit their project to their national committee overseeing genetic manipulation, the RAC (Recombinant DNA Advisory Committee). Finally, approval is also required from the Food and Drugs Administration which concerns itself with all new therapies.

In the 1980s scientists and ethicists were locked in a fierce debate on the ethical consequences of gene replacement therapy. They were concerned primarily because they were worried that the society might come under the control of some totalitarian dictator who would set out to create a master race. People were worried whether it will lead to commercial eugenics.

In the early 1970s, there were many ethical questions raised about *in vitro* fertilization in humans. In the last few years, clinics, on the whole have adhered to very high professional standards and they have been very responsible. Thus if scientists, doctors and the public are morally sound, upright and responsible, then the pitfalls of gene replacement therapy as mentioned earlier can be avoided. And if somatic cell gene replacement therapy turns out to be a real boon, and it can really help patients, then it will succeed. But if somatic cell gene replacement therapy turns out to be of little real value, and the risks from it turn out to be greater than expected, then it will not be acceptable.

12.5 Bioethics: Facing Problems and Finding Solutions

Life on this planet is a 'finely tuned delicate balance' of all forms of life, a balance created by millions of years of life, by millions of years of evolution. We must have a commensurate understanding to foresee the consequences. We should develop a comparable sense of human dignity and freedom and a broadened, philosophical, comprehensive vision far beyond mere impulses and stunts.

Technical innovations and their possible repercussions require ethical reflection on what it means to be human. Ethics is not a theory for action. It is concerned with the not-to-be transgressed limits of that action. Plato cautioned that man cannot follow his scientific desires without destroying himself.

The following questions may serve as criteria for ethical judgments on biotechnological research:

(1) Should we be involved in changing the course of nature to the full extent thai biotechnology makes this possible?
(2) To whom are the researchers responsible and who exercises responsibility for checks and controls?
(3) Are means proportioned to achieving limited goals or does the end justify the means?
(4) Are the results responsibly foreseen or pursued out of scientific curiosity for fame and recognition?

When we are involved in research, we should guard and protect life and contribute to human dignity. The preservation of human life and the environment in the present and future must be the supreme motivation of all research. Biotechnological research can be justified only by reason of specific goals pursued and foreseen results produced. The goal of biotechnological research should be to preserve, protect and revere life.

Biological processes generally lead to the welfare of persons and can be further followed and developed. It is the duty of human beings to experiment and find out the means to improve and enhance the completeness and integrity of human persons. We must go ahead with our involvement in biotechnology provided we are happy to exercise a delegated authority with due reverence for the dignity of man, made in the image of God.

We are at the cross-road, just like with the use of nuclear energy. The benefits arid hazards are to be weighed not only by scientists but also by the society at large. Immediate benefits are to be weighed against long range effects on man and the world of life as a whole. Hence science has to necessarily interact with value systems.

To conclude, human nature being what it is, our tendency is to grab every new discovery and any new technique, if not for the immediate benefit it confers, at least for the 'kick' of it. This is unworthy of human beings who are supposed to reason and judge, discern and then decide. We are only familiar with the deterioration of environment as a result of rapid, indiscriminate and hasty adoption of technologies. With indiscriminate and irrational application of biotechnology, we run the risk of damaging the most prized possession of human beings, namely, our biological inheritance. Hence with deep respect for human dignity and at the same time with an urge to fight all that is negative and evil in human persons, we must go forward in the pursuit of newer biotechnological discoveries.

In 1975, an international group of scientists took the unprecedented step of convening a meeting to consider the ethical and safety implications of the then newly discovered recombinant DNA technology. One outcome of the meeting held at California, was the development of a series of guidelines that regulated and in some cases prohibited, recombinant DNA experiments. In the United States the guidelines were produced under the aegis of the National Institutes of Health (NIH). The guidelines required, among other things, that all NIH-funded experiments that involve recombinant DNA be submitted to the NIH Recombinant DNA Advisory Committee for approval. Other countries developed their own guidelines, although these were often similar to those promulgated by NIH.

In 1982, an advisory panel of the NIH, the Recombinant DNA Advisory Committee (RAC) published revised guidelines. According to new regulations, of the five classes of experiments that were severely controlled under the former guidelines, three must still obtain NIH approval before initiation; these are resistance of microorganisms to drugs, genes encoding the synthesis of toxins and operations involving the release of genetically engineered organisms into the environment (such as those used in pest control).

In Strasbury, on 26 January 1982, the Parliamentary Assembly of the Council of Europe recommended certain provisions aimed at protecting the individual from the inherent dangers of genetic manipulation. Three areas were specifically mentioned: genetic map of human cells, gene therapy of somatic cells, gene therapy of germ cells. In spite of certain advantages of genetic engineering techniques, the report concluded that man-made decisions should not substitute the free play of nature and that every one's right not to be genetically manipulated should be affirmed.

These recommendations represented the first attempt, at an international level, to establish legal protection against the consequences of genetic manipulation.

Outside the United States, variations and inconsistencies in biotechnology regulation. exist. Unsettled jurisdictional questions among government agencies within several countries similar to uncertainties in the United States, threaten to affect development of coherent international policies. Although most countries have liberalised their recombinant DNA research guidelines, France and Germany are considering whether to restrict biotechnology because of ethical questions associated with gene therapy protocols.

France's recombinant DNA guidelines is a bit ambiguous about the deliberate release of genetically engineered organisms. In Germany, the deliberate release of genetically engineered organisms is expressly prohibited. The Green Party has opposed gene therapy due to its possible misuse. Japan's biotechnology regulations are considered 'most extensive'.

Study Outline

Biotechnology is the most controversial scientific discovery in recent times due to its good and. bad effects on the ethical and social aspects of human beings. '

Medical and Chemical

Biotechnology has revolutionized the medical field by providing new and efficient tools to combat diseases. Human insulin, interferon, monoclonal antibody, growth hormones are some examples. Many new chemicals such as amino acids, vitamins, enzymes and the biological molecules are available in greater amount. In spite of all these, if left alone, pharmaceutical and chemical companies will direct their research only towards profit forgetting human dignity. Some scientists say AIDS virus was created by scientists in laboratory.

Agriculture and Food

There has been a great improvement of plants and animals in relation to pest control and food stuff. Development of protoplast fusion, single cell protein, biofertilizers and transgenic animals are same examples. Friends of animals are concerned at the idea of using animals simply as guinea pigs.

Energy and Environment

New kinds of energy sources have been developed. Oil eating bacteria have been designed. Fermenters and biocatalysts have been found. At the same time there are biohazards especially if some pathogens and toxins are developed for use in wars. The concern related to biological weapons is a real one.

Humans

Many helpful discoveries have been made with a direct aim of helping infertile couples such as artificial insemination, *in vitro* fertilization, embryo transfer, surrogate motherhood etc. All these are helpful; at the same time there are possibilities of making it a business without respect to human sexuality and human dignity. Prenatal diagnosis helps to identify any genetic disorder of the child already at the pregnancy stage. Gene therapy is helpful to correct the genetic defect. In spite of their good intentions, these techniques can be misused to carry out abortion and karyotypic changes for benefit and business. Stem cells are useful to generate organs for transplantation.

Bioethics: Facing Problems and Finding Solutions

Life is a finely tuned delicate balance. We have to develop a comparable sense of human dignity, freedom and a broadened, philosophical comprehensive vision far beyond mere impulses and stunts. Ethics is not a theory for action. It is concerned with the not-to-be transgressed limits of that action. Biotechnological research can be justified only by reason of specific goals pursued and foreseen results produced. The preservation of human life and dignity and the environment in the present and future must be the supreme motivation of all research.

Questions

(1) What are the dangers of medical and chemical applications of biotechnology?
(2) Do you justify animals being used as guinea pigs for research?
(3) What are the dangers of biological weapons if developed by some country?

(4) What is the moral objection for *in vitro* fertilization and embryo transfer?
(5) Is euthanasia ethically correct?
(6) How far can we justify gene replacement therapy?
(7) What are the basic ethical norms to be observed in biotechnological research?
(8) What are stem cells?
(9) What do we mean by human cloning?

Further Readings

Agarwal, S.K. (2005). *Advanced Environmental Biotechnology.* A.P.H. Publishing Corporation, New Delhi.

Ahmed, N. (2004). *Industrial and Environmental Biotechnology*. New Horizons Press, New York.

Balasubramanian, D., Bryce, C.F.A., Dharmalingam, K., Green, J. and Kunthala Jayaraman (eds) (2002). *Concepts in Biotechnology.* University Press, Hyderabad.

Baltimore, L. (2000). *Molecular Cell Biology.* W.H. Freeman & Co., New York.

Banerjee, M. (2005). *Biotechnology*. A.P.H. Publishing Corporation, New Delhi.

Beier, F.K. (2000). *Biotechnology and Patent Protection.* Oxford & IBH Publishing Company, New Delhi.

Berg, J.M. and Stryer, T. (2002). Biochemistry (5th edition). W.H. Freeman and Company.

Brown, T.A. (1999). *Principles of Genetic Engineering*. Wiley, New York.

Chawla, H.S. (2002). *Introduction to Plant Biotechnology.* Oxford & IBH Publishing Company, New Delhi.

D'Souza, L., Anuradha, M., Nivas, S., Hegde, S. and Rajendra, K. (2004). *Biotechnology for a Better Future*. SAC Publications, Mangalore.

Das, H.K. (2004). *Text Book of Biotechnology.* John Wiley and Sons, New Delhi.

De, K.K. (2004). *An Introduction to plant Tissue Culture.* New Central Book Agency, kolkata

Drlica, K. (1984). *Understanding DNA and Gene Cloning- guide for the curious*. John Wiley and Sons, New York.

Dubey, R.C. (2004). *Text Book of Biotechnology.* S. Chand & Company, New Delhi

Eric Grace (1997). *Biotechnology unzipped: Promises & Realities*. Universities Press India Ltd., Hyderabad.

Flickinger, M.C. and Drew, S.W. (2002). *Encyclopeadia of Bioprocess technology: Fermentation, Biocatalysis and Bioseparation*. Volume 1, A Wiley interscience publication, New York.

Freshey, R.I. (2000). *Culture of Animal Cells*. Wiley, New York.

Ghosh, T.K. (2005). *Biotechnology in Environmental Management.* Vol. 1&2. A.P.H. Publishing Corporation, New Delhi.

Gilbert (2003). Developmental Biology, 7th edition. Sinaeur Associates Inc., Sunderland.

Glick, B.R. and Pasternak, J.J. (2003). *Molecular Biotechnology: Principles and Applications of Recombinant DNA.* ASM Press. Washington D.C.

Glover, D.M. (1984). *Gene cloning: The Mechanics of DNA Manipulation.* Chapman and Hall, London.

Goodenough, U. (1984). *Genetics.* Saunders College Publishing, Philadelphia.

Gupta, P.K. (2004). *Cell and Molecular Biology.* Rastogi Publications, Meerut.

Gupta, P.K. (2004). *Elements of Biotechnology.* Rastogi Publications, Meerut.

Hartl, D.L., Freifelder, D. and Snyder, L.A. (1988). *Basic Genetics*. Jones and Bartlett Publisher, Boston.

Ignacimuthu, S. (1996). *Applied Plant Biotechnology.* Tata McGraw-Hill, New Delhi.

Ignacimuthu, S. (1998). *Plant Biotechnology.* Oxford & IBH, New Delhi.

Ignacimuthu, S. (2005). *Basic Bioinformatics.* Narosa Publishing House, New Delhi.

Ignacimuthu, S. (2006). *Methods in Biotechnology.* Elite Publishing House, New Delhi.

John E. Smith (1996). *Biotechnology.* Cambridge University Press, London.

Kumar, H.D. (2005). *Text Book on Biotechnology.* Affiliated East-West Press, New Delhi.

Lilia Alberghina (2003). *Protein Engineering in Industrial Biotechnology.* Harwood Academic Publishers, New York.

Lohar, P.S. (2005). *Biotechnology.* MJP Publishers, Chennai.

Mansi, M.E. and Bryce, C. (2003). *Fermentation Microbiology and Biotechnology.* Taylor & Francis Ltd., London.

Munshi, M. and Sopory, S.K. (2004). *Biotechnology: Applications and Careers.* Viva Books Ltd., New Delhi.

Nitchall, C. (2002). *Introduction to Genetic Engineering.* Cambridge University Press, London.

Old, R.W. and Primrose, S.B. (1985). *Principles of gene Manipulation: An introduction to Genetic Engineering,* Blackwell, Oxford.

Old, R.W., Twyman, R.M. and Primrose, S.B. (2001). *Principles of Gene Manipulation* (6th edn.). Blackwell Scientific Publications Ltd, Oxford.

Olguin, E.J., Sanchez, G. and Hernaudez, E. (eds) (2003). *Environmental Biotechnology and Cleaner Bioprocesses.* Taylor & Francis Ltd., London.

Pasternak, J.J. (2001). Molecular Biotechnology – Principles and Applications of Recombinant DNA (II Edition), Replica Press Pvt. Ltd., New Delhi 110040.

Primrose, S.B. (1987). *Modern Biotechnology*. Blackwell, Oxford.

Primrose, S.B. (1988). *Principles of Genome Analysis*. Blackwell Science Ltd, Oxford.

Primrose, S.B. (2002). *Molecular Biotechnology*. Panima Books Ltd., New Delhi.

Ranga, M.M. (2002). *Animal Biotechnology*. Agrobios (India), Jodhpur.

Ratledge, C. and Kristiansen, B. (2004). *Basic Biotechnology*. Cambridge University Press, London.

Rema, L.P. (2006). *Applied Biotechnology*. MJP Publishers, Chennai.

Rita Singh. (2003). *Introduction to Biotechnology*, Vol.I & II. Global Vision Publishing House, Delhi.

Royal Society of Chemistry, Burlington House, London.

Schmauder, H.P. (ed) (2002). *Methods in Biotechnology*. Taylor & Francis Ltd., London.

Smith, J.E. (2003). *Biotechnology*. Cambridge University Press, London.

Thomas, J.A. (2003). *Biotechnology and Safety Assessment*. Taylor & Francis Ltd., London.

Twyman, R.M. (1998). *Advanced Molecular Biology*. Viva Books Ltd., New Delhi.

Walker, M. and Gingold, E.B. (1988). *Molecular Biology & Biotechnology*.

The Royal Socety of Chemistry, London.

Watson, J.D., Tooze, J. and Kurtz, D.T. (1998). *Recombinant DNA*, 2nd Edn. W.H.

W. H. Freeman & Co., New York

Whitford, D. (2005). *Protein Structure and Function*. Lasewords Pvt. Ltd.,

Wu, W. (1997). *Methods in Gene Biotechnology*. CRC Press, Florida.

Annexure

NOBEL PRIZE WINNERS

Year	Scientist/s	Research
2006	Andrew Z. Fire and Craig C. Melo	Discovery of RNA interference-gene silencing by double-stranded RNA.
2005	Barry J. Marshall and Robin Warren	work on peptic ulcer disease, - discovery of the bacterium *Helicobacter pylori* and its role in gastritis and peptic ulcer disease.
2004	Richard Axel and Linda B Buck	Discoveries of odorant receptors and the organization of the olfactory system.
2003	Paul C. Lauterbur and Sir P. Mansfield	Magnetic resonance imaging (MRI).
2002	Sydney Brenner, H. Robert and John E. Sulston	Genetic regulation of organ development and programmed cell death.
2001	Leland H. Hartwell, R. Timothy and P.M. Nurse	Key regulators of the cell cycle.
2000	Arvid Carlsson, Paul Greengard and Eric Knadel	Signal transduction in the nervous system.
1999	Gunter Blobel	Proteins have intrinsic signals that govern their transport and localization in the cell.
1998	Robert F. Furchgott, Louis J. Ignarro and Ferid Murad	Nitric oxide as a signaling molecule in the cardiovascular system.
1997	Stanley Prusiner	Prions – a new biological principle of infection.
1996	P.C. Doherty and R.F. Zinkernagel	Specificity of the cell-mediated immune defence.

Year	Scientist/s	Research
1995	E.B. Lewis, C.N. Volhard and E.F. Wieschaus	Genetic control of early embryonic development.
1994	Alfred G. Gilman and M. Rodbell	G-proteins and the role of these protcins in signal transduction in cells
1993	R.J. Robrets and P.A. Sharp	Split genes and RNA processing.
1993	K. Mullis	Polymerase Chain Reaction.
1993	K. Smith	Site directed mutagenesis.
1992	E.H. Fisher and E.G. Krebs	Reversible protein phosphorylation as a biological regulatory mechanism.
1991	E. Neher and B. Sakmann	Function of single ion channels in cells.
1990	J.E. Murray and E.D. Thomas	Organ and cell transplantation in the treatment of human desease.
1989	J.E. Bishop and H.E. Varmus	Cellular origin of retroviral oncogenes.
1989	T.R. Cech and S. Altman	Ribozyme.
1988	Sir J.W. Black, G.B. Elion and G.H. Hitchings	Important principles for drug treatment.
1988	J. Deisenhofer, R. Huber and H. Michel	Bacterial photosynthetic reaction centre.
1987	Susumu Tonegawa	Genetic principle for generation of antibody diversity.
1986	Stanley C. and Rita Levi-Montalcini	Growth factors.
1985	M.S. Brown and J.L Goldstein	Regulation of cholesterol metabolism.

Year	Scientist/s	Research
1984	N.K. Jerne, G.G.F. Kohaler and Cesar Milstein	Specificity in the development and control of the immune system and the discovery of the principle for production of monoclonal antibodies.
1983	Barbara McClintock	Mobile genetic elements.
1982	A. Klug	Structure of virus and components of life.
1981	David H. Huble and T.N.Wiesel	Information processing in the visual system.
1981	Roger W. Sperry	Functional specification of cerebral hemisphere.
1980	Baruj B., J. Dausset and G.D. Snell	Genetically determined structures on the cell surface that regulate immunological reactions.
1979	A.M. Cormack and Sir G.N. Hounsfield	Computer assisted tomography, CAT-scan
1978	Warner A., Daniel N. and Hamilton O. Smith	Restriction enzymes and their application to problems of molecular genetics.
1977	R. Guillemin and Andrew V. Schally	Peptide hormone production of the brain.
1977	Rosalyn Yalow	Radioimmuno assays of peptide hormones.
1976	B.S. Blumberg and D.C. Gajdusk	New mechanisms for the origin and dissemination of infectious diseases.
1975	D. Baltmore, R. Dulbecco and H.M. Temin	Interaction between tumour viruses and the genetic material of the cell.
1974	A. Claude, C. De Duve and G.E. Palade	Structural and functional organization of the cell.
1973	KV. Frisch and T. Nikolaas	Organization and elicitation of individual and social behaviour patterns.

Year	Scientist/s	Research
1972	G.M. Edelman and R.R. Porter	Chemical structure of antibodies.
1971	E.W. Jr. Sutherland	Mechanism of the action of hormones.
1970	Sir B. Katz, U.V. Euler and Julius Axelford	Humoral transmitters in the nerve terminals and the mechanisms of release and inactivation.
1969	Max Delbruck, A.D. Hershey and S.E. Luria	Replication mechanism and he genetic structure of viruses.
1968	H.G. Khorana, R.W. Holley and M.W. Nirenberg	Interpretation of the genetic code and its function in protein synthesis.
1967	R. Granit, H.K. Hartline and W. George	Primary physiological and chemical visual processes in the eye.
1966	Preyton Rous	Tumour inducing viruses.
1966	C.B. Huggins	Hormonal treatment of prostatic cancer.
1965	F. Jacob, L. Andre and J. Monod	Genetic control of enzyme and virus synthesis.
1964	K. Bloch and F. Lynen	Mechanism and regulation of cholesterol and fatty acid metabolism.
1963	Sir C.E. John, Sir A.L. Hodegkin and Sir A.F. Huxley	Ionic mechanisms involved in excitation and inhibition in the peripheral and central portions of the nerve cell membrane.
1962	Francis H.C. Crick, J.D. Watson and M.H.F. Wilkins	Molecular structure of nucleic acid and its significance in information transfer in living material.
1961	G.V. Bekesy	Physical mechanism of stimulation within the cochlea.

Year	Scientist/s	Research
1960	Sir F.M. Burent and Sir Peter B. Medawar	Acquired immunological tolerance.
1959	S. Ochoa and A. Kornberg	Mechanisms in the biological synthesis of ribonucleic acid and deoxyribonucleic acid.
1958	F. Sanger	Primary structure of protein.
1958	G.W. Beadle and E.L. Tatum	Genes act by regulating definite chemical events.
1958	Joshua Lederberg	Genetic recombination and organization of the genetic material of bacteria.
1957	Daniel Bovet	Synthetic compounds that inhibit the action of certain body substances, especially their action on the vascular system and the skeletal muscles.

Glossary

Adventitious Developing from unusual points of origin, such as shoots, root tissues; developing from callus or embryos; developing from sources other than zygotes.

Agar A polysaccharide having gel-forming capacity obtained mainly from certain species of red algae.

Amino acid The building block molecules that are linked together to make peptides and proteins; contains amino group (NHz) and acid group.

Amniocentesis A procedure in which fluid containing foetal cells is withdawn from the uterus of a pregnant woman by a needle inserted through the abdominal wall. The cells can be analyzed for indications of the presence of certain genetic diseases in the foetus.

Ampicillin resistance When plasmid mediated, this means presence of a degrading enzyme B-lactamase which inactivates the antibiotic ampicillin.

Amplification Refers to the production of additional copies of a chromosomal sequence, found as either intra chromosomal or extrachromosomal DNA.

Androgenesis Male parthenogenesis i.e., the development of haploid embryo from a male.

Antibiotic Any of a group of structurally diverse chemicals produced by microorganisms, including bacteria and moulds, that kill other microorganisms. Antibiotics are used to treat bacterial diseases and some of the agents have proved valuable in cancer chemotherapy.

Antibody Antibodies are proteins produced by the B lymphocytes of the immune system. They help to defend the body against foreign invaders, including pathogenic viruses and bacteria, by searching out and binding to foreign molecules.

Antigen Strictly speaking, any molecule that is recognized and bound by an antibody. Usually this is the molecule used to elicit production of the antibody.

Antigenicity The ability to be recognized and bound by an antibody.

Anti-idiotype antibody An antibody made in response to, and recognizing the iodiotype of, another antibody. Anti-idiotype antibodies are under investigation as possible vaccines.

Aseptic With reference to *in vitro* procedures, it indicates a condition which is free from all microorganisms. Aseptic culture Culture of various explants under aseptic conditions.

Autoradiography Detection of radioactivity labelled molecules by their effect in creating an image on a photographic plate.

Autosome Any chromosome other than those that determine the sex of an organism. The human species, for example, has 46 chromosomes, two of which (the X and Y chromosomes) determine the sex of an individual and the rest of which are autosomes.

Autotroph An organism that can grow on carbon dioxide as its sole source of carbon.

Auxin A class of plant growth regulators chemically and functionally related to the natural plant hormone IAA.

Auxotroph A mutan,t organism that will not grow on a minimal medium but requires the addition of some growth factor.

Axenic Totally free from association with other organisms.

Bacillus thuringiensis A species of bacteria that infects insects and its toxin is used as a biological insecticide.

Bacteria Small, prokaryotic organisms that lack a nucleus and usually have rigid cell walls. Although some bacterial species cause disease in man, most are useful both in nature (for example those that carry out nitrogen fixation or break down organic matter) and in the biotechnology industry.

Bacteroid The form taken by the bacteria of the genus *Rhizobium* in the nitrogen-fixing nodules on the roots of legume plants.

Baculovirus A type of virus that infects insects and is used as a biological insecticide.

Base-pairing In the DNA double helix the two strands are held together by weak bonds that join the bases protruding from one chain to those of the other chain. The bases are paired so that adenine joins with thymine, and guanine with cytosine. Thus, the sequence of one DNA strand specifies the sequence of the second.

Bifunctionai vector; Bifuq.ctional plasmid (Shuttle vector) A DNA molecule capable of replicating in two different organisms. e.g. in *E. coli* and *B. subtilis* or in *E.coli* and yeast.

Biochemical Oxygen Demand (BOD) A measure of the amount of oxygen consumed in biological processes that break down organic matter in water, a measu(e of the organic pollutant load.

Bioleaching The use of solutions containing bacteria to dissolve and recover valuable metals from ores.

Biomining The use of bacteria to recover valuable metals from ores. As the biomining methods are currently constituted, they are generally applied to ores of such poor quality that metal recovery by more traditional operations is not economically feasible.

Bioreactor A vessel or tank in which fermentation reactions are carried out. Bioreactors are equipped with a variety of instruments for monitoring and adjusting the conditions in the tank so that the reaction proceeds efficiently.

Biotechnology The application of living organisms or of substances made by living organisms to make products of value to human beings.

Biotransformation Transformation of a metabolite of lower order to one of higher scientific or commercial values by a cell.

B lymphocyte A type of white blood cell that produces antibodies when appropriately activated. 'B' refers to the bursa of fabricius, the organ where the B cells mature in the chicken. The comparable organ in mammals is unknown.

Callus An undifferentiated mass of cells that forms on plant wounds and is also produced by plant tissues growing in cell culture.

Capsomere An individual protein subunit of capsid.

Carbohydrate Biological compounds containing carbon, hydrogen and oxygen, usually with two hydrogens and one oxygen for every carbon atom. The carbohydrates include the simple sugars, such as glucose, and *more* complex molecules, such as starch and cellulose, in which many sugars have been joined together *to* form large polymers.

Carcinogen Cancer inducing substance.

Carrier An individual who carries and can transmit a gene for a hereditary disease, but who does not have the disease. Many genetic diseases are caused by recessive genes, two copies of which must be inherited for the condition to develop; a carrier, who has only one copy, will not show any symptoms.

cDNA A duplex DNA complementary *to* an RNA, synthesized from it by in *vitro* reverse transcription.

Cell The fundamental unit of which living organisms are composed. Some organisms, such as bacteria, consist only of one cell, whereas others, such as man, contain billions.

Cell culture Growing cells of tissues on appropriate nutrients in laboratory dishes.

Chimaeric antibodies Antibodies in which the individual protein chains are composed of segments from two different species. The most common combination today is mouse with human.

Chloroplast A type of membranous part;icle that occurs in plant cells and is the site of photosynthesis.

Chorionic villus biospsy A procedure in which a small sample of tissue is removed from the chorion (one of the membranes of the foetus) and examined for foetal abnormalities, especially those of genetic origin.

Chromatin The complex of protein and DNA of which the chromosomes are composed.

Chromosomes The thread-like structures in the cell nucleus that contain the genes in a linear array. Each somatic cell in a eukaryote has a double set of chromosomes.

Clone A group of genetically identical cells or organisms that are all descended asexually from the same individual. (See also gene cloning).

Cloning vector Any plasmid or phage into which foreign DNA may be inserted *to* be cloned.

Codon A sequence of three successive nucleotides in DNA or RNA that either specifies a single amino acid in a protein or serves as a stop signal marking the end of a gene.

Cofactor A small molecule necessary for the catalytic activity of an enzyme.

Colony hybridization A technique for using in *situ* hybridization to identify bacteria carrying chimaeric vectors whose inserted DNA is homologous with some particular sequence.

Cosmids Plasmids into which phage lambda Cos sites have been inserted; as a result, the plasmid DNA can be packaged *in vitro* in the phage coat. This vector is designed to clone large fragments of eukaryotic DNA.

Cross-protection A situation in which infection of a cell with one viral strain protects the cell against infection by another related strain.

Crown gall A tumour formed on dicotyledonous plants as a result of infection by *Agrobacterium tumefaciens.* The tumour is caused by transfer of *DNA* from the Ti plasmid of the bacterium to the plant cell.

Cryopreservation Storage and preservation at ultra low temperatures, usually at –196°C.

Cultivar A uniform group of cultivated plants obtained by breeding or selection and propagated as a pure line.

Cybrid A fusion product arising out of a fusion between a protoplast containing nucleus and a sub-protoplast/protoplast without nucleus.

Cytokinins A class of plant growth regulators chemically and functionally related to the natural plant hormone zeatin.

Deoxyribonucleic acid (DNA) One of the two types of nucleic acid and the material of which genes are composed. A strand of DNA is formed by linking together many individual building blocks called nucleotides in a large molecule. The linear sequence of the nucleotides specifies the linear sequence of amino acids in the protein of a product gene.

Deoxyribose A sugar occurring in nucleic acids, specifically in deoxyribonucleic acids.

DNA polymerase The enzyme that copies the DNA of the genetic material when it duplicates before cell division.

Differentiation Developmental change of a cell which leads to its perfoffi1ing specialized functions.

Dimorphism Occurrence of two distinctly different external forms.

Dominant gene One in which inheritance of single copy of the gene is sufficient to confer the trait specified.

Double helix The three-dimensional stmcture of DNA in which the two strands of the molecule are twined together in a regular helical structure.

Embryo A young sporophytic plant, as yet retained in the gametophyte or in the seed.

Embryoid Embryo-like structure derived from cells of the vegetative plant body grown *in vitro.*

Enhancer A regulatory DNA sequence associated with a gene that increases transcription of that gene into messenger RNA.

Enzyme Proteins that act as biological catalysts, speeding up the rates of chemical reactions in living organisms. Most enzymes are extremely specific and act on a very limited range of molecules.

Escherichia coli (*E. coli*) A common bacterium that lives, among other places, in the human intestinal tract. Much of the fundamental work in understanding the biochemical basis of life was performed on *E. coli.* Laboratory strains of the bacterium are now used in biotechnology for gene cloning and making recombinant proteins.

Eukaryote Any organism in which the cells have a true nucleus enclosed by a membrane. The chromosomes are contained within the cell nucleus. Eukaryotes are generally considered to be more advanced forms of life than prokaryotes.

Evolution The development of new forms of life from pre-existing species.

Explant A part of an entire plant used for *in vitro* culture.

Expression vector A vector containing a promoter sequence which facilitates very efficient transcription of an inserted gene.

F-factor Fertility factor in a bacterium, an episome that determines the sex of a bacterium; F+ and F- cells function as male and female respectively.

Fatty acid Organic acids found in fats and also as intermediates in such energy-producing pathways as the tricarboxylic acid cycle. Fatty acids have a number of diverse applications. They can be used, for example, as flavouring agents and lubricants.

Feedstock chemicals Chemicals used in large quantities as starting materials for the manufacture of other chemicals.

Fermentation The use of microorganisms, or in some cases of enzymes extracted from microorganisms, to carry out any of a wide variety of chemical reactions. The classic example of fermentation is the conversion of sugar to alcohol by yeast.

Fermenter The tank or other apparatus in which fermentation reactions are carried out. The fermentor is usually equipped with devices for monitoring and adjusting the conditions of the reaction it contains.

Gene The basic unit of heredity; a gene encodes a specific trait that can be passed on from one generation to the next. In molecular terms, a gene is a segment of nucleic acid, usually deoxyribonucleic acid, that specifies the structure of a single protein chain.

Gene bank A collection of a cloned gene fragments from a single genome.

Gene cloning The use of recombinant DNA technology to isolate and produce large quantities of an individual gene.

Gene library A set of cell clones, now usually clones of bacterial cells, each of which contains a DNA fragment from a particular source. A human gene library, for example, consists of cell clones containing fragments of human DNA.

Generalised transduction; Unrestricted transduction A transduction in which transducers do not have a specific site of attachement to the chromosome and have equal probability of transducing any gene.

Gene therapy Treatment of a human genetic disease by introducing a new gene into the patient to take over the function of the defective gene that is causing the disease.

Gene splicing joining of two cleaved gene segments, created through the action of restriction endonucleases, by interweaving of strands at two ends with the help of ligases.

Genetic disease A disease that is caused by a defective gene and can be transmitted from one generation to the next.

Genetic engineering The application of recombinant DNA methods to confer new traits on organisms by introducing new genes into their cells.

Genome The complete set of chromosomes with gene composjtion of an organism.

Germ cells The cells that give rise to the sperm in males and the eggs in females.

Glycolysis The series of reactions that begins the breakdown of the sugar glucose and results in the release of a small quantity of energy for use by the cell. The fermentation of sugar to alcohol in yeast occurs through the glycolytic pathway.

Graft-versus-host disease A condition that occurs in persons who have received bone marrow transplants. It is caused by the transplanted marrow (the graft) producing immune cells that attack the recipient's tissues as foreign.

Haemoglobin This is the oxygen-carrying molecule of red blood cells. Haemoglobin consists of four protein chains, two each of the protein alpha-globin and two each of beta-globin, plus the red-coloured pigment haem.

Haploid Having a single complete set of chromosomes per cell, usually a gametophyte.

Hereditary disease A disease that can be transmitted from one generation to the next and is the result of a defective gene.

HeLa Cells A pure cell line of human cancer cells used for the cultivation of viruses.

Heterotroph An organism that cannot grow on carbon dioxide but must have more complex carbon sources such as sugars.

Heterozygote Genes are inherited in pairs, with one member of the pair coming from the mother and one from the father. A heterozygote is an individual in which the pair consists of two different variants of the gene in question. For example, a normal beta-globin gene might be paired with a sickle cell gene.

Homozygote An individual in which the two members of a particular gene pair are the same.

Hormone A biologically active substance produced in one part of the body and carded by the blood to another part where it exerts its effects.

Hybridization 1. In molecular biology, a procedure in which single-stranded nucleic acid molecules, from either DNA or RNA, are mixed. If the molecules have similar structures they will hybridize, that is, bind to one another by the base-pairing rules. The procedure can be used to give an indication of the degree of relatedness of two genes, ono detect RNAs or DNAs using a specific nucleic acid probe. 2. The crossing of two species to form hybrids that have some of the characteristics of each parent.

Hybridoma A hybrid cell made by fusing an antibody-producing B lymphocyte with a myeloma cell. Hybridomas are the source of monoclonal antibodies.

Hypqxanthlnel-guanine phosphoribosyl transferase (IIPRT) An enzyme needed for the synthesis of the building blocks of nucleic acids. An HPRT deficiency that results from a gene defect is the cause of Lesch-Nyhan disease.

Idiotype Region characteristic of a particular antibody. The idiotype, which is located in or near the antigen-binding site of the antibody, can itself stimulate antibody production and may'have a shape complementary to that of the antigen recognized by the antibody.

Immobilization Method used to restrict free movement of cells usually by entrapment on a suitable matrix.

Immunogenicity The ability to elicit an immune response.

Immunoglobulin Any of the serum proteins with antibody activity.

Interferons A group of related proteins having a variety of activities in the body. These include fighting viral infections and stimulating the cell-killing abilities of certain types of immune cells. The interferons are being tested in therapies for cancer and acquired immune deficiency syndrome (AIDS).

Interleukins A group of proteins that transmit signals for growth and development among immune cells and are necessary for mounting normal immune responses. Interleukin-2, for example, is undergoing clinical trials for treating cancer and acquired immune deficiency syndrome (AIDS).

In vitro Literally means 'in glass' e.g. a test tube. Now applied to growth of a tissue in any type of culture container.

Isoenzyme Multiple molecular forms of an enzyme exhibiting similar or identical catalytic properties.

Leghaemoglobin A type of haemoglobin found in the nitrogen fixing nodules on the roots of legume plants. Leghaemoglobin tightly binds oxygen, which would otherwise poison the nitrogen fixing enzymes.

Legume Member of a group of plants that includes peas, beans and alfalfa. Legumes can form symbiotic relationships with nitrogen-fixing bacteria of the genus Rhizobium.

Lesch-Nyhan disease A genetic disease caused by a defective gene for the enzyme hypoxanthine-guanine phosphoribosyl transferase. The condition is characterized by increased concentrations of uric acid in the blood and neurological symptoms, including mental retardation and a compulsion for self-mutilation.

Ligase An enzyme capable of joining two segments of a broken strand of double-stranded DNA, polynucleotide ligase.

Linkage analysis The association of a particular structural variation in DNA with the presence of a mutant gene that can cause a genetic disease. Linkage analysis can be used for diagnosing genetic diseases and detecting the gene carriers.

Linker A synthetic oligonucleotide which contains a restriction site.

Long terminal repeats (LTRs) Duplicated DNA sequences found at the ends of the genomes of certain viruses. They carry signals needed for the expression of the viral genes.

Meiosis Nuclear division in the germ cells, which results in. the halving of the number of chromosomes so that the egg cells or sperm that are produced receive just one set of chromosomes instead of the double set found in each somatic cell.

Messenger RNA (mRNA) A form of RNA that is copied from the DNA of the genes so that its structure contains the 'message' encoded in the gene. The messenger RNA carries that message to the ribosomes where it directs protein synthesis.

Metabolism The sum total of all the biochemical reactions in the cell.

Micropropagation Another term for *in vitro* propagation.

Mitosis Nuclear division in the somatic cells. Before the nucleus divides, the chromosomes are duplicated so that each daughter cell that will be formed receives a complete double set of chromosomes.

Monoclonal antibody An antibody produced by a hybridoma clone. Because all the cells in a clone are identical, they all produce the same antibody molecule. Monoclonal antibody technology provides a way of producing essentially unlimited quantities of a pure antibody.

Mutagenesis The introduction of changes into an organism genes.

Mutant An organism that has undergone some change as a result of a gene mutation.

Mutation Any change in the DNA of a gene that produces some alteration in the organism carrying that gene.

Myeloma A tumour of the antibody-producing B lymphocyte. Myeloma cells are used to make hybridomas for the production of monoclonal antibodies.

nif genes A complex of genes needed for nitrogen fixation. Only prokaryotes, including certain bacteria and blue-green algae, carry nif genes, but some of these organisms can form close symbiotic relationships with green plants, especially legumes.

Nitrogenase An enzyme complex needed for the reduction of atmospheric nitrogen to ammonia during biological nitrogen fixation.

Nitrogen fixation The reduction of atmospheric nitrogen to ammonia. The reaction, which requires a great deal of energy, can be carried out chemically or biologically.

Nodulation The formation of nitrogen-fixing nodules on the roots of plants by bacteria, such as those of the genus *Rhizobium* that form symbiotic relationships with legumes.

Nucleic acid Molecules consisting of a backbone of alternating sugar and phosphate groups from which protrude certain organic bases, which are attached to the sugars. The nucleic acids are so called because they were originally isolated from cell nuclei. They include deoxyribonucleic acid, which forms the genetic material and the ribonucleic acids.

Nucleotide A molecule consisting of a sugar to which is attached a phosphate group and an organic base. Nucleotides are the building blocks of the nucleic acids.

Nucleus The most prominent structure within the cell of eukaryotes; the nucleus is bound by a membrane and contains the chromosomes.

Oncogene A gene that can cause cells to undergo cancerous transformation. Oncogenes are aberrant forms of normal cellular genes that are needed for growth and differentiatiol).

Organogenesis Differentiation of organs like roots, shoots, flowers etc.

Papain A proteolytic enzyme produced in the juice of fruit and leaves of the papaya plant.

Pathogen Any microorganism or virus that causes disease.

Peptide A molecule formed by the linking together of two to perhaps 100 amino acids. (See also protein)

Photosynthesis The conversion of carbon dioxide and water to carbohydrates by plants, using light as the energy source.

Plasmid A small, usually circular, molecule of DNA that occurs in bacteria and is not part of the bacterial chromosome. Plasmids, which carry small numbers of genes, have been adapted as vectors for transferring genes between species.

Polymer A large molecule formed by linking together many simple building blocks. Proteins, nucleic adds and polysaccharides are examples of naturally occurring polymers.

Polysaccharide Large carbohydrates formed by linking together many sugar molecules. Starch and cellulose are examples.

Prokaryote Organisms, including the bacteria, that consist of usually a single cell that does not have a nucleus. prokaryotes are usually considered to be less advanced forms of life than eukaryotes.

Promoter A regulatory DNA sequence that is associated with a gene and is necessary for the accurate initiation of the gene's transcription.

Protein A biological polymer formed by linking together many amino acids. The principal distinction between peptides and proteins is size; proteins usually have molecular weights greater than 10,000 whereas the molecular weights of peptides are less than 10,000. The categories may overlap, however. Proteins serve as enzymes and also help to form cellular structures.

Protoplast A plant cell that has been denuded of its rigid cellulose wall. Protoplasts are used to produce somatic cell hybrids and also as targets for gene transfer in plant genetic engineering.

Provirus The state of a virus in which it is integrated into a host cell chromosome in order to be transmitted through many cell generations.

Receptor A molecule, usually a protein, that is present on a cell's outer membrane. A receptor recognizes and binds a specific intercellular messenger such as a hormone or growth factor, thereby initiating the messenger's effects within the cell.

Recessive gene One encoding a trait that will not be evident unless two copies of the gene are present. Many genetic diseases are caused by recessive genes.

Recombinant DNA A DNA molecule formed by joining DNA segments from two or more sources.

Recombinant protein A protein made, usually in bacteria, yeast or other cultured cells, as the product of a gene in a recombinant DNA molecule. Many human proteins of potential clinical importance are now made as recombinant proteins.

Regeneration The development and formation of new organs.

Restriction enzyme A bacterial enzyme that cuts DNA at a specific nucleotide sequence. Restriction enzymes are used for making recombinant DNA, for gene mapping, and in the diagnosis of genetic diseases.

Restriction fragment length polymorphism (RFLP) A change in the size of the fragments produced when a DNA sample is digested by a restriction enzyme that is the result of a change in the DNA sequence. RFLPs are used in diagnosing genetic diseases.

Restriction mapping The mapping of a DNA molecule by digesting it with restriction enzymes. Each DNA molecule will have its own characteristic pattern of sites recognized by the enzymes, and the maps can therefore be used to compare the relatedness of DNAs from different sources.

Retrovirus Any of a group of virsuses that have RNA, instead of DNA, as their genetic material and the life-cycles of which include a step in which the viral RNA is copied into DNA. Retroviruses are being developed as vectors for gene transfer.

Rhizobium A genus of bacteria that includes the nitrogen-fixing species that form symbiotic relationships with legume plants.

Ribonucleic acid (RNA) One of the two major types of nucleic acid. RNA is similar in structure to DNA, but contains the sugar ribose instead of deoxyribose. The RNAs include messenger RNA, ribosomal RNA and transfer RNA.

Ribose A sugar occurring in the ribonucleic acids.

Ribosomal RNA (rRNA) The type of RNA that combines with several proteins to form the ribosomes.

Ribosome An intracellular particle composed of protein and ribosomal RNA. Ribosomes are the sites of protein synthesis.

Shot-gun cloning Cloning of an entire genome in the form of randomly generated fragments.

Sickle cell anaemia A hereditary form of anemia caused by a defect in the gene coding for beta-globin, one of the two proteins of haemoglobin.

Single-cell protein Proteins made by single-celled organisms such as bacteria, fungi or algae for use in animal or human foods.

Somaclonal variation Genetic variability occurring in plants that have been regenerated from cells maintained in culture. The variability can arise even in cells that originally came from the same plant and would be expected to have identical genetic compositions.

Somatic cell Any of the cells of an organism except the germcells

Somatic cell hybrid A hybrid produced by fusing somatic cells from two different species, especially plant species.

Somatic embryogenesis Formation of embryos from asexual cells.

Southern blotting Procedure for transferring denatured DNA from an agarose get to a nitrocellulose paper where it can be hybridized with a complementary nucleic acid.

Splicing Gene splicing manipulation, the object of which is to attach one DNA molecule to another.

RNA splicing Removal of introns from RNA precursors.

Stem cell An immature form of bone marrow cell. It divides to form progeny some of which serve to maintain the stem cell population while. others give rise to all the major cell lineages originating in the bone marrow.

Steroid A member of a class of compounds that have a core structure of one five-carbon arid three six-carbon rings. Cholesterol is a steroid, as are the male and female sex hormones and a number of additional hormones that regulate salt and water balance and metabolism.

Substrate A compound that is acted on by an enzyme and thus converted to another compound.

Sugar A simple, usually sweet, form of carbohydrate. Some sugars, such as glucose, are energy sources for cells. They are also building blocks for polysaccharides such as starch and cellulose.

Surface sterilization Destruction of microorganisms from the surface of plant parts with the help of chemical agents e.g. mercuric chloride.

Suspension culture A susperision of free cells and cell aggregates capable of growth in a liquid nutrient medium.

Symbiosis A relationship in which individuals of two different species live together to their mutual benefit. The relationship between nitrogen-fixing *Rhizobium* bacteria and legume plants is an example.

T DNA DNA present in transformed plant cells after transfer through Ti plasmid.

T lymphocyte A type of white blood cell that performs several functions needed for normal immune responses. Some T lymphocytes are killers that destroy cells recognized as foreign (virus-infected cells. for example). Other T cells act as regulators—either helpers or suppressors—of other immune cells, including the antibody-producing B lymphocytes. 'T' refers to the thymus gland, the organ in which T lymphocytes mature.

Temperate bacteriophage A bacteriophage capable of replicating in step with its host bacterium, being thus transmitted through cell divisions without necessarily causing lysis.

Thalassaemia A type of hereditary anaemia in which a gene defect results in a deficiency or complete absence of one of the two proteins of the haemoglobin molecule.

Thiobacillus ferrooxidans A species of bacteria that is used for biomining.

Ti plasmid A plasmid carried by the bacterium *Agrobacterium tumefaciens*. The bacteria transfer the plasmid into plant cells where it induces the formation of crown galls. Modified forms of the Ti plasmid are now being used for the genetic engineering of plants.

Tissue culture The maintenance or growth of tissues, in vitro, in a way that may allow differentiation and preservation of their architecture and/ or function.

Tissue plasminogen activator (TPA) An enzyme that converts the inactive enzyme precursor plasminogen to the active enzyme plasmin, which acts to dissolve blood clots. TP A that is made by recombinant DNA technology is being tested clinically for dissolving the blood clots in the coronary arteries of heart attack victims.

Transcription The copying of the DNA of genes into 'messenger RNA, which is the first step in gene expression.

Transfer RNA (tRNA) A type of RNA that picks up amino acids, carries them to the ribosomes where protein synthesis is taking place, and lines them up in the proper position on the messenger RNA so that they can be joined together to form a protein.

Transformation 1. The introduction of foreign genes into cells, which acquire some new characteristic as a result. 2. The conversion of normal cells to cancer cells.

Transit peptide A peptide containing about 15 to 25 amino acids that are attached to a protein. A transit peptide directs the protein to its final destination inside or outside the cell and is then removed.

Translation The conversion of the nucleotide sequence of a messenger RNA into .the amino acid sequence of a protein during protein synthesis.

Vitamins Naturally occurring organic substances, necessary in small amounts for the normal metabolism of plants.

Transposable element A piece of DNA that can move about the genome and can cause mutations if it inserts into a gene. Transposable elements, which are also called transposons, are being investigated as potential vectors for gene transfer.

Vaccine A prepation introduced into the body to stimulate immunity against a pathogen, usually a bacterium or virus. Most vaccines are made from the pathogen itself, which is killed or attenuated so that it no longer causes disease.

Vector In biotechnology, a DNA molecule, usually a plasmid or viral DNA, used to transfer genes into cells.

Virus Particles consisting of a nucleic acid core, which may be either DNA or RNA, surrounded by a protein coat. Viruses are parasites that reproduce by entering cells and taking over the cells' own synthetic machinery.

Index

About the Author

Rev. Fr. Dr. S. Ignacimuthu, s.j., is a Jesuit priest teaching and guiding research in the field of Biotechnology and Entomology. He completed his B.Sc. and M.Sc. from the University of Madras and his M.Phil. and Ph.D. from the University of Delhi, with outstanding merit. He obtained his D.Sc. from the University of Madras. A fellow of several national international scientific associations, he has also been the principal investigator for several major research projects supported by government scientific agencies. He has published more than 220 research papers and 30 books, some of which are used as text books all over India. The other books by the same author are: Basic Biotechnology, Plant Biotechnology, Applied Plant Biotechnology and Basic Bioinformatics.

He has been the Vice Chancellor of Bharathiar University, Coimbatore and University of Madras, Chennai. Presently he is the Director, Entomology Research Institute, Loyola College, Chennai.

